# MEDICAL APHORISMS

## TREATISES 22–25

THE MEDICAL WORKS
OF MOSES MAIMONIDES

Medical Aphorisms: Treatises 1–5

Medical Aphorisms: Treatises 6–9

Medical Aphorisms: Treatises 10–15

Medical Aphorisms: Treatises 16–21

Medical Aphorisms: Treatises 22–25

On Asthma

On Asthma, Volume 2

On Hemorrhoids

On Poisons and the Protection against Lethal Drugs

On Rules Regarding the Practical Part of the Medical Art

◆ ◆ ◆

*Forthcoming Titles*

Commentary on Hippocrates' Aphorisms

Medical Aphorisms: Hebrew Translations
by Nathan ha-Meʾati and Zeraḥyah Ḥen

Medical Aphorisms: Indexes and Glossaries

On Coitus

On the Elucidation of Some Symptoms and the
Response to Them (On the Causes of Symptoms)

The Regimen of Health

NEAL A. MAXWELL INSTITUTE
FOR RELIGIOUS SCHOLARSHIP

BRIGHAM YOUNG UNIVERSITY

*Maimonides*

# Medical Aphorisms
# Treatises 22–25

# كتاب الفصول في الطبّ

*A parallel Arabic-English edition*
*edited, translated, and annotated by*

Gerrit Bos

⬩ ⬩ ⬩

PART OF THE MEDICAL WORKS
OF MOSES MAIMONIDES

*Brigham Young University Press ⬩ Provo, Utah*

Library of Congress Cataloging-in-Publication Data

Names: Bos, Gerrit, 1948– editor, translator. | Maimonides, Moses, 1138–1204. Kitāb al-fuṣūl fī al-ṭibb. Treatises 22–25. | Maimonides, Moses, 1138–1204. Kitāb al-fuṣūl fī al-ṭibb. Treatises 22–25. English. | Middle Eastern Texts Initiative (Brigham Young University), sponsoring body. | Brigham Young University, issuing body. | Maimonides, Moses, 1138–1204. Medical works of Moses Maimonides.
Title: Medical aphorisms. Treatises 22–25 : a parallel Arabic-English edition / Maimonides ; edited, translated, and annotated by Gerrit Bos.
Description: First edition. | Provo, Utah : Brigham Young University Press, [2017] | Series: Medical works of Moses Maimonides | Middle Eastern Texts Initiative. | Includes bibliographical references and index. | In Arabic and English.
Identifiers: LCCN 2016043645 | ISBN 9780842528764 (cloth : alk. paper)
Subjects: | MESH: Medicine | Aphorisms and Proverbs
Classification: LCC R733 | NLM WZ 290 | DDC 610—dc23
LC record available at https://lccn.loc.gov/2016043645

Printed in the United States of America.

First Edition

To my beloved mother, Gerritje Brouwer (1922–2011)

# Contents

❖ ❖ ❖

### *Kitāb al fuṣūl fī al-ṭibb* (Medical Aphorisms)

❖ ❖ ❖

# Sigla and Abbreviations

## Arabic Manuscripts of Maimonides' *Medical Aphorisms* (*Kitāb al-fuṣul fī al-ṭibb*)

**B** Oxford, Bodleian, Uri 412, Poc. 319, cat. Neubauer 2113; fols. 1–123.

**E** Escorial, Real Biblioteca de El Escorial 868, fols. 117–26 (numbered in reverse order).

**G** Gotha, orient. 1937, fols. 6–273.

**L** Leiden, Bibliotheek der Rijksuniversiteit 1344, Or. 128.1, fols. 1–140.

**O** Oxford, Bodleian, Hunt. Donat 33, Uri 423, cat. Neubauer 2114; fols. 1–78.

**P** Paris, Bibliothèque nationale, héb. 1210; fols. 1–130.

**S** Escorial, Real Biblioteca de El Escorial 869, fols. 176–1 (numbered in reverse order).

**U** Oxford, Bodleian, Hunt. 356, Uri 426, cat. Neubauer 2115; fols. 1–107.

## Arabic Manuscripts of Galenic Works

**A** Ayasofya 3593, fols. 48a–51b, Galen, *Fī sūʾ al-mizāj al-mukhtalif* (*De inaequali intemperie liber*), edited by Gerrit Bos, Michael R. McVaugh, and Joseph Shatzmiller.

**Be** Berlin 6231, fols. 235b–69b, Epitome of Galen, *Al-adwiya al-muqābila lil-dawā* (*De antidotis*).

**C** Cairo, Ṭal$^{c}$at ṭibb 550, *Tafsīr Jālīnūs li-kitāb Buqrāṭ fī al-ahwiya wa-al-buldān*. Arabic translation of Galen, *In Hippocratis De aere aquis locis commentarius*, forthcoming edition by G. Strohmaier.

**H** Paris, Bibliothèque nationale, arab. 2853, Galen, *Kitāb fī manāfi$^{c}$ al-a$^{c}$ḍā$^{c}$* (*De usu partium*), Arabic translation by Ḥubaysh, revised by Ḥunayn.

**W** London, Wellcome Or. 14a, Galen, *Kitāb al-mawāḍi$^{c}$ al-ālima* (*De locis affectis*), Arabic translation by Ḥunayn.

A superscripted 1 after a siglum (e.g., **G**$^{1}$) indicates a note in the margin of that manuscript. A superscripted 2 indicates a note above the line.

## Hebrew Translation

**p** Paris, Bibliothèque nationale, héb. 1173, fols. 1–92, by Nathan ha-Meʾati, titled *Sefer ha-Perakim*.

## Other

**Bo** Maimonides, *Aphorismi secundam doctrinam Galeni*, Latin translation by John of Capua, ed. Bologna 1489.

**Ka** Maimonides, *Medical Aphorisms* 25.56–72, Judeo-Arabic text (based on **G**) and Hebrew translation, ed. J. D. Kafiḥ (Maimonides, *Iggerot*).

**N** Maimonides, *Pirke Mosheh*, Hebrew translation by Nathan ha-Meʾati, ed. Bos (forthcoming).

**r** Maimonides, *The Medical Aphorisms of Moses Maimonides*, English translation by Rosner 1989.

**Ra** al-Rāzī, *Kitāb al-shukūk*, ed. Mohaghegh.

**Sch** Maimonides, *Medical Aphorisms* 25.59–68, Arabic text and English translation, ed. J. Schacht and M. Meyerhof (*Maimonides against Galen*).

**Z** Maimonides, *Pirke Mosheh*, Hebrew translation by Zeraḥyah ben Isaac ben Sheʾaltiel Ḥen, ed. Bos (forthcoming).

| | |
|---|---|
| <> | supplied by editor and translator, in Arabic text |
| [ ] | supplied by translator, in English text |
| add. | added in |
| del. | deleted in or by |
| om. | omitted in |
| emend. Bos | emendation by Bos |
| (?) | doubtful reading |
| (!) | corrupt reading |

## Transliteration and Citation Style

Transliterations from Arabic and Hebrew follow the romanization tables established by the *American Library Association and the Library of Congress (ALA-LC Romanization Tables: Transliteration Schemes for Non-Roman Scripts*. Compiled and edited by Randall K. Barry. Washington, DC: Library of Congress, 1997; available online at www.loc.gov/catdir/cpso/roman.html).

Passages from *Medical Aphorisms* are referenced by treatise and section number.

# Foreword

Brigham Young University and its Middle Eastern Texts Initiative are pleased to sponsor and publish the Medical Works of Moses Maimonides. The texts that appear in this series are among the cultural treasures of the world, representing as they do the medieval efflorescence of Arabic-Islamic civilization—a civilization in which works of impressive intellectual stature were composed not only by Muslims but also by Christians, Jews, and others in a quest for knowledge that transcended religious and ethnic boundaries. Together they not only preserved the best of Greek thought but enhanced it, added to it, and built upon it a corpus of scientific and philosophical understanding that is properly the inheritance of all the peoples of the world.

As an institution of the Church of Jesus Christ of Latter-day Saints, Brigham Young University is honored to collaborate with Gerrit Bos and other members of the academic community in bringing this series to fruition, making these texts available to many for the first time. In doing so, we at the Middle Eastern Texts Initiative hope to serve our fellow human beings of all creeds and cultures. We also follow the admonition of our own religious tradition, to "seek . . . out of the best books words of wisdom," believing, indeed, that "the glory of God is intelligence."

—Daniel C. Peterson
—D. Morgan Davis

# Preface

This edition of Maimonides' *Medical Aphorisms*, treatises 22–25, is the final volume in a series of five that covers all twenty-five treatises. In addition to these five volumes containing the original Arabic text of the aphorisms, a separate volume covering the medieval Hebrew translations by both Nathan ha-Me'ati and Zeraḥyah ben Isaac ben She'altiel Ḥen is in preparation. The same holds good for an extensive glossary of approximately five thousand terms of the Arabic text and the Hebrew translations with alphabetical Hebrew indexes.

This edition of the *Medical Aphorisms* is part of an ongoing project to critically edit Maimonides' medical works that have not been edited at all or have been edited in unreliable editions. The project started in 1995 at the University College London, with the support of the Wellcome Trust, and now enjoys the financial support of the Deutsche Forschungsgemeinschaft. So far it has resulted in the publication of critical editions of Maimonides' *On Asthma* (2 vols.); *Medical Aphorisms* (5 vols.); *Treatise on Poisons and the Protection against Lethal Drugs*, *On Hemorrhoids*, and the *Treatise on Rules Regarding the Practical Part of the Medical Art*.

The series is published by the Middle Eastern Texts Initiative at Brigham Young University's Neal A. Maxwell Institute for Religious Scholarship. On this occasion I thank Professor Daniel C. Peterson, under whose direction this series was inaugurated, and his colleague Dr. D. Morgan Davis for his continuing enthusiastic support and dedication to the project. Thanks are also due to Angela C. Barrionuevo, Felix Hedderich, Don Brugger, David Calabro, Fabian Käs, and Anne Kachergis for their diligent editing, proofreading, and typesetting. I also thank Professor Vivian Nutton for his help in correctly understanding and translating several Greek passages from the Galenic medical corpus.

# Translator's Introduction

This fifth and final volume of the critical edition of Moses Maimonides' *Medical Aphorisms* covers treatises 22–25.[1] The central subjects of these treatises are the specific properties of medicines (treatise 22), the differences between well-known diseases and the elucidation of medical technical terms (treatise 23), medical curiosities and rare occurrences (treatise 24), and doubts about Galen's words (treatise 25).[2]

The remedies that Maimonides lists in treatise 22 and that are effective through their specific properties mostly consist of all sorts of animals, their parts, excrements, and urine. In a lengthy theoretical discussion in his *Commentary on Hippocrates' Aphorisms*, Maimonides calls the specific property through which these remedies are effective their "specific form" (*al-ṣūrah al-nawʿīya*), and adds that these remedies operate through the whole of their essence, contrary to remedies that operate either through their matter, or through their quality.[3] While the pharmacological action of these remedies can be assessed by a physician, this

1. For Maimonides' biographical and bibliographical data, see Bos, introductions to Maimonides, *On Asthma* (ed. and trans. Bos), 1:xxiv–xxxiii; and to Maimonides, *Medical Aphorisms* (ed. and trans. Bos), 1:xix–xxxii.

2. I thank my colleague and friend Tzvi Langermann for his critical comments to a first draft of this introduction.

3. Maimonides, *Commentary on Hippocrates' Aphorisms* 24–27; also cf. Maimonides, *On Poisons* 15 (ed. and trans. Bos, 16): "It cannot be denied that a hot or cold remedy can be beneficial for any poison, whether hot or cold, because the action of remedies that save from fatal poisons is not dependent upon their quality but upon their whole substance, as the physicians declare, or upon their specific property, as they say. This means, as the philosophers have explained, that [these remedies] are effective through their 'specific form.'" See also Maimonides, *On Hemorrhoids* 2.3 (ed. and trans. Bos, 10). The subject is discussed in Schwartz, "Magiyah, maddaʾ nisyoni u-metodah maddaʾit," 35–38; Pseudo-Ibn Ezra, *Sefer*

is not the case with the remedies that are effective through their specific form but that lack a pharmacological basis. Their effectivity can be learned only through experience. Thus Maimonides remarks:

> As to the knowledge of what the drug does with respect to its specific form, and this is what is said [above], that it performs this action with its entire substance, we have no indication whatsoever by which to draw conclusions about this action, except by experience (*tajriba*).[4]

Although Maimonides was an eminent rationalist philosopher and physician, he allows the application of these remedies since as he says "experience has shown them to be valid even if reasoning does not require them."[5] Thus he remarks about practices that the sages allowed:

> You must not consider as a difficulty certain things that they have permitted, as for instance the nail of one who is crucified and a fox's tooth. For in those times these things were considered to derive from experience and accordingly pertained to medicine and entered into the same class as the hanging of a peony upon an epileptic and the giving of a dog's excrements in cases of the swelling of the throat and fumigation with vinegar and marcasite in cases of hard swellings of the tendons.[6]

Maimonides' position reminds one of that of the sages who held that "whatever is used as a remedy is not [forbidden] on account of the ways of the Amorite,"[7] that is, idolatry. To put it in other words: Any substance that we know by experience to be an effective remedy is allowed.

The attitude of Galen, Maimonides' major source for the list of these remedies, towards the employment of animal and human *materia medica*, is ambivalent. On the one hand he speaks, as Keyser remarks, against γοητεία (magic), but on the other hand he accepts magical remedies from authoritative predecessors while interpreting them according to his own system.[8] While authority and experience are the criteria for allowing the application of animal and human *materia medica*

---

*Hanisyonot* 17–20; Langermann, "Gersonides on the Magnet," 273–74; and Freudenthal, "Maimonides' Philosophy of Science," 151–56.

4. Maimonides, *Commentary on Hippocrates' Aphorisms,* aphorism 26.
5. Maimonides, *Guide of the Perplexed* 3.37 (ed. and trans. Pines, 2:544).
6. Maimonides, *Guide of the Perplexed* 3.37 (ed. and trans. Pines, 2:544).
7. See Babylonian Talmud, Shab 67a.
8. See Keyser, "Science and Magic in Galen's Recipes," 187.

as a remedy, Galen asserts that these substances, like all things, have natural powers and that these can be used medicinally. Thus feces have a strong expulsive force. But one does not have to use them, especially not the strong-smelling ones like those of human beings, disgusting as they are, since other medicines are available. However, those feces that do not stink, like those of cows, goats, ground-crocodiles, and dogs fed on bones, have been proven useful by himself and others.[9] Similarly urine: while he considers the drinking of the urine of wild boars as something horrid, since it is the strongest smelling of all urines, he prescribes human urine, the weakest of all urines, especially for healing suppurating sores, on the basis of his own authority and experience.[10]

Prominent Galenic sources consulted by Maimonides for the list of remedies working through their specific property are:

1. Galen's *De theriaca ad Pisonem* (aphorisms 22.1–16). The Arabic text quoted by Maimonides closely parallels that of Ḥunayn's Arabic translation, which has been edited by Richter-Bernburg. Although Richter-Bernburg assumed that this work is pseudo-Galenic, recent research has convincingly shown that it is an authentic work from the hand of Galen.[11]

2. *De simplicium medicamentorum temperamentis ac facultatibus* (aphorisms 22.18–32). In this work, consisting of a total of eleven books, Galen discusses the mineral *materia medica* in book 9, and the animal *materia medica* in books 10 and 11.

Prominent non-Galenic sources consulted by Maimonides are:

1. Abū Marwān ibn Zuhr (d. 1161) (aphorisms 22.36–56). In this lengthy section Maimonides quotes a wide variety of remedies from the *Kitāb al-taysīr fī al-mudawāt wa-al-tadbīr* (Book on the Facilitation of Treatments and Diet) and the *Kitāb al-aghdhiya* (Book on Foodstuffs). Maimonides explicitly informs us about his reason for including these remedies:

> Abū Marwān ibn Zuhr has mentioned many specific properties [of remedies] that he tested. He was one of the [great] empiricists. His

9. See aphorism 22.20 in this volume.

10. See aphorism 24.9 in this volume; Keyser, "Science and Magic in Galen's Recipes," 195; and Durling, "Excreta as a Remedy," 29–30.

11. See Nutton, "Galen on Theriac."

> son told me amazing things about his precision and diligence in matters depending upon experience. Therefore, I thought it a good thing to mention them in his name, although some of them have been mentioned by others before. However, he is the one who verified these experiential matters.[12]

Again, we see how the criterion of experience plays a major role in Maimonides' decision to quote these remedies.

2. Al-Tamīmī (d. 980) (aphorisms 22.57–70). Although Maimonides was aware of the fact that al-Tamīmī was not an original author (since he usually quoted from the works of other physicians and sometimes made mistakes), he still considered his recipes useful since al-Tamīmī "allegedly was very experienced."[13]

Treatise 23, in which Maimonides discusses the differences between well-known diseases and the elucidation of medical technical terms, is illustrative of Maimonides' expert knowledge of Galen's medical writings and of medical literature in general. We are also witnesses of his critical mind and attitude towards Galen, in spite of his high regard for him as a physician, and towards other physicians. Thus he remarks in aphorism 23.25 that some of the commentators have confused some of the technical terms, for instance, indiscriminately using the term *ṣifāqāt* for (1) the internal membranes of the organs; (2) the tunics of the eye; and (3) some of the coverings, such as the third covering of the spinal cord. Maimonides' thorough and detailed medical knowledge even in a field as difficult and complicated as that of eye diseases is borne out by his explanation of several obscure terms in this field, such as *kumna* (pus behind the horn-like tunic), *sulāq* (ptilosis), and *mūsaraj* (prolapse of the iris) in aphorism 23.71. About the illness called *damᶜa* he remarks that it occurs if most of the flesh in the inner corner of the eye disappears.

As I have noted before, Maimonides does not merely reproduce the Galenic text but often reformulates it through abbreviation or addition. Such an addition may assume the form of a definition of a certain illness, as in aphorism 23.73 for hardness of hearing and deafness. While Galen merely gives a recipe for treating this illness, Maimonides defines

---

12. Aphorism 22.35 in this volume.

13. This is the argument that Maimonides uses for quoting a variety of "natural" remedies in aphorisms 22.82–89 in this volume.

the illness as follows: "Deafness means that a person cannot hear a low voice at all and hears a loud voice with difficulty. This process continues to progress slowly until the patient becomes completely deaf in the course of time." On another occasion such an addition gives us an insight into Maimonides' medical experience: in aphorism 23.77 he adds to the Galenic text which type of angina is safe and which type is not:

> Angina is a swelling in the throat and consists of four types. The first is that the inside of the throat swells up, that is, its cavity up to the end of the larynx, whereby none of the swelling is visible externally. The second is when the throat swells up at the outside and the patient does not have a sensation of choking; this is the safest of all four types. The third is when the swelling includes both the inside of the throat and the outside, and this is the worst of all. The fourth is when no swelling is visible on the outside, but the patient has the feeling of choking. *De locis affectis* 4.

And in aphorism 23.84, where Galen remarks that "sometimes the cause of indigestion is the irregularity in which foods are taken [...], or their quantity or their quality," Maimonides adds that the irregularity concerns the order in which the food is taken, that is, "what is taken first and what is taken later." In order to prevent a misunderstanding of Galen's ambiguous statement, which might also mean that one eats at irregular times, Maimonides added that qualification and thus once more stressed a dietetic rule that also appears in his treatise *On Asthma*.[14]

Another valuable feature of the *Medical Aphorisms* pointed out before is that it preserves medical material otherwise lost and unknown. For example, aphorism 23.76 preserves the following unique quotation from Galen's lost treatise *De voce et hanelitu*, which was not noted by Baumgartner in his reconstruction of this text from secondary sources:

> The windpipe is called *ḥalqūm* (trachea). The term *ḥalqūm* is especially used for the site where the two channels, that is, the larynx and the esophagus arrive at, below the root of the tongue. In the throat there are muscles which are known as *naghānigh*. It is a plural term, meaning [the muscles at] both sides of the throat. *De voce* [*et hanelitu*].

And aphorisms 23.107–8 preserve unique quotations regarding the names of the different types of milk from Ibn al-Tilmīḏ's *Ikhtiyārāt*

---

14. Maimonides, *On Asthma* 5.4 (ed. and trans. Bos, 1:26).

*al-Ḥāwī* (Selections from [the book] *al-Ḥāwī* [composed by al-Rāzī]), which survives only in Arabic bio-bibliographical literature.

The central subject of treatise 24 is medical curiosities and rare occurrences. One unusual source consulted by Maimonides is a commentary ascribed to Hermes and Galen on Hippocrates' *Book on Women's Diseases* as preserved in MS Manissa, Kitabsaray 1815 (aphorisms 24.1–2). From Maimonides' introduction it is clear that he himself noticed that this was not a normal Galenic commentary:

> In the *Book on Women's Diseases* composed by Hippocrates, translated by Ḥunayn, and commented upon by Galen, I found an addition that is not part of Ḥunayn's translation nor of Galen's commentary. In that additional commentary there are strange things, among them that he says: Porphyry has related that there was a great eclipse of the sun in Sicily [and that] in that year women gave birth to abnormally shaped babies that had two heads. And that some women menstruated from their mouth through vomiting.[15]

Treatise 24 shows Maimonides' interest in botany and his familiarity with botanical literature current in his time. Thus he gets involved in the controversy concerning Galen's alleged familiarity with the eggplant (aphorisms 24.13–14). Contrary to Ibn Riḍwān who held that Galen did know this plant on the basis of his statement in his commentary to *Epidemics II* that the site beneath the skin where blood flows outside the vessels takes on the color of eggplant, Maimonides states that it is his firm opinion that Galen did not know this plant, an opinion shared by most Arab botanists; in modern research, however, the question is undecided. Further information about Maimonides' medical experience is provided by the information he gives in aphorism 24.40 concerning the frequency of diabetes as a comment to Galen's statement that he has observed this illness only twice (aphorism 24.39). Maimonides remarks that he never saw this illness in the Maghreb but noticed twenty cases of people suffering from it during a period of twenty years in the land of Egypt. This statement also provides valuable information about a possible date of the composition of the aphorisms, a controversial issue in current research. It seems to support the theory that the text was composed around 1185, twenty years after his arrival in Egypt from the Maghreb.

15. Aphorism 24.1 in this volume.

Aphorism 24.44 gives us another example of his open mind, critical attitude, and expertise in Galen's works and his medical terminology, as reflected in the Arabic translations. On the basis of this familiarity with Galenic terminology, he comes to the conclusion that the ascription of a treatise "on the prohibition of the burial [of the dead] within twenty-four hours" to Galen is false, and that the translator al-Biṭrīq considered the work to be authentic only because of his ignorance concerning the language typical for Galen. Maimonides' conclusion as to the pseudepigraphical character of this work is confirmed in Arabic bio-bibliographical literature. Following this introductory statement Maimonides quotes seven texts from this work (aphorisms 24.45–51), since he considers them useful. A comparison of these quotations with the text extant in MS Ayasofya 3724, fols. 140a–146a, indicates that Maimonides had a different text in front of him, since the differences between both texts are considerable, and some quotations (aphorisms 24.47, 50, and 51) cannot be identified at all. Treatise 24 also contains some material that has been lost in Galen's original Greek text. Aphorism 24.20, for instance, is a quotation from Galen's *De motibus dubiis*, which survives only in an Arabic translation by Ḥunayn and Latin translations by Niccolò da Reggio and Mark of Toledo.[16] Aphorisms 24.59–60 are valuable quotations from al-Biṭrīq's translation of Galen's *De simplicium medicamentorum temperamentis ac facultatibus*, which has otherwise been lost. The translation that survived and was consulted by most Arab physicians is the one ascribed to Ḥubaysh.

Treatise 25, devoted to doubts about Galen's words, actually consists of two parts: the first part consisting of aphorisms 25.1–58, 69–72, and the second part covering aphorisms 25.59–68. The first part contains Maimonides' critique of the medical inconsistencies found in Galen's works and the second part contains Maimonides' refutation of Galen's denial of the Mosaic doctrines of God's omnipotence and creation of the world. This last part has, not surprisingly, drawn most of the attention of the scholarly world so far; its original text was edited and translated by Schacht and Meyerhof and more recently by Joseph Kafiḥ.

Maimonides was certainly not the first to criticize Galen in his capacity as a medical theorist. In fact, there is a long tradition of

16. For a critical edition of the Arabic and medieval Latin translations, see Galen, *On Problematic Movements*, ed. Nutton and Bos.

Galenic criticism regarding medical issues.[17] The Byzantine compilator Alexander of Tralles (d. 605), for instance, criticizes Galen for prescribing warm compresses in the case of someone suffering from corruption of the stomach and indigestion. Subsequently, Symeon Seth of Antioch (eleventh century) composed a refutation of Galenic theories in physiology.[18] Among the Arab physicians, an important critic of Galen was al-Rāzī (d. 925). His criticism can be found in a special monograph devoted to the subject, entitled *Kitāb al-shukūk ʿalā Jālīnūs* (Doubts concerning Galen).[19] In this work the author sometimes continues the tradition of scholarly discussions based on the Aristotle-Galen controversy. At other times, however, his criticism is the result of his personal clinical experience. Al-Rāzī used to collect the notes of his cases and to check them against Galen's theories.

Maimonides takes al-Rāzī's criticism of Galen as the starting point for his own account of Galen's medical inconsistencies. According to Maimonides, al-Rāzī's criticism is mostly directed against Galen's way of reasoning and his logical conclusions, and not against his medical inconsistencies. These *shukūk* are therefore not medical problems but philosophical ones. He adds that Ibn Zuhr and Ibn Riḍwān already solved those problems,[20] and that he does not intend to deal with any of them because the whole topic is a waste of time. Maimonides states that his intention is to deal with medical problems, since Galen was the master (*imām*) of the art of medicine, in which field he should be followed. He should not be followed in any other field. Maimonides clearly thought that al-Rāzī should not have attacked Galen for his philosophical and logical inconsistencies, but rather for his medical ones. Moreover, he thought that al-Rāzī had no authority to attack Galen since he was

17. For a general account of the criticism of Galen, see Averroës, "Averroes 'contra Galenum,'" 278–90; Temkin, *Galenism: Rise and Decline*, 76–80; and Ullmann, *Medizin im Islam*, 67–68; see also Bos, "Medical Aphorisms: Towards a Critical Edition," 42–45; and Bos and Fontaine, "Medico-philosophical Controversies," 32–34.

18. Bouras-Vallianatos, "Galen's Reception in Byzantium," 458–69.

19. For the term *shukūk* (doubts) as a parallel to the Greek πρόβλημα, ζήτημα, ἀπορία, see Averroës, "Averroes 'contra Galenum,'" 285. For a summary of this work, see Pines, "Rāzī critique de Galien."

20. ʿAlī ibn Riḍwān (d. 1068), Abū l-ʿAlāʾ ibn Zuhr (d. 1130–31), and other physicians came to the defense of Galen against the attack of al-Rāzī and tried to solve the doubts raised by him (*ḥall al-shukūk*); see Averroës, "Averroes 'contra Galenum,'" 285.

only a physician and not a philosopher.[21] Maimonides' harsh words of criticism against al-Rāzī are certainly unjustified. Al-Rāzī criticizes Galen not only for his logical philosophical arguments but also for practical medical ones. In so doing, al-Rāzī bases his criticism on the collection of case notes he assembled as a practicing physician.[22] Moreover, although Maimonides remarks that he will not deal with al-Rāzī's criticism since it is a waste of time, he nevertheless attacks him for his criticism of Galen's theory that the Greek language was superior to all of the other languages, which in comparison sound like the grunting of pigs, the croaking of frogs, or the cawing of the raven (aphorisms 25.56–57). And Maimonides' attack on Galen for letting blind passion dominate the perceptive faculties of the mind, and thus believing in the superiority of the testicles over the heart (aphorisms 25.25–26), bears close similarity to al-Rāzī's rationale for modern scholars' criticism of the works of the ancients, namely, the occurrence of errors in their works caused by passion overwhelming their reason.

Although Maimonides' critique of Galen on medical issues is largely concentrated in treatise 25, it is certainly not lacking in the other treatises of his *Medical Aphorisms*, as I have noted before. Thus there is a certain continuity with the previous treatises, and not an absolute break, as current research has suggested. Moreover, several of the aphorisms discussed in treatise 25 already appear in the previous treatises in a different context. As to the actual critique itself, Maimonides is very careful in blaming Galen for the inconsistencies found in his works. In fact, he recognises that these inconsistencies may also go back to a mistake by the translator of Galen's works into Arabic or to his own bad understanding (aphorism 25.1). Thus he remarks in aphorism 25.11 that Galen's inconsistency in prescribing bleeding from the leg in the case of epilepsy, vertigo, or obstruction might be explained by the translator's omission of special conditions allowing for such a bleeding. And when the inconsistency obviously goes back to Galen himself, Maimonides

21. Maimonides, quoted by Marx, "Texts by and about Maimonides," 378: "Ve-sefer ḥokhmah elohit she-ḥibber al-Razi hu lo aval eyn bo toᶜelet lefi she-al-Razi hayah rofe bilvad" (The book on theology composed by Rāzī is useless since he was only a physician). See Stroumsa, "Al-Fārābī and Maimonides," esp. 247.

22. One example is his critique based on two thousand cases he assembled in the hospitals of Baghdad and Rayy and in his home that refuted Galen's remarks on the different kinds of fevers, their durations, and attacks in *De crisibus* (see al-Rāzī, *Kitāb al-shukūk*, p. 62, line 13–p. 63, line 19).

remarks that it is due to unmindfulness since nobody is free from these things except for exalted human beings (aphorism 25.1). Nevertheless, at times Maimonides criticizes Galen severely and in an ironic tone, as in the case of Galen's belief in the superiority of the testicles over the heart mentioned above, where Maimonides exclaims:

> Consider then, ye who possess insight, [whether this is correct,] because if the heart would be excised from a living being, could he remain alive to live a good life? That is, could he have sexual intercourse and show his male sexual potency and not lack any vital function? But if his testicles are cut off, he remains alive as we see [in the case of] eunuchs. Are then the testicles more eminent than the heart?[23]

And in a thorough analysis of Maimonides' criticism concerning Galen's discussion of putrefactive fevers (aphorisms 25.5, 23, and 24), Langermann has shown that Maimonides' criticism is severe and thorough.[24] Yet, sometimes his criticism is undeserved and incorrect. For instance, in aphorism 25.28 Maimonides attacks Galen for believing that a third type of epilepsy is a mere quality without any substance whatsoever that happens in the brain. Maimonides' account is not a fair reflection of the Galenic statement in this matter. In fact, Galen does not consider the third type of epilepsy to be merely a quality. He raises the question whether types two or three are the result of an insubstantial quality or of some actual substance. Like Pelops, he believes in at least some substantial change, even if the result is achieved by a sort of sympathy. The cold breeze arising to the brain is thus something physical, a symptom of ongoing changes. One might summarize Maimonides' criticism as a scholastic exercise, sometimes bordering upon casuistry. Maimonides was thus part of the medieval Arabic tradition of closely scrutinizing texts, which was surprisingly similar to the methods used in renaissance Italian universities.[25]

Just as the first part of treatise 25 of the *Medical Aphorisms* in a way builds on the previous parts, so the second part is a continuance of the first part. For, as Langermann puts it, in this first part Maimonides prepared the ground for his challenge to Galen's competence as a

23. Aphorism 25.26 in this volume.
24. Langermann, "Maimonides on the Synochous Fever," 184–89.
25. See Langermann, "Perusho shel Shelomo ibn Yaᶜish," 1332.

philosopher by demonstrating Galen's wavering and confusion even in medical matters.[26] This challenge is taken up by Maimonides in a lengthy statement in aphorism 25.59, where he rebukes Galen for overestimating his abilities and not having limited himself to the science he excels in, namely, medicine. The blind admiration of the people has turned him into a conceited person suffering from megalomania who thinks that he can speak with authority about any theme from any branch of science without having studied that particular branch seriously. Maimonides remarks:

> And this [man] Galen, the physician, was attacked by this disease in the same degree as others who were equal to him in science. That is, this man was very proficient in medicine, more than anybody we have heard about or whose words we have seen; he has achieved great things in [the field of] anatomy, and things became clear to him—and to others in his time as well—about the functions of the organs, their usefulness and structure, and about the [different] conditions of the pulse, which were not clear in Aristotle's time. He, I mean Galen, has undoubtedly trained himself in mathematics and has studied logic and the books of Aristotle on the natural and divine sciences, but he is defective in all that. His excellent intellect and acumen that he directed towards medicine, and his discoveries of some of the conditions of the pulse, anatomy, and the usefulness and functions [of organs]—which are undoubtedly more correct than what Aristotle mentions in his books, if one looks at them impartially—have induced him to speak about things in which he is very deficient and about which the experts have contradictory opinions.

Maimonides then describes in detail Galen's deficiency in logic, as this becomes especially evident from his monograph *De demonstratione*. Maimonides backs up his argument by calling as a witness the famous philosopher and scholar al-Fārābī, who wrote a devastating critique of Galen's logic evident in *De demonstratione*. According to al-Fārābī, Galen should have directed most of his attention to the so-called hypothetical syllogisms since these are most useful for a physician in extracting the different parts of the medical art and for recognizing hidden diseases and their causes in every individual patient. Unfortunately, the only syllogisms Galen discussed are the hyparctic (assertoric) syllogisms, which are useless for a physician.

---

26. Langermann, "Maimonides on the Synochous Fever," 189, esp. n. 36.

At this point Maimonides starts his major assault on Galen for his faulty opinions in the divine sciences, especially his denial of the Mosaic doctrines of God's omnipotence and his denial of the biblical account of creation. For Galen aligns himself with Plato and the other Greeks in denying God's omnipotence by asserting the irreducibility of matter and its qualities (aphorism 25.62). Galen illustrates his denial with the example of the eyelashes, the length of which is perfect for keeping things out of the eyes. He wonders how this is possible, since all the other hairs of the body keep growing, and asks his Mosaic opponent:

> Do you say, then, that the Creator has commanded this hair to remain at all times at one and the same length and not to grow longer and that the hair has accepted that order, obeyed, and remained [at the same length], without deviating from what it had been ordered either out of fear and apprehension to offend against the command of God or because of politeness and awe before God who gave this command, or that the hair itself knows that it is more appropriate and better to do so?

According to Galen it is unthinkable that God could create such eyelashes merely by his will; on the contrary, he chose the best possible course of action and provided the eyelashes with the right material principle, namely, the cartilage to stay at the right length. In other words, according to Galen, God cannot overstep the possibilities implanted in nature. Maimonides responds to Galen's attack by admitting that according to the Mosaic doctrine of God's omnipotence it is true that God can transgress the laws of nature in performing miracles. Thus, he can transform ashes into a horse or ox, a rod into a serpent, and dust into lice (aphorism 25.64). According to Maimonides, this absolute power of God to override the laws of nature is intrinsically linked to the fundamental Mosaic doctrine of the creation of the world:

> Since the first matter, according to Him, was brought into existence after nonexistence and was then shaped [into its forms], it is possible that God, who brought it into existence, will destroy it once He has made it. Likewise, it is possible that He will change its nature and the nature of everything that is composed of it and will give it instantly a nature different from the regular one, just as He brought it into existence instantly.

Now that from the account of the creation of the world he has proven that God can perform miracles and indeed did so on several occasions as related in the Torah, Maimonides uses the actual perception of these miracles as an argument for proving the creation of the world (aphorism 25.64) and thus refutes the Aristotelean doctrine of the eternity of the world. At the same time Maimonides points out that God's omnipotence was only superficially understood by Galen, for God's seemingly unlimited power is restricted by his very nature since he can do nothing in vain and by chance, but only with justice and equity. And as to Galen's position of skepticism concerning the Mosaic doctrine of the creation of the world (that is, doubt about whether it is created or uncreated), Maimonides argues that it only results from his confusion and poor logical argumentation (aphorisms 25.66–68). It seems as though Maimonides wants to say that if Galen had only reasoned according to proper logical rules, he would have come to the conclusion that the world was created after all.

## Manuscripts of the *Kitāb al-fuṣūl fī al-ṭibb* (Medical Aphorisms)

The work is extant in the following manuscripts:

1. Gotha, orient. 1937 (**G**); fols. 6–273 (fol. 7 numbered twice); Naskh script.[27] A considerable section of the text from aphorism 6.10 (beginning at *al-mawt*) to aphorism 7.16 (ending at *min amthāl*) is missing.[28] Other sections—namely, aphorisms 20.30–33, and 23.7, 13, 15, 69, and 82—seem to have been missing from the original version used by the scribe and were added by him at the end of these treatises from another version.[29] According to the colophon on fol. 273a, which appears after aphorism 25.55, the scribe copied the text from a copy of the original redaction of the work by Maimonides' nephew Abū al-Maʿālī (or

27. See Pertsch, *Arabische Handschriften*, 3:477–78; and Kahle, "Mosis Maimonidis Aphorismorum," 89–90.

28. Other sections missing are aphorisms 20.30–33 and 25.56–58.

29. Cf. the following statement on fol. 231a: وجدت عند المقابلة في هذه المقالة زيادة على ما في نسخة الأصل وهي (When collating this version with another one, I found an addition in this treatise to that featuring in the original version, namely, . . . ), and on fol. 94a: وجدت هذه الزيادة في هذه المقالة عند المقابلة من نسخة غير الأصل (I found the following addition to this treatise when collating [this version] with another not-original version).

Maʾānī) ibn Yūsuf ibn ʿAbdallāh.[30] The scribe adds that he found a note in the text at hand in which Abū al-Maʾālī remarks that, in the case of the first twenty-four treatises, Maimonides would correct his autograph notes and that he, Abū al-Maʾālī, would then make a fair copy and correct it in Maimonides' presence; however, the text of the twenty-fifth treatise was copied by him in the beginning of the year 602 AH (August 1205 CE), after the death of Maimonides, so the latter had not been able to do the redaction.[31] Although it is generally agreed that this manuscript has preserved the best readings,[32] it should be noted that in some cases the text suffers from a certain carelessness by the scribe resulting in mistakes and corruptions. Moreover, the language he employs is sometimes extremely vulgar and colloquial. Another characteristic of the text is that the central issue of many aphorisms is indicated in the margin in terminology derived from the text itself.

2. Leiden, Bibliotheek der Rijksuniversiteit 1344, Or. 128.1 (**L**); fols. 1–140; Maghribī script.[33] The manuscript ends on fol. 140b with the following colophon:

> This is the end of the treatise—praise be to God—and the completion of the *Book of Aphorisms* of the most perfect and unique scholar Mūsā ibn Maymūn ibn ʿUbaydallāh, the Israelite, from Cordova—may God be pleased with him. The copying [of the text] was completed in the month of May of the year 1362 according to the calendar of al-Ṣufr in the city of Ṭulayṭula—may God protect it—and it was written by Yūsuf ibn Isḥāq ibn Shabbathay, the Israelite.

The calendar of al-Ṣufr was common in Spain, especially among Christians, and started about thirty-eight years before the Christian

---

30. See the remark by the scribe at the end of treatise 24 (fol. 239a): "Something like the following was written at the end of this treatise: This is what I found in the copy written by Abū [. . .]: I did not make a fair copy of this treatise until after his death—may God have mercy with him—and [A]bū al-Zakāt the physician wrote: Praise be to God, who is exalted."

31. See Pertsch, *Arabische Handschriften*, 3:477–78; Kahle, "Mosis Maimonidis Aphorismorum," 90; Kaufmann, "Neveu de Maïmonide," 152–53; Meyerhof, "Medical Work," 276; Kraemer, "Six Unpublished Maimonides Letters," 79–80 n. 93; Sirat, "Liste de manuscrits," 112; and Stern in Maimonides, "*Treatise to a Prince*" (ed. and trans. Stern), 18.

32. Cf. Schacht and Meyerhof, "Maimonides against Galen," 59; and Rosner, introduction to Maimonides, *Medical Aphorisms* (trans. Rosner), xiv.

33. See Voorhoeve, *Handlist of Arabic Manuscripts*, 85.

calendar.[34] Accordingly, the manuscript was written in May 1324 in Toledo. More than that of any of the other manuscripts, the language of this manuscript conforms to the rules of classical Arabic; thus the influence of vulgarization is thus far less pronounced than in the others. Just like **G**, it has many marginal catchwords.

3. Paris, Bibliothèque nationale, héb. 1210 (**P**); fols. 1–130; Judeo-Arabic; no date.[35] The manuscript contains only treatises 1–9 (the last one incomplete), part of treatise 24, and the major part of treatise 25. Also missing are aphorisms 8.42–59. According to the inscription on fol. 1v, the manuscript was once in the possession of R. Meir ha-QNZ(?)Y. The text has been copied carefully, so that there are only a few mistakes; the top section has been so stained that the first lines are hard to read.

4. Escorial, Real Biblioteca de El Escorial 868 (**E**); fols. 117–26 (numbered in reverse order); Maghribī script.[36] According to the colophon, this text was copied in the city of of Qal$^{c}$a (Alcalá) by Mūsā ibn Sūshān al-Yahūdī in the year 1380 (read 1388), corresponding to the year 5149 since the creation. The text offers a close parallel to **L**, both having many otherwise unique readings in common, including whole paragraphs not occurring in any other manuscript, such as aphorism 3.52. Like **L**, this manuscript has several marginal catchwords, but they are not as many and they use a different terminology.

5. Escorial, Real Biblioteca de El Escorial 869 (**S**); fols. 176–1 (numbered in reverse order); Oriental script; no date.[37] The text is missing an important section between aphorisms 10.28 (beginning at المستدلّ) and 21.72 (ending at عتّاب), and finishes at aphorism 25.58. Aphorisms 23.7, 13, 15, 69, and 82—mentioned in **G** as an additional section—also appear in **S** at the end of treatise 23, but without the copyist's note. The text of this manuscript is closely related to **G**.

---

34. Dozy, *Supplément aux dictionnaires arabes*, 1:836; Kahle, "Mosis Maimonidis Aphorismorum," 90–91.

35. Zotenberg, ed., *Catalogues des manuscrits hébreux*, 223; Vajda, *Index général des manuscrits arabes musulmans*, 345.

36. See Derenbourg, comp., and Renaud, ed., *Médecine et histoire naturelle*, 74–75; and Cano Ledesma, *Manuscritos árabes de El Escorial*, 65, no. 33.

37. See Derenbourg, comp., and Renaud, ed., *Médecine et histoire naturelle*, 76; and Cano Ledesma, *Manuscritos árabes de El Escorial*, 65, no. 33.

6. Oxford, Bodleian, Uri 412, Poc. 319, cat. Neubauer 2113 (**B**); fols, 1–123; Judeo-Arabic; Sephardic semi-cursive script.[38] According to the colophon, the text was copied by Makhluf ben R. Shmuʾel he-Ḥazan DMNSY (from Mans?), and completed on the eleventh of Elul 5112 (1352 CE).[39] Numerous Hebrew versions—derived from Nathan ha-Meʾati's Hebrew translation—have been added to the text above the lines and in the margins. The text suffers from many omissions and corruptions but does provide some unique variant readings—such as, in aphorism 3.22: المركّب, a unique, correct version according to Galen's τῆς συνθέτου σαρκὸς.[40]

7. Oxford, Bodleian, Hunt. Donat 33, Uri 423, cat. Neubauer 2114 (**O**); fols. 1–78; Sephardic semicursive script; ca. 1300(?).[41] The text begins with treatise 23, continues with the end of aphorism 6.90 to the treatise 24 (which is incomplete, with large sections missing), and ends with treatise 12. The colophon found at the end of treatise 12 reads:

كملت المقالة التاسعة عشر وعدد فصولها ألف الحمد للّه على حسن ع<...> والسلام
على المألّفين من اللّه <...> تمّ الكتاب في سنت الف ט״ג לחרבן ב״ש תם

The flyleaf at the beginning reads:

הדה אלכתאב יסמא כתאב אלפצול לאן אנמזג׳ קול אטבא והו שרח אלמוג׳ז
והו כתאב יסמא אלדכיראת אלאטבא בג׳מעהון לגאלינוס ופצולהו ואבא קראט
ופצ׳להו צחא וקול אלחכים מוסא אלקורטבי ופצול אבן זהר ועדד ופצולהון אללף
פצל פי אלטב ואמראץ׳ אלבדן מן אלראס ללקדם פי עלם אלאבדאן מנלראס לחד
אלאקדאם ופצול באלאכואץ לעלאג׳ אל נאס

The flyleaf at the end by the same hand reads:

כתאב אלדי כאן ענתי פי מצר נאקלתו פי סאלופכי׳ פי זמאן צלטן עצמן תריך
ע׳ה׳ע׳ס׳ סנת אלדי כונת פי אליגורנא מע דודור מורין ורחונא לאליגורנא קדנא

38. See Neubauer, *Hebrew Manuscripts in the Bodleian Library*, 721; see also Beit-Arié, comp., and May, ed., *Supplement of Addenda and Corrigenda*, col. 392.

39. May, in Beit-Arié, comp., and May, ed., *Supplement of Addenda and Corrigenda*, col. 392, state that Steinschneider refers to "a physician by the name of Makhluf of Marsala, Syracuse (Sicily)."

40. Galen, *De usu partium* 12.3 (ed. Helmreich, 2:188, line 4).

41. See Neubauer, *Hebrew Manuscripts in the Bodleian Library*, 722; and Beit-Arié, comp., and May, ed., *Supplement of Addenda and Corrigenda*, col. 392.

שהירין ורחות אנא ומעלמי לאנגלאתירא קדנא סני וג׳ינא עלא ויניזיא קדנא שהר
וג׳ינא לשיו פי סנת ה׳ ותלאתמיי״ ותלאתין וכמס׳. תאריך

The text has a few catchwords, some in Judeo-Arabic and some in Arabic. The beginning and end have been falsified, and the original figures of the chapters have been altered. This manuscript is closely related to **E** and **L**, sharing many characteristic readings.

8. Oxford, Bodleian, Hunt. 356, Uri 426, cat. Neubauer 2115 (**U**); fols. 1–107; Oriental semicursive script; late thirteenth century.[42] The manuscript itself provides us with two dates on fol. 106b: 1535 and a second date that is hard to decipher—possibly the year 1500. The text runs from aphorism 10.5 (at الضرورة) until aphorism 24.27 and has the following colophon:

תמת אלמקאלה י״ה בעון מאלך אלדוניה אלחכים עלא אל ספלייה ואלעלאויה
וחאכים עלא עלאוייה ואל ספלייה צחיב אל דוניה אל מצ״ייא. שנת ה׳ר״צ׳ה

The text on the flyleaf at the beginning reads:

האדא לשמעון אלחכים אלמערוף באבן חנין אלראיס פי מדינת בגדאד
אלמערוף בל עלם פל טב כתאב כט אבי עזרא רחמהו אלה קד נקלו מן כתאב קדים

A second text on the same flyleaf reads:

האדא אלכתאב אלעזיז אלשריף לחביש אלתפליסי ומפראתו פל אדויה מתעלקה
באכואץ אלצחיחה ואלמעדין ועדד אלפצול סתמאיה וסתה וסבעון בעון אלחי אלחק
אלקיום קד אן כתאב פי מדינה באביל פי שנת ה׳ק׳ג׳ה׳. כתבתו(?) באיבירייא
ובאירחמן ארחם [...].[43]

The text on the flyleaf at the end (fol. 107a) reads:

תמאת מקאלה חביש אלתפליסי אלמערוף אבן חבש אלחכים אלעריף אלזאהיר
אלמאהיר אלעריף באלתקים ואלתלטיף אלכביר אלחריף עדד מקאלתהו סתה מאיה

42. See Neubauer, *Hebrew Manuscripts in the Bodleian Library*, 722; and Beit-Arié, comp., and May, ed., *Supplement of Addenda and Corrigenda*, col. 392.

43. כתבתו(?) באיבירייא ובאירחמן ארחם [...]: Missing in Neubauer, *Hebrew Manuscripts in the Bodleian Library*, 722; and Beit-Arié, comp., and May, ed., *Supplement of Addenda and Corrigenda*, col. 392.

וסתה וסבעין פל אדויה ואלמפרדאת [...] אלמקאלת ועדד אלפצול מגמוע גמיע סימן
תהעו בעון [...] רחמאן.[44]

Just as in the previous manuscript, the beginning and end have been falsified. Similarly, the headings and figures of the chapters have been altered.

9. Göttingen 99. This manuscript was copied by Antonius Deussingius in the year 1635 in Leiden from **L**.[45]

10. Istanbul, Velieddin 2525.[46]

For the edition of Maimonides' *Medical Aphorisms: Treatises 22–25* in this volume, the following manuscripts have been consulted: Gotha 1937 (**G**), Leiden 1344 (**L**), Paris 1210 (**P**), Escorial 868 (**E**) and 869 (**S**), and Oxford 2113 (**B**), 2114 (**O**), and 2115 (**U**). These manuscripts can be divided into two main groups, namely, **GS** and **BELOPU**. The edition is mainly based on **G**.

The decision to edit Maimonides' *Medical Aphorisms* in Arabic characters, rather than in Hebrew ones, has been inspired by Maimonides' own practice. Recent scholarship gives reason to assume that Maimonides usually composed a first draft of his medical works—intended for private use—in Arabic, written in Hebrew characters, and that these works were subsequently transcribed into Arabic characters when intended for public use. Thus Stern remarks that "all of Maimonides' medical works were naturally published in Arabic script, since otherwise they would have been of no use to the non-Jewish public," and adds that Maimonides first drafted the text in Hebrew script, because the Hebrew script was easier for him, and then had it transcribed into the Arabic script.[47] Stern's point of view has been endorsed by Hopkins, who remarks that although we have sporadic autograph examples of his Arabic handwriting, Maimonides always used the Hebrew script when writing privately.[48] Other scholars have partly expressed different opinions in this matter. Meyerhof remarks that Maimonides composed all of his medical writings in Arabic, probably

---

44. Missing in Neubauer, *Hebrew Manuscripts in the Bodleian Library*, 722; and Beit-Arié, comp., and May, ed., *Supplement of Addenda and Corrigenda*, col. 392.

45. See Kahle, "Mosis Maimonidis Aphorismorum," 89.

46. See Ullmann, *Medizin im Islam*, 167 n. 4. I was unable to obtain photocopies of this manuscript.

47. Stern, in Maimonides, "*Treatise to a Prince*" (ed. and trans. Stern), 18. Cf. Blau, *Judaeo-Arabic*, 41 n. 6.

48. Hopkins, *Languages of Maimonides*, 90.

using Arabic characters, since he had nothing to hide from the Muslims.[49] Blau suggests that when addressing a general public, including Muslims and Christians (as in the case of medical writings), Jewish authors might have used Arabic script; but when addressing a Jewish audience, they wrote in Hebrew characters.[50] Langermann remarks that it seems likely that many of Maimonides' medical writings were originally written in Arabic characters which were only afterwards transcribed into Hebrew ones.[51]

For editing the Arabic text, which is written in Middle Arabic typical for this genre, I have adhered to the guidelines formulated by Kahl. Morphological and syntactic and even grievous offenses against the grammar of classical Arabic have been neither included in the apparatus nor changed or corrected at all. Orthographic peculiarities have not been included in the critical apparatus. They have been either adjusted to the conventional spelling or adopted in their given forms.[52]

## Hebrew translations of the *Kitāb al-fuṣūl fī al-ṭibb* (Medical Aphorisms)

As with volumes 1–4 of *Medical Aphorisms*, this edition is supplemented by a list of faulty readings and translations selected from Muntner's edition[53] of Nathan ha-Meʾati's Hebrew translation[54] and from Rosner's English translation of that edition (**r**).[55] Muntner's edition is based on a corrupt manuscript—Paris, Bibliothèque nationale, héb. 1173 (**p**)[56]—and therefore has many errors. Since Rosner's translation

49. Meyerhof, "Medical Work," 272.

50. Blau, *Judaeo-Arabic*, 41. Cf. Baron, *Social and Religious History of the Jews*, 8:403 n. 42.

51. Langermann, "Arabic Writings in Hebrew Manuscripts," 139.

52. See Kahl in Ibn Sahl, *Dispensatorium Parvum* (ed. Kahl), 35–38.

53. Maimonides, *Pirḳe Mosheh bi-refuʾah*, (ed. Muntner).

54. Nathan ha-Meʾati (from Cento) prepared this translation in Rome between 1279 and 1283 CE. For his data see Vogelstein and Rieger, *Geschichte der Juden in Rom*, 1:398–400; and Steinschneider, *Hebräische Übersetzungen des Mittelalters*, 766; and Freudenthal, "Sciences dans les communautés juives," 69–70; Bos, *Novel Medical and General Hebrew Terminology*, 2:21–27, 95–99.

55. Maimonides, *Medical Aphorisms* (trans. Rosner).

56. See Zotenberg, *Catalogues des manuscrits hébreux*, 215.

follows Muntner's edition, it suffers from many mistakes as well. The list also provides versions of these particular readings by Zeraḥyah ben Isaac ben She'altiel Ḥen, derived from his translation of the *Medical Aphorisms* (**Z**).[57] I also note a few examples of faulty readings by Zeraḥyah and correct ones by Nathan. It is my hope that on the basis of this list and ideally on the basis of future critical editions of these translations, it will be possible to provide critical evaluations of the translation activity of these two prominent translators. With this goal in mind, a supplemental volume containing a comparative Arabic-Hebrew-English glossary of technical terms used in the *Medical Aphorisms* is being planned. The Hebrew terms will also be listed alphabetically in separate indexes with reference to the comparative glossary. Thus, the glossary and indexes may contribute to our knowledge of medieval Hebrew medical terminology. They may also be used to amplify dictionaries of the Hebrew language or, ideally, to create a dictionary devoted to this particular area.[58] During the compilation of the glossary, it became increasingly clear that both Hebrew translations are based on an Arabic text represented by manuscripts **E** and **L**, since they share several unique readings.

57. Zeraḥyah's versions are derived from my forthcoming critical edition that is based on MS Florence, Biblioteca Mediceo-Laurenziana, MS Plut. LXXXVIII. 29, which was copied in the fourteenth century. On Zeraḥyah, who was active as a translator in Rome and who prepared the translation of the *Medical Aphorisms* in 1279, see Vogelstein and Rieger, *Geschichte der Juden in Rom*, 1:271–75, 409–18; Ravitzky, "Mishnato shel Rabi Zeraḥyah," 69–75; Bos in Aristotle, *De Anima* (ed. Bos), ch. 7: "Zeraḥyah's technique of translation;" Freudenthal, "Sciences dans les communautés juives," 67–69; and Zonta, "Hebrew translation of Hippocrates' *De superfoetatione*," 104–9; Bos, *Novel Medical and General Hebrew Terminology*, 1:121–27; Maimonides, *Medical Aphorisms: Medieval Hebrew Translations* (ed. Bos, forthcoming).

58. As a further step to such a dictionary devoted to the medieval Hebrew medical terminology, see my *Novel Medical and General Hebrew Terminology* (*Journal of Semitic Studies*, Suppl. 27, 30, 37), 3 vols. (Oxford: Oxford University Press, 2011–2016).

MEDICAL APHORISMS

TREATISES 22–25

◆

*In the name of God,*
*the Merciful, the Compassionate.*
*O Lord, make [our task] easy.*

# The Twenty-Second Treatise

## *Containing aphorisms concerning the specific properties [of remedies]*

(1) We[1] find medicines that are effective through their powers, and we find [other] medicines that are effective through their total substance, as I will describe now. *De theriaca ad Pisonem.*[2]

(2) Mouse heads, burned and kneaded with honey and rubbed on [the spot affected by] alopecia, stimulate hair growth. Similarly, mouse excrement, if pulverized in vinegar, is beneficial for alopecia. Viper skin is also good for [alopecia] if it is ground with honey. *De theriaca ad Pisonem.*[3]

(3) If the brain of a camel is dried and imbibed with vinegar, it is beneficial for epilepsy. The brain of a weasel has a similar effect. *Ibidem.*[4]

(4) The brain of a bat with honey is beneficial for a cataract in the eye. The brain of a sheep has a similar effect.[5]

بسم الله الرحمن الرحيم

ربّ يسّر

# المقالة الثانية والعشرون

تشتمل على فصول تتعلّق بخواصّ

(١) نجد أدوية تفعل بقواها فنجد أدوية تفعل بجملة جوهرها مثل ما أنا ذاكره الآن. في مقالته في الترياق إلى قيصر.

(٢) رؤوس الفيران تحرق وتعجن بعسل ويلطخ بها داء الثعلب فينبت الشعر. وكذلك خرء الفأر إذا سحق بالخلّ نفع من داء الثعلب. وكذلك ينفع منه جلد الأفاعي إذا سحق بعسل. في مقالته في الدرياق إلى قيصر.

(٣) دماغ البعير إذا جفّف وسقي بخلّ نفع من الصرع وكذلك يفعل دماغ ابن عرس. في تلك المقالة.

(٤) دماغ الخفّاش مع العسل ينفع من الماء النازل في العين. وكذلك يفعل دماغ الشاة.

١ بسم الله الرحمن الرحيم ربّ يسّر] om. BELU بسم الله الرحمن الرحيم O || ٤ بخواصّ] بالخواصّ BOSU || ٩ بعسل] نفع add. GS | في مقالته في الدرياق إلى قيصر] في تلك مقالة ELB | الدرياق] الترياق SBU

(5) The gall of a female hyena, if mixed with honey and applied as an eye salve, is beneficial for a cataract in the eye.[6] If a falcon is cooked in lily oil, it is good for weak vision.[7]

(6) If one rubs the gums of children with the brain of a sheep, it eases the growth of the teeth without pain.[8]

(7) If the horn of a stag is burned and pulverized with wine, it is beneficial for pain and weakness of the teeth. The anklebone of a cow, if burned and pulverized with wine, is good for pain and weakness of the teeth. *Ibidem*.[9]

(8) If one drinks the filings of the horn of a bull with water, it stops a nosebleed. Its thighbones have a similar effect. *Ibidem*.[10]

(9) Shrimp[11] empty [the body] of tapeworms.[12] Similarly, the anklebone of a cow, if burned and drunk with honey, evacuates tapeworms from the belly. *Ibidem*.[13]

(10) Excrements of a mouse crumble bladder stones.[14] Similarly, a scorpion—if eaten with bread—crumbles [bladder] stones.[15] Earthworms [*Lumbricus terrestris*] have the same effect. *Ibidem*.[16]

(11) If earthworms are pulverized and administered to a jaundice patient, his body will be cleansed immediately.[17]

(12) If dung beetles are boiled in olive oil and that oil is dripped into the ear, it will alleviate the pain immediately.[18]

(13) If the anklebone of a cow is burned and imbibed with oxymel, it[19] reduces the swelling of the spleen; it also stimulates the libido. *Ibidem*.[20]

(14) If goose fat is melted in rose oil, it is beneficial for inflamed tumors.[21]

(15) The burned skin of a hippopotamus is beneficial for hard tumors.[22] If a river crab is pulverized and put on a hard tumor, it dispels [the tumor]. *Ibidem*.[23]

(٥) مرارة الضبعة العرجاء إذا خلطت بعسل واكتحل بها نفعت من الماء النازل في العين. البازي إذا طبخ بدهن السوسن نفع من ضعف البصر. في تلك المقالة.

(٦) دماغ الشاة إذا مسح به درادر الصبيان سهّل نبات الأسنان بلا ألم.

(٧) قرن الأيّل إذا أحرق وسحق بالخمر نفع من وجع الأسنان وضعفها. كعب البقر إذا أحرق وسحق بالخمر نفع من وجع الأسنان وضعفها. في تلك المقالة.

(٨) برادة قرن الثور إذا شرب بالماء حبس الرعاف وكذلك تفعل عظام فخذيه. في تلك المقالة.

(٩) الإربيان تستفرغ حبّ القرع. وكذلك كعب البقر إذا أحرق وشرب بعسل استفرغ حبّ القرع من البطن. في تلك المقالة.

(١٠) خرء الفأر يفتّت حصاة المثانة وكذلك العقرب إذا أكلت مع الخبز يفتّت الحصاة وكذلك تفعل الخراطين. في تلك المقالة.

(١١) الخراطين إذا سحقت وسقيت صاحب اليرقان نقي بدنه على المكان.

(١٢) الخنفساء إذا غليت في الزيت وقطّر ذلك الزيت في الأذن سكّن وجعها من ساعته.

(١٣) كعب البقر إذا أحرق وشرب بسكنجبين أذبل الطحال العظيم وهو مهيج للباه. في تلك المقالة.

(١٤) شحم الإوزّ إذا أذيب بدهن الورد نفع من الأورام الملتهبة.

(١٥) جلد فرس البحر محرق ينفع من الأورام الجاسية. السرطان النهري إذا سحق وجعل على الورم الجاسي فشّه. في تلك المقالة.

---

١ الضبعة] الضبع B الضبعا U || ١٢ وسقيت صاحب] وسقيت لصاحب L وسقت لصاحب EB

(16) Cow's milk is clearly beneficial for[24] intestinal ulcers. Castoreum[25] is clearly beneficial for shivers.[26] *Ibidem.*[27]

If crocodile fat is put on the spot of its bite, it heals immediately. Similarly, if one takes a weasel and rubs it on the spot of its bite, it is healed immediately. And if one takes a viper, pulverizes it, and puts it on the spot of its bite, [this[28] remedy] somewhat alleviates the pain. *Ibidem.*[29]

(17) If one heats marcasite[30] stone and sprinkles vinegar on it and then places the limb that has a hard tumor above the vapor that arises from it, you will see it dissolve in an amazing way, as[31] if it is an act of magic. *Ad Glauconem* [*de medendi methodo*] 2.[32]

(18) If peony [*Paeonia officinalis* Retz.] root is tied with something and hung on [the neck] of children suffering from epilepsy, it cures them. I have tested and tried this and found a similar [effect].[33]

(19) Asafetida[34] [gum resin of *Ferula assa-foetida*] is beneficial for a swollen uvula in the same way. Similarly, roasted nigella [*Nigella sativa* and var.], if it is tied with a finely woven cloth and then [its hot vapor] is inhaled, [will[35] dry up] the rheum of someone suffering from it. Similarly, if[36] one takes some of the threads that were dyed with the purple hailing[37] from the purple-fish, and that were used for choking a viper, and wraps them around the neck of someone who suffers from an inflammation of the tonsils or from any other inflammation in the neck, you see that it is beneficial for it in an amazing way. *De* [*simplicium*] *medicamentorum* [*temperamentis ac facultatibus*] 6.[38]

(20) Excrements[39] of a dog that has been nourished with bones—namely, those [excrements] that appear white and dry and free from stench—should be dried and pulverized and then given as a drink to patients suffering from angina[40] and inflammation of the throat, together with another medicine beneficial for this [disease]. It may also be given as a drink to those suffering from dysentery, in milk that was boiled with [red-hot][41] stones or iron. Inveterate ulcers can also be treated with it if it is mixed with some other medicine that is good for this. It may also be mixed with medications that dissolve tumors. *De* [*simplicium*] *medicamentorum* [*temperamentis ac facultatibus*] 10.[42]

(١٦) لبن البقر نافع من قروح الأمعاء والجندبادستر ينفع من الكزاز نفعا بيّنا. في تلك المقالة.

شحم التمساح يوضع على موضع عضّته فيبرأ من ساعته. وكذلك ابن عرس إذا أخذت تلك الدابّة ودلك بها موضع عضّتها برئ من ساعته و إذا أخذت الأفعى ودقّت ووضعت على موضع نهشتها سكّنت الألم قليلا. في تلك المقالة.

(١٧) حجر المرقشيثا إذا حمّي ورشّ عليه الخلّ وجعل العضو الذي فيه ورم صلب على البخار المتراقي فيه رأيت من تحلّله عجبا وكأنّه فعل السحر. في ثانية أغلوقن.

(١٨) أصل الفاوانيا إذا شدّ في شيء وعلّق على الصبيان الذين يصرعون شفاهم وقد امتحنت ذلك وجرّبته وقد نجد نظير ذلك.

(١٩) الحلتيت ينفع اللهاة الوارمة على هذا الوجه. وكذلك الشونيز المقلو إذا شدّ في خرقة مهلهلة وهو حارّ واستنشقه المزكوم. وكذلك خيوط الأرجوان التي تخرج من البحر إذا صبغ وخنقت بها الأفعى وأخذ من تلك الخيوط فلفّ كما يدور على عنق إنسان به ورم النغانغ أو غيره من جميع الأورام الحادثة في العنق رأيت منه العجب العجيب في نفعه إيّاه. سادسة الأدوية.

(٢٠) زبل الكلاب التي تغتذي بالعظام وهو الذي تراه أبيض اللون يابسا بريئا من النتن يجفّف ويسحق ويسقى لأصحاب الخوانيق وأورام الحلق مع أحد الأدوية النافعة لذلك. ويسقى لصاحب دوسنطريا باللبن المطبوخ بالحجارة أو بالحديد وتعالج به أيضا القروح المتقادمة إذا خلط ببعض أدويتها ويخلط أيضا بالأدوية المحلّلة للأورام. عاشرة الأدوية.

---

٣ و كذلك] $G^1$ || ٦ العضو] للعضو G على العضو EO || ٧ فعل] من فعل ESOU || ٨ أصل] om. G || ٩ نجد] وجد G يوجد B || ١١ مهلهلة] سلسة LBU ملسة O || ١٣ في] يوم add. L || ١٥ الكلاب التي تغتذي] الكلب الذي يغتذي L || ١٧ دوسنطريا] دوسنطاريا SU دوسطرايا L دشنطريا E دوسنطارية B دشونطريا O

(21) A child [suffering from an inflammation of the throat] should be treated for three days with a diet of oven bread and white lupine [*Lupinus albus*] and should be given slightly diluted wine to drink and should beware of indigestions. On the third day one should take his stool, dry it, pulverize it, knead it with honey, and smear it on the throat of [the child] that suffers from such an inflammation of the throat that it endangers his life. *De* [*simplicium*] *medicamentorum* [*temperamentis ac facultatibus*] 10.[43]

(22) If the excrements of a wolf that is nourished with bones—that is, white excrements—are given as a drink to someone afflicted by the pain of a colic, [the pain] will subside. Sometimes it [prevents] a colic before it [actually] occurs, and it does not occur in someone who is used [to taking this remedy] or [the attack] is milder than usual. [The excrements] may also be hung on [the neck of] someone suffering from a colic, for [this] brings clear benefit.[44] *De* [*simplicium*] *medicamentorum* [*temperamentis ac facultatibus*] 10.[45]

(23) The excrements of a goat [mixed] with barley meal and kneaded with vinegar dissolve hard tumors, tumors of the knee[46] and spleen. Do[47]not use this therapy for those with a soft [body], like women, children, and eunuchs.[48]

(24) If cow's dung is smeared on dropsy patients, it is of great benefit to them. If it is kneaded with vinegar, it dissolves hard tumors. *De* [*simplicium*] *medicamentorum* [*temperamentis ac facultatibus*] 10.[49]

(25) Sheep excrement, dried and kneaded with vinegar, heals warts, fleshy excrescences, ulcers that develop from burning with fire, and shingles in which one has the sensation of crawling ants. *De* [*simplicium*] *medicamentorum* [*temperamentis ac facultatibus*] 10.[50]

(26) Pigeon dung should be pulverized, filtered, and smeared on chronically [painful] limbs that one wants to heat. Similarly, [it is good as a cataplasm for] chronic cold pains, such as podagra, migraine, headache, pain in the back, abdomen, kidneys, and joints. *De* [*simplicium*] *medicamentorum* [*temperamentis ac facultatibus*] 10.[51]

(27) I know someone in our times who [treated patients] by giving them burned human bones to drink without informing them about this, lest they turn away from [taking] it. This man used to cure with these burned bones many [patients] suffering from epilepsy and pain in the joints. *De* [*simplicium*] *medicamentorum* [*temperamentis ac facultatibus*] 10.[52]

(٢١) يتقدّم إلى صبي ويغذى ثلثة أيّام بخبز تنّوري وترمس ويشرب شراب قليل المزج ويتحفّظ من التخم. ويؤخذ زبله في اليوم الثالث ويجفّف ويسحق ويعجن بعسل ويطلى على حلق من يرم حلقه حتّى يشرف على الموت فيبرأ. عاشرة الأدوية.

(٢٢) زبل الذئب الذي يغتذي بالعظام وهو الزبل الأبيض إذا سقي منه لمن هاج به وجع القولنج سكن. وربّما شفى من القولنج من قبل حدوثه ولا يحدث لمن اعتاده أو يكون أخفّ من المعتاد. وقد يعلّق على من به قولنج فينفعه منفعة بيّنة. عاشرة الأدوية.

(٢٣) بعر المعز مع دقيق الشعير معجون بالخلّ يحلّل الأورام الصلبة وأورام الركبة وصلابة الطحال. ولا يعالج به الرخص البدن كالنساء والصبيان والخصيان.

(٢٤) أخثاء البقر يطلى به المستسقين فينفعهم منفعة عظيمة. وإذا عجن بالخلّ يحلّل الأورام الصلبة. عاشرة الأدوية.

(٢٥) زبل الضأن ييبّس ويعجن بالخلّ فيبرئ الثآليل واللحم الزائد والقروح الحادثة عن حرق النار والنملة التي يحسّ فيها كدبيب النمل. عاشرة الأدوية.

(٢٦) زبل الحمام يدقّ وينخل وتطلى به الأعضاء المزمنة التي تريد تسخينها. وكذلك الأوجاع الباردة المزمنة كالنقرس والشقيقة والصداع وأوجاع الظهر والبطن والكليتين والمفاصل. عاشرة الأدوية.

(٢٧) إنّي لأعرف إنسانا ممن في دهرنا هذا يسقي عظام الناس المحرقة من غير أن يعلمهم بذلك كيلا يفرّون منها. وكان هذا الرجل يشفي بهذه العظام المحرقة خلقا كثيرا ممّن به الصرع وممّن به وجع المفاصل. عاشرة الأدوية.

---

١ أيّام] G¹ || ٢ المزج] المزاج ESO | ويسحق] G¹ || ٩ يحلّل] حلّل LB || ١١ ويعجن] ويجمع B || ١٢ كدبيب] بدبيب ELU | عاشرة الأدوية] في تلك مقالة ELO || ١٥ عاشرة الأدوية] في تلك مقالة ELO || ١٧ وكان] G¹

(28) If chicken dung is pulverized and given as a drink with vinegar to someone who chokes by [the consumption of] fungi, he will vomit thick, viscous humors and be healed.[53] *De* [*simplicium*] *medicamentorum* [*temperamentis ac facultatibus*] 10.[54]

(29) If one burns river crabs alive in a red copper pot, takes one part of their ashes, half a part of great yellow gentian [*Gentiana lutea*], and one tenth of frankincense [*Boswellia* spp.], and from this [mixture] sprinkles a large spoonful on water and gives it to someone bitten by a dog, it is of amazing benefit. Similarly, the ashes of these river crabs alone are very beneficial for such persons, but not the ashes of sea [crabs]. *De* [*simplicium*] *medicamentorum* [*temperamentis ac facultatibus*], last book.[55]

(30) The lung of a fox, if dried and imbibed, cures asthma. *De* [*simplicium*] *medicamentorum* [*temperamentis ac facultatibus*], last book.[56]

(31) If one constantly drinks the broth [prepared] from larks and eats their flesh, it cures a colic. *De* [*simplicium*] *medicamentorum* [*temperamentis ac facultatibus*], last book.[57]

(32) If earthworms—that is, the long worms that can be found in the earth when one digs or ploughs in it—are pulverized and put on nerves that have been cut off, they immediately provide an amazing benefit.[58] If one drinks them together with concentrated grape juice, they also stimulate micturition.[59] *De* [*simplicium*] *medicamentorum* [*temperamentis ac facultatibus*], last book.[60]

(33) Vinegar has a specific property that distinguishes it from other similar substances, namely, that next[61] to its cutting effect it dissolves [and at the same time] checks[62] the dissolution process. This is because its nature is partially hot, but only in a small insignificant quantity, while most of its nature is cold and fine. *Mayāmir* 1.[63]

(34) The spleen of a wild donkey or the spleen of a wild horse should be dried and pulverized and given as a drink to those suffering from a spleen disease [in a dose of] six *dirhams*[64] with five ounces[65] of diluted wine. *Mayāmir* 9.[66]

(٢٨) زبل الدجاج يسحق ويسقى بخلّ لمن خنقه الفطر فيتقيّأ أخلاطا غليظة لزجة فيبرأ. عاشرة الأدوية.

(٢٩) السرطانات النهرية تحرق أحياء في قدر نحاس أحمر ويؤخذ من رمادها جزء ومن الجنطيانا نصف جزء ومن الكندر عشر جزء ويذرّ على الماء من مجموع ذلك قدر ملعقة كبيرة ويسقى ذلك لمن نهشه الكلب فينفعه منفعة عجيبة. وكذلك رماد هذه السرطانات وحده ينفعهم جدّا ولا ينفعهم رماد البحرية. آخر الأدوية.

(٣٠) رئة الثعلب إن جفّفت وشربت شفت من الربو. آخر الأدوية.

(٣١) مرق القنابر إذا أدمن شربه وأكل أجرامها أبرأ من القولنج. آخر الأدوية.

(٣٢) الخراطين وهي الديدان الطوال التي توجد في الأرض إذا حفرت أو حرثت إذا سحقت ووضعت على العصب المقطوع نفعته من ساعته منفعة عجيبة. وإذا شربت أيضا مع عقيد العنب أدرّت البول. آخر الأدوية.

(٣٣) في الخلّ خاصّة شيء يخصّه دون نظرائه وذلك أنّه جمع مع تقطيعه أنّه محلّل مانع لتجلّب ما يتجلّب. وذلك بسبب أنّ بعض طبعه حارّ وذلك فيه وتح يسير وأمّا جلّ طبعه فبارد لطيف. أولى الميامر.

(٣٤) طحال حمار الوحش أو طحال فرس برّي يجفّف ويدقّ ويسقى منه المطحولين ستّة دراهم بشراب ممزوج خمسة أواق. تاسعة الميامر.

---

٩ الطوال] الكبار O | أو حرثت] om. ESLO || ١٢ خاصّة] om. L خاصّية B || ١٣ لتجلّب ما يتجلّب] لتحلّل ما يتحلّل ELO لتحلّل ما يتجلّب U | طبعه][1]G | وذلك] لأن [2]L add. | وتح يسير] ريحا يسيرا (?)L || ١٥ ويدقّ] ويحرق O || ١٦ تاسعة] سابعة ELBO

(35) Abū[67] Marwān ibn Zuhr has mentioned many specific properties [of remedies] that he tested. He was one of the [great] empiricists. His[68] son told me amazing things about his precision and diligence in matters depending upon experience. Therefore, I thought it a good thing to mention them in his name, although some of them have been mentioned by others before. However, he is the one who verified these experiential matters. All those specific properties are mentioned by him in his *Book*[69] *on the Facilitation [of Treatment and Diet]* and in the *Book*[70] *on Foodstuffs*, which he composed for one[71] of the Andalusian kings. His father, Abū[72] al-ʿAlāʾ, mentions some of these [remedies] in his [book entitled] *al-Tadhkira*. They are as follows:

(36) The[73] ingestion of nine granules[74] of emerald, pulverized and filtered, in a mouthful of water on an empty stomach stops[75] the diarrhea[76] caused by poisons. If[77] it is hung [around the neck] of someone suffering from diarrhea or lientery, it cures him. If[78] the emerald is hung [around the neck], it strengthens the stomach and is beneficial for epilepsy. If it is kept in the mouth, it strengthens the teeth and the stomach, and if one puts it on as a ring, it strengthens the cardia of the stomach and stops emesis and brings [the person] around. The[79] criteria for [the application of] the emerald are the same as those for the theriac. It should not be taken together with food, but there should be an interval of nine[80] hours between them.

(37) Looking in the eyes of a wild ass gives a lasting healthy vision and is beneficial for the formation of a cataract [in the eyes]. He says: This is true without any doubt.[81]

(38) The[82] consumption of the heads of hares, as much as one is able to eat them, is beneficial for trembling. I found by experience that it is also beneficial for numbness and hemiplegia. The consumption of hare meat crumbles [kidney] stones.

(39) I[83] found by experience that the drinking of water in which mastic has been cooked protects against diseases of the liver and stomach, and that the drinking of water in which watermelon seed has been cooked protects against [kidney] stones, and that the anointment of the eyelids with gold[84] strengthens vision, and[85] that if one cooks therewith or throws [some of it] into a cooked dish, it strengthens the body in general. [I[86] also found by experience] that the application of a poultice of fresh rose blossoms to the eyes protects against ophthalmia.

(٣٥) ذكر أبو مروان بن زهر خواصّا كثيرة جرّبها وكان من المجرّبين. أخبرني ولده بعجائب من تحريره واجتهاده في التجربة فلذلك رأيت أن أذكرها منسوبة إليه وإن كان قد ذكر بعضها غيره لكنّه هو الذي صحّح تجربة ذلك. وتلك الخواصّ كلّها ذكرها في كتابه في التيسير وفي كتابه الذي ألّفه في الأغذية لبعض ملوك الأندلس. وذكر أبو العلاء أبوه بعضها في التذكرة له وهي هذه:

(٣٦) شرب تسع حبّات من الزمرّد مسحوقا منخولا بجرعة ماء على الريق يقطع إسهال السموم وإن علّق على من به إسهال أو زلق الأمعاء أبرأه وإن علّق الزمرّد قوّى المعدة ونفع من الصرع وإمساكه في الفم يقوّي الأسنان والمعدة والتختّم به يقوّي فم المعدة ويقطع القيء وينعش من الغشي. وحكم الزمرّد كحكم الترياق لا يجمع بينه وبين الطعام ويكون بينهما تسع ساعات.

(٣٧) النظر إلى أعين حمر الوحش يديم صحّة البصر وينفع من نزول الماء. قال: صحّ ذلك صحّة لا شكّ فيها.

(٣٨) أكل رؤوس الأرانب كلّما يمكن أكله من الرأس ينفع من الارتعاش. ووجدت بالتجربة أيضا أنّها تنفع من الخدر والفالج. وأكل لحم الأرنب يفتّت الحصاة.

(٣٩) وجدت بالتجربة أنّ شرب الماء الذي طبخ فيه المصطكى أمان من علل الكبد والمعدة. وأنّ شرب الماء الذي يطبخ فيه بزر بطّيخ أمان من الحصى وأنّ الاكتحال بالذهب يقوّي البصر وأنّ الطبخ فيه أو إلقاء الذهب في الطبيخ يقوّي البدن على العموم وأنّ تضميد العينين بزهر الورد الطريء أمان من الرمد.

---

٦ إسهال] آفة L || ٧ أبرأه] حبسه B || ١١ أعين] $G^1$ | حمر] حمار ELBO | قال] om. ELO || ١٥ شرب . . . والمعدة. و] om. B || ١٧ الطبخ فيه أو] om. L || ١٨ أمان] نافع B

(40) The[87] anointment of the eyelids with rose syrup made with sugar strengthens vision. Its permanent use cures dilatation of the palpebral membrane. This has been verified by experience; I have not ceased to use it for strengthening vision. I have found that pulverized and filtered clove [*Syzygium aromaticum*], sprinkled every night on the forehead during winter, protects against catarrhs, while mace[88] is of a similar effect in all the seasons [of the year]. But the different kinds of mint[89] [*Mentha*] are less beneficial than clove, and similarly citron [*Citrus medica*] peel is less beneficial than mace.[90]

(41) Constant[91] anointing of the spine of the back with sweet almond oil, lukewarm, protects against the bending [of the body] that occurs to the elderly. It[92] has been verified by experience that the consumption of turnip[93] [*Brassica rapa*], boiled, sharpens vision.

(42) The[94] consumption of the heads of sparrows[95] and especially the male ones, and similarly the consumption of turnips cooked either in meat or alone, and similarly [the consumption of] carrots, and similarly the consumption of young pigeons that are able to fly, and similarly the ingestion of juice of chickpeas [*Cicer arietinum* and var.]—each of these substances on its own is good for strengthening [the lust for] sexual intercourse, let alone when they are eaten together in one dish.

(43) The consumption of male domesticated pigeons cures hemiplegia, paralysis, numbness, apoplexy, and trembling. The inhalation of the odorous breath of pigeons and [the inhalation] of that which dissolves from their bodies into the air protects against all these diseases, and[96] washing the bottom after defecation with lukewarm sweet water protects against hemorrhoids.[97]

(44) The wearing of hare furs strengthens the bodies of old and young people, and the wearing of lambskin strengthens the bodies of children. The proximity to cats causes marasmus and phthisis.[98]

(45) The[99] consumption of garden radish [*Raphanus sativus* and var.] and cabbage [*Brassica oleracea*] eliminates hoarseness and the[100] consumption of roasted quince [*Cydonia oblonga*] after meals gives energy and joy. The[101] consumption of citron [*Citrus medica*] peel strengthens the heart, and its seeds are beneficial against poisons. Lemon [*Citrus limon*] peel is [also] beneficial against poisons, as are the leaves of its tree.[102]

(٤٠) الاكتحال بشراب الورد السكّري يقوّي البصر ويبرئ مداومة ذلك من الانتشار. صحّ ذلك بالتجربة ولم أزل أستعمله في تقوية البصر. وجدت أنّ القرنفل المسحوق المنخول ذرورا على مقدّم الرأس كلّ ليلة في زمن الشتاء أمان من النزلات والبسباسة تنفع كذلك في جميع الفصول. وأمّا الفوذنجات فهي دون القرنفل في النفع وكذلك قشر الأترجّ دون البسباسة.

(٤١) لزوم دهن فقار الظهر بدهن اللوز الحلو مفترّا أمان من الانحناء الحادث للشيوخ. وصحّ بالتجربة أنّ أكل اللفت مطبوخا يحدّ البصر.

(٤٢) أكل رؤوس العصافير وبخاصّة ذكورها وكذلك أكل اللفت مطبوخا بلحم أو وحده وكذلك الجزر وكذلك أكل فرّاخ الحمام النواهض وكذلك شرب ماء الحمّص كلّ واحد من هذه بمفرده معين على الجماع فناهيك إن جمعت في طعام واحد.

(٤٣) أكل ذكران حمام الأبراج شفاء من الفالج والاسترخاء والخدر والسكتة والرعشة. وشمّ روائح أنفاس الحمام وما يتحلّل من جرمها في الهواء أمان من تلك العلل كلّها والاستنجاء بالماء العذب الفاتر أمان من البواسير.

(٤٤) لباس أفرية الأرانب مقوّية لأبدان الشيوخ والشبّان ولباس أفرية الخرفان مقوّية لأبدان الصبيان. ومقاربة القطّات تورث الذبول والسلّ.

(٤٥) أكل الفجل والكرنب يذهب بالبحح وأكل السفرجل المشوي بعد الطعام ينشط ويفرح. وأكل قشر الأترجّ يقوّي القلب وحبّه ينفع من السموم وقشر الليمون ينفع من السموم وكذلك ورقة شجرته.

---

٣ تنفع كذلك] تفعل ذلك B تنفع من ذلك E || ٧ أكل . . . وكذلك] om. B | يحدّ] يقوّي SG || ١٠ الجماع] النساء ELBOU || ١١ الفالج والاسترخاء] الاسترخاء ELOU أمراض الاسترخاء B | والسكتة] om. LB || ١٦ بالبحح] بالبحة ELO || ١٧ وقشر الليمون ينفع من السموم] om. B

(46) The[103] consumption of *al-murrī al-naqīʿ*[104] and vinegar removes the causes for the development of worms in the abdomen. The[105] consumption of peaches [*Amygdalus persica*], in spite of their harmful effects, is beneficial against vapor [arising] from the stomach. Similarly, field eryngo [*Eryngium campestre*] has about the same effect. The[106] smelling of peaches brings [someone] around, and the drinking of the juice of their leaves kills worms.

(47) If[107] black mustard [*Brassica nigra*] oil is dripped into a deaf ear, hearing returns, and[108] the immersion in lukewarm olive oil is beneficial for all pains of the body.

(48) If[109] the inner coat of the stomach of the male bustard is dried and mixed with collyria, it has the specific property of being beneficial against a cataract in the eye. The[110] coat of the stomach of the ostrich has the specific property, if one takes thereof, of being beneficial for those suffering from a stomach disease and for crumbling [kidney] stones.

(49) Young hawks and falcons have a delicious taste and strengthen the soul and have the specific property of being beneficial against hypochondriac melancholy and other corruptions of the mind.[111]

(50) If[112] the penis is rubbed with hedgehog fat, it gives a strong erection and provides increased pleasure during sexual intercourse. If[113] the penis of a hedgehog is dried, pulverized, and ingested, it gives a strong erection. The penis of a male deer has a similar effect [if dried, pulverized, and ingested] by its specific property.

(51) Common jujube [*Ziziphus jujuba*] has the specific property of being beneficial for diseases of the lung, esophagus, chest, and urinary bladder; it is moist and tends slightly towards heat.[114]

(52) The[115] acidic inner part of the citron eliminates thirst, vigorously subdues yellow bile, and[116] strengthens the soul. Myrobalan[117] has the specific property of being beneficial for the stomach. The[118] drinking[119] of half a *dirham* of balsam of Mecca [*Commiphora opobalsamum*] counter-acts all poisons.

(53) If a carnelian is pulverized and the teeth are rubbed with it, it makes them white and prevents their corrosion.[120]

(٤٦) أكل المرّي النقيع والخلّ يقطع أسباب تولّد الديدان في البطن. وأكل الخوخ مع مضرّته ينفع من بخر المعدة. وكذلك القرصعنة تفعل قريبا من فعله. وشمّ الخوخ ينعش من الغشي وشرب عصارة ورقه يقتل الديدان.

(٤٧) دهن الخردل يقطّر في الأذن الصمّاء فيعود السمع والانغماس في الزيت الفاتر ينفع من أوجاع البدن كلّها.

(٤٨) قشر قانصة الحبارى الداخل إذا جفّف له خاصّية في النفع من نزول الماء في العين إذا خلط في الأكحال وقشر قانصة النعام له خاصّية إذا تنوّلت في نفع المعودين وتفتيت الحصى.

(٤٩) فراخ البزاة والصقور لذيذة الطعم يشجّع النفس ولها خاصّية في النفع من المالنخونيا والمراقية وغيرها من فسادات الذهن.

(٥٠) شحم القنفذ إذا دهن به الذكر أنعظ إنعاظا قويا وأكسب لذّة زائدة عند الجماع. وذكر القنفذ إذا جفّف وسحق وشرب أنعظ إنعاظا قويا. وكذلك يفعل ذكر الأيّل بخاصّية فيها.

(٥١) العنّاب له خصوصية بالنفع من أمراض الرئة والمريء والصدر والمثانة وهو رطب يميل إلى الحرّ قليلا.

(٥٢) حمّاض الأترجّ يذهب العطش وهو شديد القمع للصفراء مقوّ للنفس. وللهليلج خاصّية في نفع المعدة. وشرب نصف درهم من البلسان يقاوم جميع السموم.

(٥٣) والعقيق إذا سحق وحكّت به الأسنان بيّضها ومنع تأكّلها.

---

٧ تنوّلت] تناولت O || ١١ وأكسب . . . إنعاظا قويا] $G^{1}$ | لذّة] لذاذة ELBOU || ١٦ العطش] بالعطش EBO

(54) Broad beans[121] [*Vicia faba*] have the specific property of corrupting the mind. Milk has the specific property of being harmful for the brain. Aloe[122] [*Aloe vera*] [has the specific property] of being harmful for the anus. Colocynth[123] [*Citrullus colocynthis*] [has the specific property] of being harmful for the liver. Figs[124] [*Ficus carica*] have the specific property of producing lice. Service tree [*Sorbus domestica*] [has the specific property of being beneficial] for weakness of the liver.

(55) Almonds[125] [*Prunus dulcis*] have the specific property of preserving the substance of the brain, while their moisture preserves the organs in an amazing way, without producing abnormal moisture. Rose[126] jam has the specific property of strengthening the lungs.[127]

(56) Agarwood[128] [*Aquilaria malaccensis*] has the specific property of being beneficial for the stomach and of strengthening it, and it eliminates a bad smell from the mouth. Artichoke [*Cynara cardunculus* and var.] perfumes winds [and] breath[129] from the body. Smelling narcissus[130] eliminates children's epilepsy. Its smell has the same effect as that which Galen[131] attributes to peony [*Paeonia officinalis*]. This is the end of the words of Ibn Zuhr.[132]

(57) From the words of al-Tamīmī[133] on the specific properties of drugs: He said: If one drinks a decoction of black chickpeas [*Cicer arietinum*] with bees' honey for three consecutive days, it cures the severe pain [caused by] gout. Opium poppy [*Papaver somniferum* and var.] prevents a defluxion of [superfluous] matter, whether warm or cold. Common purslane [*Portulaca oleracea*] stops the craving[134] for clay.

(58) He further said: Hemp [*Cannabis sativa*] oil has the specific property of being beneficial for earaches caused by cold and cures chronic illnesses of the ear and dissolves its obstructions. If[135] beef is boiled with vinegar, it has the specific property of being beneficial for jaundice, of expelling yellow bile, and of stopping diarrhea of bilious matter.

(59) Hedgehog meat, if dried and imbibed in oxymel, is beneficial for pains in the kidneys, elephantiasis, and dropsy of the flesh. If children feed themselves with its flesh, it is beneficial for them against epilepsy and bed-wetting.

(٥٤) للباقّلي خصوصية في إفساد الذهن وللبن خاصّية في إضرار الدماغ وللصبر في إضرار المقعدة وللحنظل في إضرار الكبد. والتين له خاصّية في توليد القمل وللغبيراء في ضعف الكبد.

(٥٥) للوز خاصّية في حفظ جوهر الدماغ ويحفظ على الأعضاء رطوبتها حفظا بديعا ولا يحدث رطوبة غريبة. وللورد المربّى خاصّية في تقوية الرئة.

(٥٦) العود الهندي له خصوصية في نفع المعدة وتقويتها ويذهب نتن الفم. والخرشف يعطّر رياح أرواح البدن. شمّ النرجس يذهب بصرع الصبيان. ويفعل شمّه ما ذكره جالينوس في الفاونيا. انتهى كلام بن زهر.

(٥٧) من كلام التميمي في خواصّ الأدوية. قال: ماء سليق الحمّص الأسود مع عسل النحل إذا شرب ثلثة أيام متوالية شفى من وجع النقرس الشديد. والخشخاش يمنع الهطل كانت المادّة حارّة أو باردة. والرجلة قاطعة لشهوة الطين.

(٥٨) وقال لدهن القنّب خاصّية في النفع من أوجاع الأذن الباردة ويشفي أمراضها المتقادمة ويحلّل سددها. ولحم البقر إذا طبخ بالخلّ كانت له خاصّية في النفع من اليرقان ودفع المرّة الصفراء وقطع الإسهال الصفراوي.

(٥٩) لحم القنفذ إذا جفّف وسقي منه بالسكنجبين نفع أوجاع الكلى والجذام والاستسقاء اللحمي. وإذا اغتذى الصبيان بلحمه نفعهم من الصرع والبول في الفراش.

---

١ خاصّية] خصوصية LBOU | الدماغ] الذهن L || ٢ المقعدة] المعدة L | والتين له خاصّية] وللغبيراء خاصّية ELBOU | وللغبيراء] وللتين ELBOU || ٤ للوز . . . الرئة] $G^1$ | بديعا] بليغا B || ٦ نتن] بريح B || ٨ الفاونيا] الفاوانية B الفاوينا U الفاوانا EO | انتهى كلام بن زهر] om. L || ٩ الأدوية] الأدويته G || ١٣ المتقادمة] المتقدمة L || ١٥ نفع] من add. L

(60) He further said: Money cowries [*Cypraea moneta*] or tellin[136] [*Tellinae*] shells, if burned and ingested in a dose of two *dirhams* with an astringent beverage, are beneficial for intestinal ulcers and dysentery. They also have a strong effect in reducing anal [prolapse]; if sprinkled thereon, it recedes.

(61) He further said: If one cooks an egg in vinegar, removes the yolk therefrom, and then seasons it with gallnuts [of *Quercus* spp.], sumac [*Rhus coriaria*], and a little bit of salt and eats it, it is beneficial for severe diarrhea and intestinal ulcers. If rocket [*Eruca sativa*] seed is pulverized and put into soft-boiled eggs with a little bit of salted skink and then sipped, it increases the sperm and greatly strengthens the erection.[137]

(62) He further said: If one takes one part of the flour of dried arum[138] root and three parts of white flour and pounds all this with sesame [*Sesamum indicum*] oil and kneads it with yeast and salt and makes a bread from it and dries this bread and pulverizes it and takes ten *dirhams* therefrom every morning with a spiced honey drink, it stops and eliminates hemorrhoids within three days. Its benefit against external and internal winds is clear and manifest.

(63) He further said: If one takes the resin of the olive tree [*Olea europaea* and var.] and of Socotra aloe [*Aloe perryi* Baker] and kneads this with the juice from peach leaves and makes suppositories from this, it cures chronic hemorrhoids, especially those surrounding the anus.

(64) He further said: Juice from the leaves of the sour apple tree averts the harm caused by fatal poisons and by the bite and sting of all vermin. If one takes three *dirhams* of the leaves of the sour apple tree—once they have been dried—and drinks it with three ounces of sour apple juice, one is saved from [the poison of] a viper bite and is healed therefrom.

(65) He said: The blossoms of the service tree [*Sorbus domestica* and var.] arouse women to desire sexual intercourse to a point that what happens to cats happens to them, namely, that they scream with joy, even when only smelling this blossom.[139]

(٦٠) وقال: الودع أو قشر الدلّينس إذا أحرق وشرب منه وزن درهمين بأحد الأشربة القابضة نفع من قروح الأمعاء والدوسنطاريا وله فعل قوي في ردّ المقعدة إذا ذرّ عليها وردّت.

(٦١) وقال: إذا سلق البيض بالخلّ وأخرجت مخاخه وتبّلت بعفص وسمّاق ويسير ملح وأكل ذلك نفع من الذرب المفرط وقرحة الأمعاء. وإذا سحق بزر الجرجير وألقي على بيض نيمبرشت مع يسير ملح سقنقور وتحسى زاد في المني وقوّى الإنعاظ جدًّا.

(٦٢) وقال: إذا أخذ جزء من دقيق أصول اللوف المجفّف وثلاثة أجزاء من دقيق الحوارى ولتّ الجميع بشيرج وعجن بخمير وملح وخبز وجفّف خبزه وسحق واستفّ منه كلّ غدوة وزن عشرة دراهم بشراب العسل المفوّه قطع البواسير وأخرجها في ثلاثة أيام ومنفعة ذلك في الأرواح الظاهرة والباطنة بيّنة ظاهرة.

(٦٣) وقال: إذا أخذ صمغ الزيتون والصبر الاسقوطري وعجن ذلك بماء ورق الخوخ واتّخذ منه فتائل أبرأت النواصير المزمنة وبخاصّة التي حول المقعدة.

(٦٤) وقال: عصارة ورق شجرة التفّاح الحامض تدفع مضرّة السموم القاتلة ولسع الهوامّ كلّها. وإذا استفّ وزن ثلثة دراهم من ورق شجرة التفّاح الحامض بعد تجفيفه وشرب بثلاثة أواق من عصارة التفّاح الحامض يخلّص من لسع الأفعى وأبرأ منه.

(٦٥) قال: نوّار شجرة الغبيراء يهيج النساء بطلب الجماع حتّى يعرض لهنّ ما يعرض للسنانير ويصحن ويفرحن ولو بشمّ هذه الزهرة.

---

٤ وأكل ذلك] om. ELBOU G[1] | على] في ELBOU || ٥ نيمبرشت] نيمرشت EGLO نمرشت SB | الإنعاظ] الإنعاض SG الانشاط B || ١٢ مضرّة] ضرر ELBOU | الهوامّ] السموم G

(66) He further said: Greater galangal [*Alpinia galanga*] has the specific property of being beneficial for internal hemorrhoids, especially if it is imbibed together with St. John's wort[140] [*Hypericum perforatum*]. Similarly, lichen[141] [*Alectoria usneoides*] is beneficial for palpitation of the heart caused by black bile. Women should sit in a decoction [prepared] therefrom [for[142] uterine diseases]. Galingale[143] [*Cyperus longus*] has the specific property of liquefying, dissolving, and crumbling [kidney] stones, and it stimulates micturition.

(67) He further said: Autumn crocus [*Colchicum autumnale* and var.] dissolves inflammations from gout when applied as a salve through its specific property. It also has the specific property of being beneficial for hemorrhoids if half a *dirham* of it is kneaded with cow's butter; if it is applied as a suppository in cotton for two nights, one does not need a third night.

(68) He further said: If one extinguishes [the heat of] gold in vinegar for some time and then rinses one's mouth with that vinegar, it removes any fetid odor from the mouth and improves the smell of the breath. It has the same effect if it is kept in the mouth.

(69) He also said: If kidney and bladder stones are burned and used as an eye powder, it cleanses a leucoma, whether it is old or recent. Sherds of transparent white Chinese earthenware, burned and mixed with one of the cleansing drugs, have the same effect.

(70) He further said: If[144] rock crystal is burned, pulverized, washed, and imbibed [in a dose of] one ounce with two *mithqāls*[145] of the milk of a donkey, it is beneficial for trembling, tremor, and phthisis. If a salve therefrom [prepared] with water is put on the breast, it makes the milk flow. It also cleanses a leucoma. It has all these [effects] because of its specific property.

(٦٦) وقال: الخولنجان له خاصّية في النفع من البواسير الباطنة ولا سيّما إذا شرب مع الداذي. وكذلك الأشنة تنفع من الخفقان السوداوي وتجلس النساء في طبيخها. وللسعد خاصّية في إذابة الحصى وتحليله وتفتيته و يدرّ البول.

(٦٧) وقال: السورنجان يحلّل أورام النقرس طلاء بخاصّية فيه. وله أيضا خاصّية في النفع من البواسير الباطنة إذا عجن منه نصف درهم بسمن بقر واحتمل بقطنة ليلتين لا يحتاج لثالثة.

(٦٨) وقال: الذهب إذا طفئ في الخلّ مرارا وتمضمض بذلك الخلّ أزال كلّ رائحة كريهة من الفم و يطيّب النكهة وكذلك إمساكه في الفم.

(٦٩) وقال أيضا: الحصى الموجود في الكلى والمثانة يحرق و يكتحل به فيجلو البياض القديم والحديث. وكذلك شقاف الصيني الأبيض الشفّاف محرقة مصوّلة مع بعض الأدوية الجلاة.

(٧٠) وقال: البلّور إذا أحرق وسحق وصوّل وشرب منه مثقالين بلبن أتن أوقية نفع من الرعشة والرعدة والسلّ و إذا طلي بالماء على الثدي أدرّ اللبن ويجلو البياض. كلّ ذلك بخاصّية فيه.

تمّت المقالة الثانية والعشرون ولله الحمد والمنّة.

---

٢ وتجلس] وتجلسن ELOU || ٤ بخاصّية فيه] بخاصّيه SLOV | خاصّية] عجيبة add. ELBOU || ٥ نصف درهم] نصفم SG وزن درهم O | بقر] الغنم العتيق LB || ٧ مرارا] مرّات ELBOU || ١٠ مصوّلة] مصلبة LO || ١٢ مثقالين] مثقال LB || ١٤ فيه] قضيب الضبع يجفّف ويسحق ويسقى للمرأة العاقر منه كلّ يوم درهمين نافع مجرّب add. G || ١٥ تمّت المقالة الثانية والعشرون ولله الحمد والمنّة] تمت المقالة الثانية والعشرون وعدد فصولها ستين فصلا والحمد لله كثيرا E تمّت المقالة الثانية والعشرين B تمّت المقالة الثانية والعشرون وعدد فصولها ستون فصلا والحمد لله على حسن عونه ولا ربّ سواه O تمّت المقالة الرابع عشر والحمد لله U

*This is the end of the twenty-second treatise, by the grace of God, praise be to Him.*

*In the name of God,*
*the Merciful, the Compassionate.*
*O Lord, make [our task] easy.*

# The Twenty-Third Treatise

## *Containing aphorisms concerning the differences between well-known diseases and the elucidation of [technical] terms that are well known to the physicians but whose [exact] meanings are sometimes unknown[1] [to them]*

(1) Overfilling in relation to the vessels means that the blood is markedly increased in quantity but that its quality is good according to its nature. Overfilling in relation to strength means that the quality of the blood has changed either into sharpness and has become biting or into crude, raw humors; even if its quantity is small [but] the strength of the surrounding organ is weak, it is burdensome to the strength. This matter is repeated in several books. It also appears in [Galen's] *De venae sectione*[2] and in his *De plenitudine*.[3]

بسم اللّه الرحمن الرحيم

ربّ يسّر

# المقالة الثالثة والعشرون

تشتمل على فصول تتضمّن فروقا بين
أمراض مشهورة أسماءها
وتبيين معاني أسماء مشهورة عند الأطبّاء
قد يجهل معناها

(١) الإمتلاء الذي بحسب الأوعية هو أن يكون الدم قد زادت كمّيته كثرة كثيرة وكيفيته جيّدة على طبيعتها. والإمتلاء الذي بحسب القوة هو أن يكون كيفية الدم تغيّرت إمّا إلى حدّة ولذع أو إلى أخلاط نيئة فجّة ولو كان مقداره قليلا أو يكون قوة العضو الحاوي ضعيفة فيثقل ذلك على القوة. تكرّر هذا المعنى في عدّة كتب وهو أيضا في مقالته في الفصد وفي مقالته في الكثرة.

١ بسم اللّه الرحمن الرحيم ربّ يسّر ] ELB بسم اللّه الرحمن الرحيم O فالأمراض لحبيس U || ٣ المقالة الثالثة والعشرون ] مقالة الرابع عشر التفليسي U || ٧ يجهل ] يغفل ELBO | معناها ] على التحرير add. ELO

(2) It is impossible that the vessels should always contain absolutely pure blood to the point that it is not mixed with some yellow bile, phlegm, or watery chyme. Therefore,[4] understand that [this is what I mean] when I speak of a surplus of chymes and of a surplus of blood.

(3) The[5] chyme that Galen calls "raw" in his *De multitidune*, and of which he says that dropsy[6] of the flesh develops from this chyme, and that it is this chyme that settles in the urine similar to cooked broad bean [*Vicia faba*] groats, is a kind of phlegm that he calls "crude" in several places.

(4) Serous blood is thin, watery blood with detrimental, biting, toxic power. What comes from the watery part of the blood is hot, calm, and tranquil. *In Hippocratis Epidemiarum librum* 6 *commentarius* 2.[7]

(5) Chyme is a liquid that is found in the body of living beings, and chyle is that which is found in fruits when they are eaten or squeezed. *In Hippocratis De humoribus commentarius* 1.[8]

(6) The liquids one finds in plants are of two kinds: The first is expressed through squeezing, and the second is that which [spontaneously] flows from plants. The [liquid] expressed by squeezing is [also] of two kinds and results either from squeezing fruits as is done with grapes, pomegranates, quinces, mulberries, and the like or from pounding the twigs and fresh leaves of a plant and then squeezing them. Each of these two types was called "chyle" by the ancients. The kind [of liquid] that flows [spontaneously] from the fruit or from the tree and that has the consistency of water is called "tear" by them. And that [liquid] whose consistency is thicker than a tear such as that which streams from some twigs if one cuts into them is called "milk." And that which is thicker than milk is called "gum." *In Timaeum commentarius* 2.[9]

(٢) محال أن يكون أبدا في العروق دم محض خالص حتّى لا يشوبه شيء من المرّة الصفراء والبلغم والكيموس المائي. ولذلك يفهم عني إذا ما قلت زيادة الكيموسات ما يفهم عني إذا ما قلت زيادة الدم. في مقالته في الكثرة.

(٣) الكيموس الذي سمّاه جالينوس في مقالته في الكثرة الفجّ وقال إنّ منه يتولّد الاستسقاء اللحمي وهو الذي يرسب في البول شبه كشك الفول المطبوخ هو النوع من البلغم الذي يسمّيه في عدّة مواضع الخام.

(٤) الدم الصديدي هو الدم الرقيق المائي الذي فيه قوة سمّية رديئة لذّاعة. أمّا ما كان من مائية الدم فهو حارّ هادئ ساكن. في الثانية من شرحه لسادسة أبيديميا.

(٥) الكيموس هو الرطوبة التي توجد في بدن الحيوان والكيلوس هو ما يوجد في الثمار إذا أكلت أو عصرت. في شرحه للأولى من الأخلاط.

(٦) الرطوبات الموجودة في النبات صنفان: أحدهما ما يخرج بالعصر والثاني ما يسيل من النبات. والذي يخرج بالعصر على ضربين إمّا بأن يعصر الثمرة كما يفعل بالعنب والرمّان والسفرجل والتوت ونحوها أو بأن تدقّ أغصان النبات وورقه الرطبة وتعصر. وكلّ واحد من هذين الضربين يسمّونه القدماء كيلوسا. وأمّا الصنف الذي يسيل من الثمر أو الشجرة وهو في قوام الماء فيسمّونه دمعة. وما كان أغلظ قوام من الدمعة مثل ما يسيل من بعض الأغصان إذا شقّت يسمّى لبنا. وما كان أغلظ من اللبن يسمّى صمغا. في مقالته الثانية من تفسير جالينوس لكتاب طيماوس.

---

٥ كشك] om. L || ٨ حارّ] om. SG | هادئ] om. ELO ساد add. S | أبيديميا] أفيديميا LOU || ١٤ كيلوسا] كيلوسات ESGBU || ١٥ في قوام] رقيق كقوام ELBOU

(7) Wheat of a good quality is that in which the pith dominates; inferior wheat is that in which the bran dominates. *Ad Glauconem* [*de medendi methodo*] 2.[10]

(8) The difference between perspiration and odor is that perspiration is the fine moisture [that exudes] from the humors, while the odors that emanate from the body are the vapors dissolving from the humors. *In Hippocratis De humoribus commentarius* 2.[11]

(9) Food that arrives in the stomach should not be said to have been digested when it has been ground and turned into small pieces, but one should say that it has been digested when it is transformed into a quality that is similar and peculiar to the body that wants to be nurtured by it. *De usis*.[12]

(10) It is a habit of physicians that when they speak of "bile" or "biles" in an absolute sense, they mean by it the bile whose color is yellow or red and do not add to this term [any further qualification] indicating its color. But if they want [to speak about] any of the other kinds of bile, they add the name of its color to its description. *De alimentorum* [*facultatibus*], end.[13]

(11) One should not say of everything that becomes corrupted of the organs of the body and its humors that it has putrefied. We should only say that it has putrefied if its corruption is accompanied by a foul smell. *De* [*simplicium*] *medicamentorum* [*temperamentis ac facultatibus*] 5.[14]

(12) Inhalation is the entrance of the air into the larynx and trachea. Respiration is the activity that occurs in the entire body through the dilation and contraction of the pulsatile vessels. *De* [*morborum*] *causis et symptomatibus* 3.[15]

(13) The knowledge of that which happens in the organs as a result of a minor, insignificant dyscrasia escapes many people, and for this reason they call it "weakness." *De* [*morborum*] *causis et symptomatibus* 1.[16]

(٧) الحنطة الكريمة هي التي الغالب عليها اللبّ والحنطة الوضيعة هي التي الغالب عليها النخالة. في ثانية أغلوقن.

(٨) الفرق بين العرق والرائحة أنّ العرق الرطوبة الرقيقة من الأخلاط والروائح التي تفوح من البدن هي البخار المتحلّل من الأخلاط. في شرحه لثانية الأخلاط.

(٩) الطعام الذي يرد المعدة لا يقال فيه عندما ينطحن ويصير أجزاء صغارا إنّه قد انهضم وإنّما يقال فيه إنّه قد انهضم عندما يستحيل إلى كيفية مشاكلة خاصّية للبدن الذي يريد أن يغتذي به. في مقالته في العادات.

(١٠) عادة الأطبّاء قد جرت بأن يعنوا بقولهم مرّة أو مرارا بقول مطلق المرّة التي لونها صفراء أو حمراء ولا يلحقون مع هذا الاسم زيادة تدلّ على لونها. فإذا أرادوا واحدا من سائر أنواع المرار الآخر ألحقوا مع ذكرها اسم لونه. آخر الأغذية.

(١١) ليس كلّ ما يفسد من أعضاء البدن وأخلاطه يقال إنّه قد عفن. وإنّما نسمّيه عفنا إذا اقترن مع فساده نتن رائحة. خامسة الأغذية.

(١٢) التنفّس دخول الهواء من الحنجرة وقصبة الرئة والنفس الفعل الذي يكون في البدن كلّه بانبساط العروق الضوارب وانقباضها. في ثالثة العلل والأعراض.

(١٣) ما يحدث في الأعضاء من سوء المزاج الحقير اليسير فمعرفته تفوت خلقا كثيرا فيسمّونه بهذا السبب ضعفا. في الأولى من العلل والأعراض.

---

٩ الاسم om. SG

(14) The illness that occurs in all joints is called "arthritis"; this very illness is called "ischias" if it occurs in the hip joint only and "podagra" if it occurs in the feet. If podagra becomes chronic and persists for a long time, the illness spreads into all joints. In all these [illnesses] much chyme develops in the joints and spreads to the nerves surrounding them. The chyme that mostly flows in the case of arthritis is that which is called "crude." *Mayāmir* 10.[17]

(15)[18] The diseases that are called "endemic" are those illnesses that are specific for most people of that city. They occur among them either in a well-known season of the year or often occur among them in every season of the year. These last diseases depend on the air and the water in that city and on the general nutrition of its inhabitants. *In Hippocratis De [aeris] aquis [locis] commentarius* 1.

(16) The diseases that are called "epidemic" are general diseases that occur to the inhabitants of a certain city in certain years. These [diseases] are consequential upon a change occurring in the air or in the water or in the usual nutrition, or in all three of these. *De [aeris] aquis [locis] commentarius* 1.

(17) Sometimes phthisis is associated with anyone whose body wastes away [and] becomes lean and meager to such a degree that he dies, regardless whether it is due to an ulcer in the lung, a dyscrasia, or something else. However, the name "phthisis" is especially used for an ulcer of the lung because phthisis mostly develops from such a condition. [*In Hippocratis*] *Epidemiarum librum* 1 *commentarius* 2.[19]

(18) The uterus is especially called "nervous" and similarly the vulva and the penis because every single one of these organs resembles a nerve in regard to stretching, dilatation, contraction, whiteness, and lack of blood [therein]; not[20] because of the fact that their substance [actually] consists of nerves, ligaments, or tendons. [*In Hippocratis*] *Epidemiarum librum* 6 *commentarius* 1.[21]

(١٤) العلّة التي إذا كانت في المفاصل كلّها سمّيت وجع المفاصل هي بعينها إذا كانت في مفصل الورك وحده سمّيت عرق النساء و إذا كانت في القدم سمّيت نقرس. والنقرس إذا عتق وطال مكثه انتشرت العلّة في المفاصل كلّها وهي كلّها كيموس يكثر في المفصل فيمدّد ما يطيف به من العصب. والذي ينصبّ في أكثر الأمر في وجع المفاصل الكيموس الذي يسمّى الخام. عاشرة الميامر.

(١٥) الأمراض التي تسمّى البلدية هي الأمراض الخصيصة بأكثر أهل ذلك البلد وهي تحدث بهم إمّا في فصل معلوم أو هي كثيرة الوقوع بهم في كلّ فصل وهذه تابعة لهواء البلد ومائه والغذاء العامّ لأهله. في شرحه للأولى من الأهوية والمياه.

(١٦) الأمراض التي تسمّى الوافدة هي أمراض عامّة تحدث بأهل بلد ما في بعض السنين وهذه تابعة لتغيّر يحدث في الهواء أو في الماء أو في الأغذية المعتادة أو في ثلاثتها. في تلك المقالة.

(١٧) قد ينسب السلّ إلى كلّ من يذوب بدنه و يقضف و يهزل حتّى يموت سواء كان ذلك عن قرحة الرئة أو عن سوء مزاج أو غيره. و إنّما جعل اسم السلّ خاصّة لقرحة الرئة لأنّها أكثر ما يحدث السلّ عنها. في الثانية من شرحه للأولى من أبيديميا.

(١٨) إنّما سمّي الرحم عصبيا وكذلك الفرج والقضيب لكون كلّ واحد من هذه الأعضاء يشبه العصب في التمدّد والانبساط والانقباض والبياض وعدم الدم لا لأنّ أجرامها من العصب أو من الرباط أو من الوتر. في الأولى من شرحه لسادسة أبيديميا.

---

١ التي] om. SG || ٣ المفصل] المفاصل B || ١٠ في تلك المقالة] في شرحه للأولى من الأهوية SG || ١٢ ويقضف] ويضعف L || ١٤ لأنّها] لأنّه L | أبيديميا] أفيديميا LOU || ١٥ و كذلك . . . هذه الأعضاء] om. B || ١٦ لأنّ] أنّ G

(19) The simple [kind of] marasmus is that which develops from the predominance of heat alone. Sometimes it is thought to occur during the abstention from food, whether intentionally or whether due to actual lack [of food]. If predominance of heat is associated with predominance of cold, one is dealing with a complex marasmus, and this is the [marasmus] that occurs to the elderly or to someone who suffers from an illness that resembles old age. If predominance of dryness is associated with heat, one is dealing with marasmus that occurs in[22] the case of fevers that are related to the substance of the organs. Such[23] a temperament unavoidably affects the heart, and in that case real marasmus occurs. *De marcore.*[24]

(20) The marasmus called "burning" is one that arises from ardent fevers, and[25] the marasmus called "syncopal" occurs in someone who suffered from syncope and then escaped this severe affliction but still retains some [of the initial syncopal condition]. [The[26] cold marasmus, on the other hand, which is a condition similar to old age, results in cases where] fevers were not cooled properly, namely, through letting the [patient] drink cold water in the beginning of the illness. What Galen calls "the hearth of fever" is the organ that initially becomes only mildly hot [but then increases in heat] so much that hectic fevers arise from its heat. *De marcore.*[27]

(21) Says Moses: If you consider what Galen mentions in his treatise *De*[28] *tremore, palpitatione, rigore et convulsione*, it will be clear to you that the terms *riʿda* [tremor] and *riʿsha* are synonyms.[29] However, it has become common practice in the field of medicine, and actually for all physicians,[30] to call *riʿda* [a tremor] whose cause is related to weakness of strength, as is the case in someone who carries a heavy load or walks on a high spot or is frightened or is emaciated by the length of his illness. And they use the term *riʿsha* for the case of someone whose tremor is caused by afflictions that subsist in the nerves and that may be caused by various factors.

(22) The discontinuation and complete cessation of voluntary activities is called "paralysis," and their diminution is called "torpor" [numbness]. A bad execution of these activities is called "convulsion." *De [morborum] causis et symptomatibus* 5.[31]

In his *De pulsu parva* he says: Paralysis means loss of sensation and movement.[32]

(١٩) الذبول البسيط هو العارض عن غلبة اليبس وحده. وقد يظنّ أنّه يعرض في الإمساك عن الغذاء كان ذلك بقصد أو من عدم وجوده. فإن اقترن مع غلبة اليبس غلبة البرد كان ذبولا مركّبا وهو العارض للشيوخ أو لمن وقع في علّة تشبه الشيخوخة. وإن اقترن مع غلبة اليبس غلبة الحرارة كان الذبول العارض في الحمّيات المتعلّقة بجرم الأعضاء وهذا المزاج لا بدّ أن يكون حاصلا في القلب وحينئذ يكون الذبول الحقيقي. في مقالته في الذبول.

(٢٠) الذبول المسمّى المحترق هو الكائن من الحمّيات المحرقة والذبول المسمّى ذا الغشي يكون بعد أن يعرض لصاحبه الغشي والتفلّت في ذلك الوقت من شدّة البلاء وتبقى فيه بقية من <...> الحمّيات بردت على ما لا ينبغي بأن سقي الماء البارد في أوّل المرض. والذي يسمّيه جالينوس مستوقد الحمّى هو العضو الذي يسخن أوّلا سخونة دون مادّة حتّى تكون من سخونته حمّيات الدقّ. في مقالته في الذبول.

(٢١) قال موسى: إذا تأمّلت ما يذكره جالينوس في مقالته في الرعدة والاختلاج والنافض والتشنّج يتبيّن لك أنّ اسم الرعدة والرعشة اسمان مترادفان. لكنّ قد جرت عادة الطبّ بل الناس كلّهم أن يسمّوا الرعدة ما سببه تابع لضعف القوة كما يجري لمن يحمل حملا ثقيلا أو يمشي على موضع عال أو لمن يجزع أو لمن أنهكه طول من المرض. ويسمّون الرعشة لمن كان سبب رعدته آفات ثابتة في العصب على اختلاف أسبابه.

(٢٢) الأفعال الإرادية بطلان ذلك الفعل وتعطيله جملة يسمّى استرخاء ونقصانه يسمّى خدرا وجريانه المنكر يسمّى تشنّجا. في خامسة العلل والأعراض. وقال في النبض الصغير: معنى الاسترخاء ذهاب الحسّ والحركة.

---

٣ وهو] نحو L || ٦ الذبول المسمّى . . . الذبول] om. B || ٧ والتفلّت] emendation editor والتقلّب MSS || ٨ في] من L || ١٢ الطبّ] الأطبّاء B || ١٤ طول من المرض] طول المرض طول الأمراض ELBOU || ١٥ لمن] لما L | رعدته] مادّته ELOU | ثابتة] تابعة B || ١٨ معنى] يعني SG

(23) Numbness is something composed of difficulty of sensation and difficulty of movement. It arises from coldness of the air, from compression of the nervous parts of the body, or from [the shock caused by] contact with a sea creature. The bodily parts first turn numb, then lose their sensation and movement. This kind of harm is called "paralysis." *De* [*morborum*] *causis et symptomatibus* 4.[33]

(24) "Throat"—by this I mean the windpipe. When I speak to you of "organs of the voice," understand from me that by this I mean only the windpipe,[34] larynx,[35] pharynx,[36] and the membrane covering the pharynx, larynx, and windpipe from the inside, and this is one continuous, thick membrane. *Mayāmir* 7.[37]

(25) Says Moses: The commentators to Galen's writings have confused some of the [technical] terms, and it is necessary to point this out. Namely, the internal membranes of the organs are called by them *ṣifāqāt* in [their commentary on] *De usu partium*. Thus they speak of the *ṣifāq* of the stomach and the internal and external *ṣifāq* of the esophagus. They use this terminology frequently in [their commentary on] that book. Similarly, they call the tunics of the eye *ṣifāqāt* in [their commentary on] the same book. Some of the coverings (i.e., membranes) are also called *ṣifāqāt*; thus they call the third covering (i.e., membrane) of the coverings (i.e., membranes) of the spinal cord *ṣifāq*. Do not let this mislead you.[38]

(26) "Pulse compression," as it is usually called by the physicians, means that the pulse is extremely weak and unequal in the beginning of a fever attack. "Heat compression" means that the heat flames up and becomes strong and is not uniform throughout the body, after it was preceded by shivering, cold of the extremities, clear indolence, and a tendency to sleep. *De febrium* [*differentiis*] 1.[39]

(٢٣) الخدر هو شيء مركّب من عسر الحسّ وعسر الحركة ويكون من برد الهواء ومن ضغط الأجسام العصبية ومن ملامسة الحيوان البحري. والأعضاء يعرض لها أوّلا أن تخدر ثمّ تصير لا حسّ لها ولا حركة ويقال لهذا النوع من المضارّ استرخاء. رابع العلل والأعراض.

(٢٤) الحلقوم وهو قصبة الرئة وإذا أنا قلت لك آلات الصوت فافهم عني أنّي إنّما أعني قصبة الرئة والحنجرة والحلق والصفاق الملبس من داخل الحلق والحنجرة وقصبة الرئة وهو صفاق واحد متّصل ثخين. سابعة الميامر.

(٢٥) قال موسى: هاؤلاء الشارحون لكتب جالينوس قد غلطوا في بعض أسماء فيجب التنبيه عليها. وذلك أنّ طبقات الأعضاء الباطنة قد سمّوها في منافع الأعضاء صفاقات فيقولون صفاق المعدة وصفاق المريء الداخل والصفاق الخارج وكثرت هذه التسمية في ذلك الكتاب. وكذلك سمّوا أيضا طبقات العين صفاقات في ذلك الكتاب. وسمّوا أيضا بعض الأغشية صفاقات وسمّوا الغشاء الثالث من أغشية النخاع صفاقا. فلا يغلطك ذلك.

(٢٦) تضاغط النبض فيما جرت به عادة الأطبّاء هو أن يكون النبض في ابتداء نوبة الحمّى صغيرا جدّا مختلفا. وتضاغط الحرارة هو أن تلتهب الحرارة وتقوى ولا تكون مستوية في الجسم كلّه بعد أن يتقدّمها اقشعرار وبرد أطراف وكسل بيّن وميل إلى النوم. في الأولى من الحمّيات.

---

٩ صفاق] صفاقي SG | صفاق] صفاقي G || ١٠ وكذلك . . . في ذلك الكتاب] $G^1$(?) || ١١ אמר המעתיק ידעתי כי להעתיק זה המאמר שלהרב ז״ל לא היה צריך כלל אחר שבלשונינו העברית לא מצאנו אלו השמות הנאמרים כי אילו הקרומות כמו שהם נמצאים בלשון הערבי שהם שלשה הנזכרים במקום זה והם בערבי אגשיה[1] וצפאקאת וטבאקאת ואע״פ שהעברי אומר קליפות וקרומות מכל מקום על אלו השלשה נופל לפי לשונינו שם הקרום בלבד כי שם הקליפה אינו נופל על אחד מאילו השלשה כלל מפני שרוב נפלו הוא על קליפות הפירות הנאכלים ועל כן ידעתי באמת כי מהעתקתי לא יתבאר כלל ולא יובן מה שרצה לומר הרב ז״ל. ודיי[2] לי התנצלותי זה עם המבוכה אשר תקרה לקורא זה המאמר לבדו ר״ל באור הקרומות add. Z

[1] אגשיה וצפאקאת וטבאקאת] אַגְשִׁיַה וצְפַאקַאת וטַבַאקַאת ב

[2] ודיי] ויספיק בדמ

(27) If you place your fingers on a [pulsatile] vessel and then lift your hand and put it back again and find that every time you put [the hand] thereon the movement of the [pulsatile] vessel diminishes, this condition is called “disappearance and loss of the pulse.” It is as if it is completely inactive when one feels it. If, on the other hand, when you place your fingers on the [pulsatile] vessel, you distinguish movement and if [only] after a prolonged application of your fingers you find that the movement diminishes and weakens little by little until it becomes completely still when one feels it, this is called a “finished pulse,” and this is the lack of activity. *De pulsu* 10.[40]

(28) A strong pulse is a powerful pulse, and a weak pulse is a faint pulse. If you place your hand on a [pulsatile] vessel and find the second pulse somewhat smaller than the first, and similarly the third smaller than the second by the same amount, and even so the fourth, and so continually, this is called a “mouse tail’s pulse.” Sometimes it remains and stays in the smallness of pulsebeats that it reached, and this is called “permanent mouse tail.” If the pulsebeats continue to get smaller until they stop completely, it is called a “finished [mouse] tail.” Sometimes the pulse returns from the smallness that it reached and becomes greater little by little until it reaches a greatness that is similar to the original pulse or not [completely] similar, [and] it is called the “recurrent mouse tail.” *De pulsu* 1.[41]

(29) The pulse that is found to be thick in the middle of the [pulsatile] vessel but becomes thinner on both sides is the one that is called “tending and inclining.” *De pulsu* 1.[42]

(30) “Continuous”[43] fevers and “perpetual” [fevers] are synonyms. Similarly, the [fever] called “synochous” is continuous, as is the continuous burning [fever]. The term “burning” has been given to it only because of its severe heat. *De crisibus* 2.[44]

(٢٧) إذا وضعت أصابعك على العرق ثمّ رفعت يدك ورددتها في كلّ مرّة توضع تجد حركة العرق قد نقصت فهذه الحالة تسمّى ذهاب النبض وتلافه وكأنّه عدم الفعل كلّه عند الحسّ. وإن كنت إذا وضعت أصابعك على العرق تبيّنت الحركة وإذا أطلت وضعها تجد الحركة تقلّ وتفتر أوّلا أوّلا حتّى تسكن البتّة عند الحسّ فإنّ هذا يسمّى نبضا منقضيا وهذا هو نقصان الفعل. عاشرة النبض.

(٢٨) النبض القوي هو الشديد والنبض الضعيف هو الخامل. فإذا وضعت يدك على العرق فوجدت النبض الثانية أصغر من الأولى قليلا وكذلك الثالثة أصغر من الثانية بذلك المقدار وكذلك الرابعة ولا يزال هكذا فهذا الذي يسمّى ذنب الفأرة. وقد يثبت ويلبث على ما انتهى إليه من صغر النبضات وهذا يسمّى ذنب الفأرة اللابث. وإن كان لا تزال النبضات تصغر حتّى تبطل بتّة فيقال ذنب منقضي. وقد يرجع ممّا انتهى إليه من الصغر ويعظم قليلا بعد قليل حتّى يعود إلى عظم ما إمّا متساوي لأوّل نبضه أو غير متساوي وهذا يسمّى ذنب الفأرة العائد. الأولى من النبض.

(٢٩) النبض الذي يوجد وسط العرق فيه غلظا ثمّ تدقّ طرفاه هو الذي يسمّى المائل والمنحني. أولى النبض.

(٣٠) الحمّيات المطبقة والدائمة اسمان مترادفان وكذلك المسمّاة سونوخس هي مطبقة وكذلك المحرقة دائمة فإنّما تخصّ باسم محرقة لشدّة حرّها. ثانية البحران.

---

١ أصابعك] إصبعك ELB | في كلّ مرّة توضع] وفي كلّ مرّة ELOU || ٢ وتلافه] وخلافه ELB وتلافه . . . (٣٩a) إذا انصبّت الأخلاط من فوهات العروق إلى] om. O || ٣ أصابعك] إصبعك ELB || ٨ يثبت ويلبث] يلبث يلبث ويثبت ELB || ١٠ فيقال] حتّى يقال إنّه SG|| ١١ ما إمّا متساوي] ما مساوي L إلى ما متساوي B | متساوي] مساوي LB || ١٣ غلظا] غلوظا O غليظاELU || ١٦ لمّا . . . في الثانية من الحمّيات] om. B

(31) When Galen stated and explained how two [different] fevers that form two [different] types can be combined—namely, phlegmatic and bilious and other ones—and said: If one fever is combined or mixed with another, he clarified [this statement] as follows: With "combined" I mean that the attacks of these two fevers start at different times, and with "mixed" I mean that the attacks of these two fevers start at the same time. *De febrium [differentiis]* 2.[45]

(32) Inflammations[46] may occur in the muscles of the ribs, after which fever arises and respiration becomes fast and superficial. This illness is similar to pleurisy, which is not accompanied by expectoration. The difference between both is that in this illness the patient does not cough at all, the pulse is not hard, the fever is not as high as the fever of pleurisy, and respiration is easier than in [the case of] pleurisy. And some patients feel pain, if one presses on the site of the illness from the outside. If that inflammation becomes ripe, either the pus in it is dissolved or it protrudes outside the skin and needs an incision. *De locis affectis* 5.[47]

(33) [The term] "hot compress" applies to everything that warms the body externally. There[48] are five kinds of it: moist, dry, biting, intermediate, and moderate. The moist one is that which is prepared with hot water with which one fills a skin or a bladder and the like. The[49] dry one is the one that is prepared with rags heated over a fire or with wormwood [*Artemisia* spp.] or with roasted millet [*Panicum miliaceum*]. The biting one is that which is prepared with salt heated in bags or with bitter vetch [*Vicia ervilia*] and the like. The[50] strength of bitter vetch is sufficient for cutting, concocting, and dissolving the thickness of the humors. The[51] moderate [hot compress] is such that one can touch with it the body of a living being, such as a child or a puppy and the like. The[52] intermediate one is that prepared with barley and bitter vetch; they should be pulverized and boiled with acid vinegar mixed with it to a degree that is stronger than could be drunk. Put this in a bag and apply it as a hot compress to the parts of the body [you want to treat]. The same [should be done] with bran. *In Hippocratis De acutorum morborum [victu et] Galeni commentarius* 2.

Moderate massage is that which one stops to apply when the body becomes hot. *De methodo [medendi]* 7.[53]

(٣١) لمّا ذكر جالينوس وبيّن كيف تتركّب حمّاتان من نوعين أعني بلغمية وصفراوية وغيرهما وقال إذا تركّبت إحدى الحمّاتين مع الأخرى أو امتزجت بها قال شارحا لقوله وأعني بالتركيب أن تكون الحمّاتان تبتدئ نوائبها في أوقات مختلفة وأعني بالامتزاج أن تكون النوائب من الحمّاتين تبتدئ في وقت واحد. في الثانية من الحمّيات.

(٣٢) تحدث الأورام في عضل الأضلاع وتتبعها حمّى ويكون التنفّس متواترا صغيرا. وهذه العلّة شبيهة بذات الجنب التي لا نفث معها. والفرق بينهما أنّ في هذه العلّة لا يسعل صاحبها أصلا ولا تكون في النبض صلابة ولا تكون الحمّى حادّة كحمّى ذات الجنب ورداءة التنفّس فيها أقلّ من ذات الجنب. وبعضهم إذا غمزت على الموضع العليل من خارج أوجعهم. فإذا نضج ذلك الورم إمّا أن يتحلّل ما فيه من القيح أو ينتأ إلى خارج الجلد ويحتاج إلى البطّ. خامسة التعرّف.

(٣٣) التكميد يقع على كلّ ما يسخن البدن من خارج وأنواعه خمسة: رطب ويابس ولذّاع ومتوسّط ومعتدل. فالرطب ما كان بماء حارّ قد ملئ منه زقّ أو مثانة ونحو ذلك. واليابس ما كان بخرق مسخنة بالنار أو بشيح أو بجاورس مقلو. واللذّاغ ما كان بملح مسخن في أكياس أو كرسنّة ونحوها وقوة الكرسنّة يكتفى بها في تقطيع غلظ الأخلاط وإنضاجها وتحليلها. والمعتدل ما كان بملاقاة جسم حيوان كصبي أو جرو كلب ونحوهما. والمتوسّط هو أن يؤخذ شعير وكرسنّة وتسحقهما وتطبخهما بخلّ حادق ممزوج مزاجا أقوى ممّا يشرب وتجعله في كيس وتكمّد به الأعضاء. وكذلك النخالة. في شرحه لثانية الأمراض الحادّة.

الدلك المعتدل هو الذي يمسك عنه عند ما يسخن البدن. في سابعة الحيلة.

---

١ لمّا . . . في الثانية من الحمّيات] om. B || ٧ أصلا] om. ELBU || ٨ ورداءة التنفّس فيها أقلّ من ذات الجنب] G$^{1}$(?) || ١٤ بها] om. B || ١٨ الدلك . . . الحيلة] om. S

(34) Cities that are facing the east are cities that lie on high mountains because the sun shines down upon them for the entire day. He also said: cities facing the east are those through which an eastern wind blows and that are protected at the western side while the eastern side is exposed. The opposite is the case with cities facing the west. *In Hippocratis De aeris [aquis locis] commentarius* 1.[54]

(35) Every ulcer that spreads on the skin but does not go any further is called by us *namla*[55] [shingles]. Every ulcer that passes beyond the skin and spreads into the flesh next to the skin is [called] *ākila*[56] [canker]. *In Hippocratis Aphorismos commentarius* 6.[57]

(36) *ᶜAbīṭ*[58] is a congelation of copious blood that is clearly visible. *De tumoribus praeter naturam.*[59]

A *nāṣūr* [sinuous ulcer] is a narrow, elongated cavity that can be closely drawn together but [whose parts] can also separate through the flow of the superfluities through it. *De tumoribus praeter naturam.*[60]

(37) When the skin is extremely thin and stays [like that] for a long time and does not adhere to the underlying flesh, this illness is sometimes called *nāṣūr* [sinuous ulcer] and sometimes *makhba* [absconsio]. *Ad Glauconem [de methodo medendi]* 2.[61]

(38) A carbuncle is an inflammation, but it is formed if the blood is affected by something similar to boiling to such a degree that the skin is burned and that an eschar is formed with it. The boil is preceded by a blister similar to a blister produced by burning with fire. This is followed by acute fever that rapidly endangers [the life] of the patient. *De tumoribus [praeter naturam].*[62]

(39) And in the first book of *De febrium [differentiis]* he remarks: Boils that are called *jamr* [carbuncles] arise from blood that is very hot and tends towards blackness.[63]

(٣٤) البلاد المشرقية هي البلاد الموضوعة في أعالي الجبال لأنّ الشمس تشرق عليها النهار كلّه. وقال أيضا المدن الشرقية هي التي تهبّ فيها ريح الصبا ويكون غربها مستورا وشرقها مكشوفا. والمدن الغربية ضدّ ذلك. في شرحه للأولى من كتاب الأهوية.

(٣٥) كلّ قرحة لا تجاوز الجلد وهي تسعى فنسمّيها نملة وكلّ قرحة تجاوز الجلد وتسعى في اللحم والجلد فهي آكلة. في شرحه لسادسة الفصول.

(٣٦) العبيط جمود دم غزير ظاهر للحسّ. في مقالته في الأورام الخارجة عن الطبيعة.

الناصور هو تجويف ضيّق إلى الطول ما هو يجتمع ثمّ يفترق عند انصباب الفضول إليه. في مقالته في الأورام.

(٣٧) متى رقّ الجلد جدّا ودام مدّة طويلة لا يلتزق بما تحته من اللحم فربّما سمّوا هذه العلّة ناصورا وربّما سمّوها مخبأ. ثانية أغلوقن.

(٣٨) الجمر هو من الأورام الحارّة إلا أنّ تولّد الجمر يكون إذا عرض للدم شبيه بالغليان حتّى يحرق الجلد ويحدث مع ذلك حشكريشة. وتتقدّم القرحة نفاخة شبيها بالنفاخة الحادثة من حرق النار ويلحق ذلك حمّى حادّة تجلب على الإنسان خطرا عاجلا. في مقالته في الأورام.

(٣٩) وفي المقالة الأولى من الحمّيات قال: القروح التي يقال لها الجمر تتولّد من دم قوي الحرارة مائل إلى السوداء.

١ البلاد . . . والمدن الغربية ضدّ ذلك] قال بقراط أنّ كلّ مدينة ناحية شرق الشمس تكون أصحّ من المدينة الموضوعة ناحية الفرقدين ومن المدينة الموصوعة ناحية الرياح الحارّة C, fol. 42r, 2–4 | البلاد] om. ELBU || ٢ الشرقية] المشرقية LB || ٦ العبيط] العبط S الغبيط GL || ٩ فربّما] om. L || ١٢ نفاخة] om. G

(39a) If[64] humors stream from the openings of the vessels into the spaces that have no flesh or muscles and the bodily part is soaked with those humors just as a sponge is soaked with liquids, this is called "inflammation." If[65] the pus corrodes parts of the flesh and the like and a cavity is formed in that place into which pus accumulates, it is called "abscess." If[66] those corrupt matters inside the abscess are surrounded by a cover similar to a membrane, it is called *dubayla* [cystic abscess]. If[67] the humor is only in the skin, it is called "furuncle," and it is very hot. If it is deep in the body, it is very malignant, and then it is similar to an abscess. The only difference between it and an abscess lies in its hardness. *De tumoribus* [*praeter naturam*].

(40) Galen says in the first book of his commentary to *Epidemics* 6: The[68] term "swelling" as used by Hippocrates indicates every[69] type of swelling. Similarly, Galen uses [the term] in a number of places for inflammations, and in a few statements he uses it for every swelling. Pustules[70] differ from tumors[71] only in the quantity of humor that produces them. Also in the case of pustules, nature strives after the cleansing of the internal [parts of the] body. If the humor that produces the pustules has only a little heat, it only produces itching. If it is very hot, it produces biting. If the humor is extremely thick or cold, it produces broad pustules. *In Hippocratis Epidemiarum librum* 6 *commentarius* 2.[72]

(٣٩a) إذا انصبّت الأخلاط من فوهات العروق إلى المواضع الخالية من اللحم أو العضل وتشرّب العضو بتلك الأخلاط كما تتشرّب الإسفنجة الرطوبات سمّي ذلك ورما. وإذا أكلت المدّة أجزاء من اللحم وغيره وصار هناك غور تجتمع فيه المدّة سمّي خراجا. فإذا كانت تلك الموادّ التي في الخراجات في داخل غشاء يحويها شبيها بالحجاب سمّيت دبيلة. ومتى كان الخلط في الجلد فقط سمي دملا وكان أسخن. ومتى كان في عمق البدن كان أردأ وهو حينئذ شبيه بالخراج. ويفرق بينه وبين الخراج بالصلابة فقط. في مقالته في الأورام.

(٤٠) قال جالينوس في المقالة الأولى من شرحه لسادسة أبيديميا إنّ اسم الخراج عند أبقراط يدلّ على كلّ ورم. وكذلك أيضا يوقّعه جالينوس في عدّة مواضع على الأورام الحارّة وفي قليل من كلامه يوقّعه على كلّ ورم. إنّما تخالف البثور الخراجات في كثرة الخلط المحدث لها فقط. وتكون الطبيعة تقصد في البثور أيضا تنقية باطن البدن. فإن كان الخلط المولّد للبثور يسير الحرارة أحدث حكّة فقط. وإن كان أشدّ حرارة أحدث لذعا. وإن كان الخلط شديد الغلظ أو شديد البرد أحدث بثورا عراضا. في الثانية من شرحه لسادسة أبيديميا.

---

٣ المدّة] المادة LBO | وغيره] وغيرته L | المدّة] المادة BO || ٥ ومتى . . . أسخن] om. G || ٧ أبيديميا] أفيديميا LO || ١١ فقط] om. L || ١٣ أبيديميا] أفيديميا L

(41) If[73] the matter streaming to a part of the body is a superfluity composed of blood and yellow bile, both of which are warmer than they should be, or if that which streams to it is only blood but blood that is boiling hot, of a fine consistency, the illness developing therefrom is called "erysipelas." "Scirrhus"[74] is the name of a hard tumor that develops from a thick, viscous humor that settles in those parts in which the [tumor] occurs.[75] It is of two types: that which is absolutely insensible and incurable and that which is a little bit sensible and is hard to cure. And[76] the sites where the tumor becomes very large and the blood is congested in it and the respiration becomes so small that one reaches a point that the patient dies are called "gangrenes" as long as they are in a stage of mortification but have not [actually] died. Their therapy consists of evacuating the blood that became congested in that part of the body by a deep scarification and by making incisions in it in [several] places until as much blood as possible is extracted. *Ad Glauconem* [*de medendi methodo*] 2.

(42) When the inflammation known as "erysipelas" becomes cold and hard and difficult to dissolve, it is called "hard[77] erysipelas." Similarly, if it is combined with a soft swelling, it is called "soft[78] erysipelas." *De methodo* [*medendi*] 14.[79]

(43) When we speak of a hard tumor, we mean any tumor that combines hardness with absence of pain. It should not be insensible and at the same time painless, for if this is the case, it cannot be cured at all. *De methodo* [*medendi*], last book.[80]

(44) Every ulcer whose healing and cicatrization is difficult because of many humors, or of hot humors streaming towards it while the bad temperament of the ulcerous part of the body is not firmly established, is called "difficult to heal." But if the bad temperament of the [ulcerous] part becomes firmly established and the illness overpowers it to a degree that the bad temperament reaches a state in which it corrupts every thing it arrives at, even if it is good, I call it with a special name: "malignant ulcer." And those ulcers that are extremely malignant I call "gangrenous ulcers." *Qaṭājānas* 1 and 4.[81]

(٤١) إن كان ما سال إلى العضو فضلا مختلطا من دم ومرّة صفراء كلاهما أسخن من المقدار الذي ينبغي أو كان ما سال إليه دما إلا أنّه دم حارّ يغلي رقيق في قوامه قيل للعلّة الحادثة عنه حمرة. وسقيروس وهو الورم الصلب الكائن من خلط غليظ لزج يرسخ في تلك الأعضاء التي يحدث فيها. وهو نوعان: ما كان منه لا حسّ له أصلا ولا بروء له وما كان حسّه قليلا فيعصر بروءه والمواضع التي يعظم فيها الورم جدّا ويحتبس فيها الدم ويعدم التنفّس حتّى يصير إلى حدّ ما يموت فهذه الأورام تسمّى طالما هي سائرة إلى الموت قبل موتها يسمّونها غانغرانا وبروءها بأن يستفرغ من الدم الذي قد اغتصّ في ذلك العضو بأن تشرطه شرطا غائرا وتبطّه في مواضع حتّى يخرج من الدم أكثر ما يمكن استخراجا. ثانية أغلوقن.

(٤٢) متى برد الورم المعروف بالحمرة وصلب وصار عسر الانحلال سمّي حمرة صلبة. وكذلك إذا اختلط مع الورم الرخو سمّي حمرة رخوة. رابعة عشر الحيلة.

(٤٣) نعني بقولنا بورم صلب كلّ ورم يجمع صلابة وعدم الوجع وليس واجب أن يكون عادم الحسّ مع عدم الوجع لأنّ ما كان كذلك لا بروء له البتّة. أخيرة الحيلة.

(٤٤) كلّ قرحة يعسر اندمالها وختمها من أجل رطوبات تتحلّب إليها إمّا كثيرة أو حارّة من غير أن يستحكم سوء مزاج العضو الذي فيه القرحة فإنّا نسمّيها عسرة الاندمال. فإن استحكم سوء مزاج العضو واستحوذ عليه العلّة إلى أن صار من سوء المزاج في حال يفسد ما يصير إليه ولو كان جيّدا فإنّي أسمّيها خاصّة قروحا خبيثة. وما كان من القروح الخبيثة خبيثا خبثا شديدا قويا جدّا سمّيناه القروح الغنغرانية الأولى والرابعة من قاطاجانس.

---

٣ وهو] هو ELBUO || ٥ ويحتبس] ويحتقن ELBUO || ٧ غانغرانا] غاناجرانا L غاناغرفنا U غاغا غانا B || ١١ وليس واجب أن يكون عادم الحسّ مع عدم الوجع] om. B || ١٢ عادم] عديم ELO || ١٧ خبيثا] om. EL | الغنغرانية] emend. editor الجبرونية G الخبرونية EL الغبرونية B الغيرونية OU

(45) A scirrhous tumor consists of two types: One of these originates from thick phlegm, and the second develops from turbid blood and its sediments. Both have in common that they are large, hard, and painless tumors. The second type has as a special feature that it is of a black color. *De tumoribus* [*praeter naturam*].[82]

(46) Cancer consists of two types, namely, a tumor that arises from black bile, and when the black bile streams into the flesh and is biting, it corrodes the entire adjacent skin and ulcerates it, and this is the ulcerous cancer. But when [the black bile] is moderate, it produces a cancer that is not ulcerous. *De tumoribus* [*praeter naturam*].[83]

(47) All cancerous tumors especially develop from a melancholic superfluity. If that superfluity tends to the lower part of the body and the expulsive faculty in the vessels expels it from the openings [of the vessels] in the anus or vagina, then [the parts from which] this evacuation [takes place] are called "hemorrhoids," and blood flows from them. Sometimes those superfluities are forced to the legs and cause varicose veins, and sometimes they are forced to the skin of the entire body, and from this elephantiasis develops. *Ad Glauconem* [*de medendi methodo*] 2.[84]

(48) Sometimes because of the severe corruption of an ulcer a malignant humor or black bile or verdigris green bile accumulates in the body and spreads and affects the parts around [the diseased part] until the healthy part adjacent to this diseased part becomes corroded. This illness is called *ākila* ["canker"]. *De tumoribus* [*praeter naturam*].[85]

(49) Canker[86] is an ulcer[ous sore] that corrodes [the flesh] deep inside, while herpes[87] is an ulcer[ous disease] that corrodes on the outside. Lanolin[88] is the wool fat [extracted from the wool], not the[89] filthy (greasy) wool [itself]. *In Hippocratis De humoribus commentarius* 3.[90]

(50) Anasarca[91] is sometimes called "leucophlegmasia."[92] It is also called *al-ḥaban*,[93] while the ascites variety is also called *jam*ᶜ *al-mā*ᵓ.[94] *De locis affectis* 5. In his commentary on *Aphorisms* 4, [Galen] says that tympanites[95] is [the illness] that Hippocrates calls "dry[96] dropsy." *In Hippocratis Aphorismos commentarius* 4.[97]

(٤٥) ورم سقيروس صنفان: أحدهما يتولّد عن البلغم الغليظ والثاني يتولّد عن عكر الدم وثفله. ويعمّهما جميعا أنّهما ورمان عظيمان صلبان غير مؤلّمين. ويخصّ الثاني أنّه أسود اللون. في مقالته في الأورام.

(٤٦) السرطان صنفان وهو ورم يتولّد عن المرّة السوداء فمتى انصبّت المرّة السوداء إلى اللحم وكانت لذّاعة أكلت جميع الجلد الذي يليه وقرّحته وهو السرطان المتقرّح. ومتى كانت معتدلة أحدثت سرطانا غير متقرّح. في مقالته في الأورام.

(٤٧) جميع الأورام السرطانية إنّما يكون تولّدها من فضلة سوداوية. فإن مالت تلك الفضلة إلى أسفل الجسم ودفعتها القوة الدافعة التي في العروق من أفواهها التي في الدبر أو في القبل سمّي ذلك الاستفراغ البواسير الذي يجري منها الدم. وربّما اندفعت إلى الرجلين فتحدث الدوالي وربّما اندفعت تلك الفضول إلى جلد البدن كلّه ومن ذلك يتولّد الجذام. ثانية أغلوقن.

(٤٨) قد يجتمع في البدن عن فساد عظيم في القرحة خلط رديء أو مرار سوداوي أو زنجاري يسعى ويلابس ما حوله من الأعضاء حتّى تأكّل العضو الصحيح الذي يلي العضو العليل. وهذه العلّة يقال لها الآكلة. في مقالته في الأورام.

(٤٩) الآكلة قرحة تأكّل من عمقها والماشرا قرحة تأكّل من ظهرها والزوفا الرطب هو الصوف الدهن لا الصوف الوسخ. في شرحه لثالثة الأخلاط.

(٥٠) الاستسقاء اللحمي قد يسمّى أيضا الاستسقاء البلغمي الأبيض ويسّمى الحبن ويسمّى أيضا النوع الزقّي منه جمع الماء. خامسة التعرّف. وقال في شرحه لرابعة الفصول إنّ الاستسقاء الطبلي هو الذي يسمّيه بقراط الاستسقاء اليابس.

---

١٢ في] مع ELBOU

(51) A[98] swelling occurs when thin phlegm accumulates. The[99] illness called "gangrene" is the beginning of the mortification of the solid parts of the body, except for the bones. If the bones perish as well, the illness is called "sphacelus."[100] *De tumoribus* [*praeter naturam*].

(52) The difference between an inflation[101] [emphysema] and a soft swelling[102] [edema] is that a soft swelling, if you press upon it, stays in its place and remains depressed, but an inflation, if you press upon it with your hand, does not remain depressed, and if you strike upon it, you hear a noise similar to that of a drum. *De methodo* [*medendi*], last book.[103]

(53) Alopecia[104] and ophiasis[105] are one and the same disease. Their names are only different because of the form of the site, since the site from which the hair comes off in the case of ophiasis is similar to the form of a snake when it is moving forward. *Mayāmir* 1.[106]

(54) The skin of the head is affected by an illness that is a type of swelling that has fine, small openings filled with a thin, viscous liquid. [This disease] is called *saʿfa*[107] [cradle cap]. [Another] illness occurs on the skin of the head [and] resembles the former in its appearance, but the openings are larger and wider than the openings of cradle cap, and they are filled with a honeylike moisture, and this [illness] is called "honeycomb."[108]

(55) Cradle cap is a small ulceration on the skin of the head from which a fluid streams that is neither watery nor as thick as honey, as is the case with that which streams from honeycomblike ulcers. It seems likely that [this ulceration] develops from salty, nitrous phlegm. *De tumoribus* [*praeter naturam*].[109]

(56) If inflammations occur in the soft flesh in the groin and armpits, and if these glands harden and become firm, that illness is called "scrofula." *De tumoribus* [*praeter naturam*].[110]

(٥١) الترهّل يحدث عند اجتماع بلغم لطيف والعلّة التي يقال لها غنغرانا فهي ابتداء موت الأعضاء الصلبة غير العظام. فإذا فسدت العظام أيضا سمّيت العلّة سفاقولس. في مقالته في الأورام

(٥٢) الفرق بين الانتفاخ والورم الرخو أنّ الورم الرخو إذا غمزت عليه لطى وانخفض والانتفاخ إذا غمزت عليه بيدك لم ينخفض وإذا ضربته سمعت له صوتا كصوت التبل. آخرة الحيلة.

(٥٣) داء الثعلب وداء الحيّة هما علّة واحدة وإنّما اختلفت أسماؤهما لموضع الشكل لأنّ الموضع الذي ينحلق شعره في داء الحيّة يكون على مثال شكل الحيّة في حال مشيها. أولى الميامر.

(٥٤) يحدث في جلدة الرأس علّة من جنس الورم تكون فيها ثقب صغار دقاق مملوءة رطوبة رقيقة لزجة يقال لها السعفة. ويحدث في جلدة الرأس علّة شبيهة بهذه في المنظر وثقبها أكبر وأوسع من ثقب السعفة وهي مملوءة رطوبة شبيهة بعسل الشهد وهذه يقال لها الشهدة. أولى الميامر.

(٥٥) السعفة هي قرحة صغيرة تكون في جلدة الرأس يجري منها صديد لا بالمائي ولا بالثخين كالعسل بمنزلة ما يجري من القروح الشهدية. ويشبه أن يكون تولّدها عن بلغم مالح بورقي. في مقالته في الأورام.

(٥٦) اللحم الرخو الذي في الحالبين والإبطين إذا حدثت فيه أورام حارّة وصلبت تلك الغدد واشتدّت سمّيت تلك العلّة خنازير. في تلك المقالة.

---

١ غنغرانا] راناعرايا L غانا غانا B غاناغرانا U ناناغرانا O || ٢ سفاقولس] سقاقولس SGOU || ٤ والورم] واللحم B | والورم] واللحم B || ٦ آخرة] أخيرة ELBU || ١٣ الشهدة] الشهدية L

(57) A hardening of the testicles is called "sarcocele,"[111] just as the watery fluid accumulated in the tunics around the testicles is called "hydrocele."[112] Epiplocele[113] and enterocele[114] and the illness consisting of both of these, that is, epiploenterocele, are names invented by more recent physicians, who call all the swellings that occur in the area of the testicles "hernia." *De tumoribus* [*praeter naturam*].[115]

(58) When humors of a bilious type dominate in the head, sleeplessness and delirium develop from it. When cold, phlegmatic humors dominate in it, stupor and forgetfulness develop from it. When the humors are in the middle between these two conditions, stupor develops next to torpor. A stupor is a mild form of delirium. *In Hippocratis Epidemiarum librum* 2 *commentarius* 2.[116]

(58a) In the first [book] of his commentary on [*Epidemics*] 3, [Galen] says that[117] raving is a mild form of delirium. One should not say that a patient suffers from stupor until it becomes difficult for him to wake up. If he sleeps for a long time and it is not difficult for him to wake up if he is prodded, it is only a long sleep but not a stupor. Both, however, are caused by coldness of the brain. *In Hippocratis Aphorismos commentarius* 2.[118]

(59) If cold dominates the brain and moisture becomes added thereto, lethargy[119] develops therefrom. If dryness is added to the cold, catalepsy develops from it. If[120] the brain only becomes warm qualitatively or in combination with [superfluous] matter, sleeplessness develops. *In Hippocratis Aphorismos commentarius* 2.[121]

(60) In *De pulsu parva* [Galen] says: The illness called "forgetfulness" arises from a phlegmatic swelling that occurs in the membranes of the brain.[122]

(٥٧) صلابة الأنثيين تسمّى قيلة اللحم كما تسمّى الرطوبة المائية التي تجتمع في الأغشية التي حول الأنثيين قيلة الماء. فأمّا قيلة الثرب وقيلة الأمعاء والعلّة المركّبة منهما أعني قيلة الثرب والأمعاء فهي أسماء مخترعة من الأطبّاء الحدث الذين يسمّون جميع الأورام الحادثة في ما يلي الأنثيين قيلة. في مقالته في الأورام.

(٥٨) متى غلب في الرأس أخلاط من جنس المرار حدث من ذلك الأرق واختلاط العقل. ومتى غلب فيه أخلاط باردة بلغمية حدث من ذلك السبات والنسيان. ومتى كانت الأخلاط متوسّطة بين الحالين حدث من ذلك مع السبات الدهش والدهش هو اختلاط عقل يسير. في الثانية من شرحه لثانية أبيديميا.

(٥٨a) وقال في الأولى من شرحه للثالثة إنّ الهذيان هو اختلاط يسير. ليس يقال إنّ بالمريض سبات حتّى يعسر انتباهه. فأمّا إذا طال نومه ولا يعسر انتباهه إذا حرّك فذلك نوم طويل لا سبات وكلاهما من برد الدماغ. في شرحه لثانية الفصول.

(٥٩) إذا قوي على الدماغ البرد وخالطته رطوبة حدث منه البرسام البارد وهو ليثرغس. وإذا خالط البرد يبس حدث منه الجمود. وإذا سخن الدماغ بكيفيته فقط أو مع مادّة حدث الأرق. في شرحه لثانية الفصول.

(٦٠) وقال في النبض الصغير العلّة التي تسمّى النسيان هذه العلّة تعرض من ورم بلغمي يكون في حجب الدماغ.

---

٢ والعلّة المركّبة منهما أعني قيلة الثرب والأمعاء] om. B || ٨ لثانية] لثالثة SG | أبيديميا] أفيديميا LO | ١١ لثانية] لثالثة G || ١٢ البرسام] الشرسام EBO || ١٤ لثانية] لثالثة G || ١٥ هذه العلّة] هي علّة L هي العلّة التي B

(61) Apoplexy [occurs] when the[123] psychical pneuma cannot pass to the parts below the head whether it is due to an illness of some sort of swelling that occurs in the brain or because the ventricles of the brain have become filled with phlegmatic moisture. The severity and graveness of the illness are according to the severity[124] of the cause effecting this disease. *In Hippocratis Aphorismos commentarius* 2.[125]

The ancients used to call epilepsy "the divine illness." Some of them called it thus because they thought that this illness comes from the demons, and others give as reason for this designation the fact that its only cause is the constellation of the moon. Plato gives as reason for this designation the fact that this illness arises in the head and harms the pure, divine part whose seat is the brain. *In Timaeum commentarius* 4.[126]

(62) Madness is a chronic mental confusion without fever whereas phrenitis is a chronic mental confusion with fever. *In Hippocratis Epidemiarum librum* 3 *commentarius* 3.[127]

(63) The "black bile" illness, that is, melancholy, is [the same as] melancholic[128] delusion. *In Hippocratis Epidemiarum librum* 6 *commentarius* 3.[129]

(64) The loss of imagination is called "torpor"[130] and "catalepsy." Its bad[131] functioning is called "delirium." Loss[132] of reasoning [power] is called "amentia," and its bad functioning is also called "mental confusion." *De [morborum] causis et symptomatibus* 3.[133]

(65) There is one type of melancholic delusion that has its origin in the stomach. Some of the ancient [physicians] call this illness the[134] "hypochondriac illness" and the "flatulent illness." It is also called "hypochondriac" and "flatulent."[135] *De locis affectis* 3.[136]

(٦١) السكتة هي إذا لم يمكن الروح النفساني أن يخرج إلى ما دون الرأس إمّا لعلّة من جنس الورم حدثت في الدماغ و إمّا لأنّ بطون الدماغ امتلأت رطوبة بلغمية. بحسب مقدار السبب الفاعل لهذا المرض يكون عظمه وشدّته. في شرحه لثانية الفصول.

القدماء كانوا يسمّون الصرع المرض الإلهي فبعضهم سمّاه كذلك لأنّهم رأوا أنّ هذه العلّة من الجنّ وبعضهم جعل علّة هذه التسمية لكون سبب هذه العلّة فأل القمر وحده. وأفلاطون يجعل علّة هذه التسمية لكون هذه العلّة تحدث في الرأس فتضرّ بالجزء الإلهي الطاهر الذي مسكنه الدماغ. في المقالة الرابعة من شرحه لطيماوس.

(٦٢) الجنون هو اختلاط ذهن دائما بلا حمّى والبرسام هو اختلاط ذهن دائما مع حمّى. في الثالثة من شرحه لثالثة أبيديميا.

(٦٣) العلّة السوداوية وهي المالنخونيا وهو الوسواس السوداوي. في الثالثة من شرحه لسادسة أبيديميا.

(٦٤) بطلان التخيّل يقال له الاستغراق والجمود وجريانه المنكر يسمّى اختلاط وبطلان الفكر يقال له عدم العقل وجريانه المنكر يقال له أيضا اختلاط. ثالثة العلل والأعراض.

(٦٥) من الوسواس السوداوي صنف يكون ابتداءه من المعدة وقوم من القدماء يسمّون هذه العلّة مرض مراقّ البطن ومرضا نافخا ويقال لها أيضا المراقّية والنافخة. في ثالثة التعرّف.

---

١ يخرج] يجري LB || ٣ يكون] من L || ٤ القدماء . . . لطيماوس] om. ELOU || ٨ دائما بلا حمّى والبرسام هو اختلاط ذهن] om. B G[1] | والبرسام] والشرسام ELO والسرسام U || ٩ أبيديميا] أفيديميا LO || ١١ أبيديميا] أفيديميا LO || ١٣ عدم العقل وجريانه المنكر يقال له] om. G

(66) The illness that the physicians call *bayḍa*[137] and *khūdha* [helmet] is an illness affecting the head; it is a chronic headache that is difficult to eliminate whereby minor causes produce attacks that are so severe that the patient does not tolerate the sound of speaking nor a bright light nor any movement. The thing he likes most is to lie down in darkness because of the severity of the pain. *De usu partium* 3.[138]

(67) Mental confusion that arises from phrenitis, which is an inflammation that occurs in the brain or its membranes, does not happen all at once, but little by little, and does not subside during the decline of the fever. But mental confusion occurring in the case of ardent fevers and caused by [illnesses] affecting other organs happens all at once and subsides when those illnesses have passed their climax. An exception is the case when the mental confusion is consequential upon an inflammation of the diaphragm, for then it is closely related to the mental confusion that is consequential upon phrenitis and that does not subside [immediately] after [the illness] has reached its climax. *De locis affectis* 5.[139]

(68) If a phlegmatic, thick, cold humor that has not yet putrefied increases in the brain, it produces [different] kinds of severe[140] stuporific attacks without fever. They are [the kinds] that are called "stupor,"[141] "torpor,"[142] and "catalepsy."[143] If the humor putrefies at some time, these things occur together with fever, and this illness is called "lethargy." *De methodo* [*medendi*] 13.[144]

(69) The cataract that occurs in the eye and[145] that the physicians call "extension" lies between the crystalline humor and the hornlike tunic. *De usu partium* 10.[146]

(70) If the membrane known as conjunctiva suffers from a bloody inflammation, namely conjunctivitis, it harms the visual ability and hinders its [normal] function accidentally. But if it is affected by chemosis[147] or pterygium,[148] the darkening of vision resulting from the covering of the pupil does not occur accidentally. *De* [*morborum*] *causis et symptomatibus* 4.[149]

(٦٦) العلّة التي يسمّيها الأطبّاء البيضة والخوذة هو مرض من أمراض الرأس وهو صداع مزمن عسر الانقلاع يصير بالأسباب اليسيرة إلى أن ينوب نوائب عظيمة حتّى أنّ صاحبه لا يحتمل صوت كلام ولا ضوء ساطعا ولا حركة وأحبّ الأشياء إليه الاستلقاء في الظلمة لعظم الوجع. ثالثة المنافع.

(٦٧) اختلاط العقل الحادث من قبل فرانيطس وهو ورم حارّ يحدث في الدماغ أو أغشيته لا يحدث دفعة بل أوّلا أوّلا ولا يسكن في وقت انحطاط الحمّى. وأمّا الاختلاط الحادث في الحمّيات المحرقة والذي يحدث من قبل أعضاء آخر فقد يحدث بغتة ويسكن إذا جاوزت تلك العلل منتهاها إلا ما كان من الاختلاط تابعا لورم الحجاب فإنّه قريب من الاختلاط التابع لفرانيطس لا يسكن عند الانتهاء. خامسة التعرّف.

(٦٨) إذا كثرت في الدماغ خلط بلغمي غليظ بارد إن لم يكن قد عفن أحدث ضروبا من السبات المستغرق من غير حمّى وهو الذي يسمّى سباتا واستغراقا وجمودا. وإن هو عفن في وقت ما حدثت هذه الأشياء مع حمّى وسمّيت هذه العلّة ليثرغس. ثالثة عشر الحيلة.

(٦٩) الماء الذي يجتمع في العين وهو الذي يسمّيه الأطبّاء انتشارا يجتمع فيما بين الرطوبة الجليدية والصفاق القرني. عاشرة المنافع.

(٧٠) الغشاء المعروف بالملتحم إذا تورّم ورما دمويا وهو الرمد أضرّ بفعل البصر وعاقه عن مجراه بطريق العرض. وأمّا إذا حدث به الوردينج وإذا حدثت به الظفرة فإنّما يحدث من ظلمة البصر بسترهما للحدقة لا يكون بطريق العرض. رابعة العلل والأعراض.

٣ لا ] يقدر add. ELBOU || ٧ قبل ] علل add. B || ٨ العلل ] العلّة L || ٩ الانتهاء ] المنتهى B || ١٠ ضروبا ] ضربا L || ١٢ هذه ] om. G

(71) If a site on the hornlike tunic becomes corroded and part of the grapelike tunic protrudes from it, this is called *mūsaraj*[150] [prolapse]. The[151] pus that originates behind the hornlike tunic is called *kumna*.[152] The[153] eyelids that become thick and hard and whose color turns red and whose hairs fall off is an illness that is called *sulāq*[154] [ptilosis]. If[155] the flesh in the inner angle of the eye disappears, it is an illness that is called *damʿa* [rhyas]. *Mayāmir* 4.

(72) A[156] fistula occurring in the inner angle of the eye is called *gharab*[157] [*Fistula lachrimalis*]. Callous[158] hardenings on the face are called *naḥīlāt*. *Mayāmir* 5.

(73) Deafness means that a person cannot hear a low voice at all and hears a loud voice with difficulty. This process continues to progress slowly until the patient becomes completely deaf in the course of time. *Mayāmir* 3.[159]

(74) The tumor that forms inside the nose as if it were a fleshy excrescence is called *nāṣūr*[160] and also "polypus." *Mayāmir* 3.[161]

(75) The term "aphthae"[162] applies to ulcers occurring on the outside of the [mucous] membrane inside the mouth and is accompanied by fiery heat. It mostly occurs to infants because of spoiled milk. The term "aphthae" is used only when the illness does not come with putrefaction. But if the aphthae last for a long time and putrefaction occurs with it, this is what the physicians call "corrosion."[163] *Mayāmir* 3.[164]

(76) The windpipe is called *ḥalqūm* [trachea]. The term *ḥalqūm* is especially used for the site where the two channels, that is, the larynx and the esophagus, arrive at, below the root of the tongue. In the throat there are muscles that are known as *naghānigh*.[165] It is a plural term, meaning [the muscles at] both sides of the throat. *De voce* [*et hanelitu*].[166]

(٧١) إذا تأكّل موضع من الطبقة القرنية ونتأ منه شيء من الطبقة العنبية فهو الذي يسمّى موسرج. والقيح المتولّد تحت الطبقة القرنية هو الذي يسمّى الكمنة. والأجفان التي تغلظ وتصلب ويصير لونها أحمر وتتناثر أشفارها هي العلّة التي تعرف بالسلاق. وذهاب اللحم الذي في المأق الأكبر يقال لهذه العلّة الدمعة. رابعة الميامر.

(٧٢) الناصور الذي يكون في مأق العين هو الذي يسمّى الغرب. والجساء الصلب الذي يكون في الوجه يسمّى النخيلات. خامسة الميامر.

(٧٣) الطرش هو أن يكون الإنسان لا يسمع بتّة الصوت المنخفض ويسمع الصوت المرتفع بكدّ. ولا يزال ذلك يزيد أوّلا أوّلا حتّى يصير صاحبه على طول الزمان إلى الصمم التامّ. ثالثة الميامر.

(٧٤) الورم الذي يحدث في داخل الأنف وكأنّه لحم زائد هو الذي يقال له الناصور ويقال له الكثير الأرجل. ثالثة الميامر.

(٧٥) اسم القلاع يقع على قروح تحدث في ظاهر الصفاق الذي من داخل الفم ويكون معها حرارة نارية. وأكثر حدوث ذلك للأطفال لرداءة اللبن. ولا يسمّى قلاعا إلا ما لا عفونة معه. فأمّا إن حدث في القلاع إذا طال به الزمان عفونة فهي التي يسمّيها الأطبّاء الآكلة. سادسة الميامر.

(٧٦) سمّيت قصبة الرئة الحلقوم وخصصت باسم الحلقوم الموضع الذي يفضي إليه المجريان الحنجرة والمريء من دون أصل اللسان. وفي الحلق العضل الذي يعرف بعضل النغانغ والنغانغ اسم جمع وإنّما هما جنبتا الحلق. في الأوّل من كتابه في الصوت.

---

٥ الغرب] الجرب L || ٦ النخيلات] الخيالات E || ٨ حتى] إلى أن B || ١٦ الحلقوم] الحلق B

(77) Angina is a swelling in the throat and consists of four types. The first is that the inside of the throat swells up, that is, its cavity up to the end of the larynx, whereby none of the swelling is visible externally. The second is when the throat swells up at the outside and the patient does not have a sensation of choking; this is the safest of all four types. The third is when the swelling includes both the inside of the throat and the outside, and this is the worst of all. The fourth is when no swelling is visible on the outside, but the patient has the feeling of choking. *De locis affectis* 4.[167]

(78) All types of asthma that occur suddenly are [called] "acute asthma," and the pulse of those suffering from acute asthma is always irregularly unequal. *De pulsu* 12.[168]

(79) If it happens to someone that he breathes uninterruptedly[169] like someone who has run fast without his suffering from fever, the physicians used to call this affliction "asthma." They also call it "orthopnea" because the patient suffering from this ailment keeps his chest erect during respiration. It is caused by narrowness occurring in the chest either because of inflammations in the organs there or because of viscous humors that flowed between the chest and the lungs or thick, viscous humors in the [different] parts of the windpipe. *Mayāmir* 7.[170]

The illness that is called "dyspnea"[171] in particular is that which originates from thick, viscous humors that are stuck in the [different] parts of the windpipe. This term is indeed used for this illness in particular. *Mayāmir* 7.[172]

(80) If the foods change in the stomach into a quality different from the natural one, it is called "dyspepsia," that is, bad digestion. If the retentive faculty of the stomach becomes inactive, it means that the stomach does not contract at all and does not wrap itself around the foods in a tight and firm manner. This happens to the stomach in the illness called "lientery." *De [morborum] causis et symptomatibus* 3.[173]

(٧٧) الذبحة هي ورم يكون في الحلق وهو أربعة أنواع: أحدها أن يرم داخل الحلق أعني تجويفه الذي ينتهي عند طرف الحنجرة ولا يظهر من الورم شيء إلى خارج. والثاني إذا ورم خارج الحلق ولا يحسّ المريض باختناق وهذا أسلمها. والثالث إذا عمّ الورم تجويف الحلق وظاهره من خارج وهذه شرّها. والرابع عندما لا يرى شيء ممّا هو خارج وارما لكن يجد العليل حسّ الاختناق. رابعة التعرّف.

(٧٨) جميع أنواع الربو الذي يحدث بغتة هو الربو الحادّ ونبض أصحاب الربو الحادّ أبدا مختلف غير منتظم. ثانية عشر النبض.

(٧٩) من عرض له أن يتنفّس تنفّسا متواليا بمنزلة ما يتنفّس من قد أحضر إحضارا شديدا من غير أن يكون محموما فقد جرت عادة الأطبّاء أن يسمّوا هذا العارض ربوا. ويسمّونه أيضا نفس الانتصاب لكون صاحب هذه العلّة ينتصب صدره عند التنفّس. وعلّة ذلك ضيق يعرض في الصدر إمّا من أورام هناك في تلك الأعضاء أو أخلاط لزجة مصبوبة بين الصدر والرئة أو أخلاط غليظة لزجة في أقسام قصبة الرئة. سابعة الميامر.

العلّة التي يقال لها خاصّة ضيق النفس وعسر النفس هي العلّة التي تحدث عن رطوبات غليظة لزجة تلحج في أقسام قصبة الرئة وهذا الاسم إنّما يقع على هذه العلّة خاصّة. سابعة الميامر.

(٨٠) أمّا تغيّر الأغذية في المعدة إلى كيفية أخرى لا إلى تلك التي في الطبع فيقال له سوء الاستمراء وهو التخمة. وبطلان القوة الماسكة من المعدة هو أن لا تجتمع المعدة أصلا ولا تلتحف على الأغذية التحاف ضمّ ولزوم. وذلك يعرض لها في العلّة المعروفة بزلق الأمعاء. ثالثة العلل والأعراض.

---

٣ وهذا] وهذه ELBUO || ٩ العارض] العرض B || ١٠ التنفّس] النفس B || ١٢ سابعة . . . الرئة] om. L || ١٦ أمّا] إنّما B || ١٨ بزلق] بلزق B

(81) A bad craving for food, if unusually severe, is called "canine appetite." It happens when a detrimental acid humor burns the stomach or when the entire body suffers from excessive[174] dissolution. *De [morborum] causis et symptomatibus* 4.[175]

(82) Just as emesis is preceded by nausea,[176] so too coughing is preceded and induced by distress.[177] And just as someone's soul[178] is upset and he is nauseous but does not vomit, so too he feels distress[179] that may prompt coughing, but he does not cough because the cause is [too] mild. *De [morborum] causis et symptomatibus* 5.[180]

(83) The stomach employs for the expulsion of a harmful substance the opening towards which that superfluity has the strongest inclination [to stream to]. If this type of disturbance[181] occurs in the entire stomach, it employs for its expulsion the two openings together and expels it both through vomiting and diarrhea, just as in the case of cholera. *De [morborum] causis et symptomatibus* 6.[182]

(84) Sometimes the cause of indigestion is the irregularity in which foods are taken in[183] terms of what is taken first and what is taken later, or their quantity or their quality. *De locis affectis* 5.[184]

(85) The illness called "bulimia" is a [form of] syncope that is caused by excessive cold of the cardia of the stomach. *De pulsu parva*.[185]

(86) One calls a "stomach patient" someone who has no tumor in his stomach but whose appetite has disappeared, or someone who feels after taking food a heaviness, pressure, anxiety, or nausea that he can hardly bear. One also calls a "stomach patient" someone who has an[186] upset stomach after having food, especially if it requires that person to vomit. *Mayāmir* 8.[187]

(٨١) أمّا الشهوة الرديئة للطعام فما كان منها مفرطا فهي الشهوة الكلبية وتكون عندما يكون خلط رديء حامض يلذع المعدة أو عندما يتحلّل البدن كلّه تحلّلا مفرطا. رابعة العلل والأعراض.

(٨٢) كما أنّ القيء يتقدّمه التهوّع كذلك يتقدّم السعال المضض الذي يدعو إلى السعال. وكما تتقلّب نفس الإنسان و يتهوّع من غير أن يتقيّأ كذلك يجد مضضا يدعو إلى السعال ولا يسعل لأنّ السبب يكون يسيرا. خامسة العلل والأعراض.

(٨٣) المعدة تستعمل في دفع الشيء المؤذي الفم الذي ذلك الفضل أميل إليه. فإن عرض مثل هذا السبب في المعدة كلّها استعملت في دفعها الفمين جميعا فتخرج بالقيء والإسهال معا بمنزلة ما يعرض ذلك في الهيضة. سادسة العلل والأعراض.

(٨٤) قد يكون سبب التخمة سوء ترتيب الطعام في ما يقدّم ويؤخّر أو مقداره أو كيفيته. خامسة التعرّف.

(٨٥) العلّة التي تسمّى بوليموس هي غشي يعرض من إفراط برد فم المعدة. في النبض الصغير.

(٨٦) إنّما يسمّى ممعودا من لا ورم في معدته وقد ذهبت شهوته للطعام أو لمن يجد بعد تناول الطعام ثقلا وضغطا وقلقا وغثيانا لا يحتمله إلا بشدّة. وكذلك يسمّون ممعودا من تتقلّب نفسه بعد الطعام وبخاصة إن أحوجه ذلك إلى القيء. ثامنة الميامر.

١٢ فم] في B || ١٦ أحوجه] أخرجه LBU

(87) Part of the stomach ailments is that ailment that is called *inqilāb* [upset stomach], which is a lack of appetite without a tumor, nausea, feeling of sickness, or vomiting. The ailment called "bulimia" is a devouring [hunger associated with] a burning [pain] occurring in the stomach that can become so severe that the patient suffers from syncope. The general treatment of all these ailments consists of astringent medicines, many of which are mixed with heating and drying medicines. *Mayāmir* 8.[188]

(88) The illness that the physicians call "liver ailment" and whose patient they call "a patient with a liver illness" is an illness of a bad temperament without a tumor, just as they speak of a "stomach illness" and a "stomach patient" in the case of someone whose stomach is ill without a tumor. It is well known that a bad temperament sometimes occurs in the substance of the liver itself and is peculiar to it, whereas at other times it occurs in the pulsatile and nonpulsatile vessels that the liver contains. At [yet] other times the bad temperament occurs in the matters that those vessels encompass. *Mayāmir* 8.[189]

(89) When[190] speaking of "spleen patients," physicians mean those patients whose spleen is affected by induration and calcification without an inflammation. The[191] illness that is really called "dysentery" is an ulceration of the intestines, and this ulceration is either simple without putrefaction or with putrefaction. [The[192] illness] that the physicians usually call "spreading[193] ulcer" is a cankerous sore. Lanolin[194] is the wool fat. *Mayāmir* 9.[195]

(90) Lientery means that the food is discharged quickly and unchanged,[196] and diarrhea means softness of the stools and their continuous discharge. *In Hippocratis Epidemiarum librum* 1 *commentarius* 2.[197]

(91) Ulceration of the rectum, which is called "tenesmus," produces a[198] severe pricking pain and an[199] urge to relieve oneself, while only a small amount is discharged from the patient. In the beginning [the discharge] is phlegmatic and fatty. As time passes, something like shreds of intestinal tissue is discharged from [these patients]. *De locis affectis* 6.[200]

(٨٧) من علل المعدة العلّة التي يقال لها انقلاب وهو ذهاب الشهوة من غير ورم أو غثيان أو تهوّع أو قيء. والعلّة التي يقال لها بوليموس وهو اللحس هو لذع يحدث في المعدة حتّى يغشى على صاحبه. وعلاج هذه العلل كلّها عامّة أدوية قابضة ويخلط في كثير منها أدوية تسخن وتجفّف. ثامنة الميامر.

(٨٨) العلّة التي يسمّيها الأطبّاء علّة الكبد ويسمّون من أصابته مكبودا هي علّة سوء مزاج من غير ورم كما يسمّون علّة المعدة وممعود لمن اعتلّت معدته من غير ورم. ومعلوم أنّ سوء المزاج مرّة يكون في نفس جوهر الكبد الخاصّ بها ومرّة يكون في العروق الضوارب وغير الضوارب التي تحتوي عليها الكبد ومرّة يكون سوء المزاج في الموادّ التي تحتوي عليها تلك العروق. ثامنة الميامر.

(٨٩) الأطبّاء يذهبون في قولهم مطحولين إلى من يصيبه في طحاله صلابة وتحجّر من غير ورم. والعلّة التي تسمّى بالحقيقة دوسنطاريا هي قرحة الأمعاء وهذه القرحة إمّا أن تكون ساذجة دون عفونة أو تكون مع عفونة. وهي التي عادة الأطبّاء أن يسمّونها قرحة تسعى وهي الآكلة. والزوفا الرطب هو وسخ الصوف. تاسعة الميامر.

(٩٠) زلق الأمعاء هو أن يكون الطعام يخرج بسرعة من غير أن يتغيّر والذرب هو لين الطبع وخروجه متواترا. في الثانية من شرحه للأولى من أبيديميا.

(٩١) القروح التي تكون في المعاء المستقيم يقال لها الزحير تحدث لصاحبها وخزا شديدا وشهوة للقيام ولا يخرج منه إلا الشيء اليسير وهو يكون في أوّل الأمر بلغميا ودكيا. فإذا طالت المدّة انحدر منهم شيء من جنس الخراطة. سادسة التعرّف.

---

٢ اللحس] om. LB عدم الحس E || ٦ كما . . . ورم] G[1] || ١١ دوسنطاريا] دوسنطارية B دوشنطارية O || ١٢ مع] معه L معها E || ١٣ ودخ] ودك ESG ورق ال . . . (?) L || ١٨ شيء] يسير add. B

(92) If the superfluities that are harmful for nature are moist, the expulsive faculty eliminates them by the severe and violent shaking that happens during a rigor or cough, and then they go to all the sites that have the property to receive them. Thus some of them go to the upper part of the abdomen, namely the stomach, and arrive there, and others go to the lower part of the abdomen, namely the intestines, and arrive there. Yet other [superfluities] go to the outside of the skin. *De [morborum] causis et symptomatibus* 5.[201]

(93) If the small intestines are affected by a hard tumor or by a severe obstruction of feces so that the patient vomits his feces, that illness is called "ileus," and hardly anyone can be saved from it. If all [parts of] the intestines and the stomach fall ill and cannot retain their contents even for a short time, or if the illness does not come with biting [pain], that illness is called "lientery." It is also called "abdominal[202] affections." The patient suffering therefrom is called an "abdominal patient." *De locis affectis* 6.[203]

What[204] is really called "dysentery" is [the illness] caused by an ulceration of the intestines. *De locis affectis* 6.[205]

(94) The illness called "polyuria" is called by some "diabetes" and by others "polydipsia"; a patient with this illness suffers from severe thirst and drinks a lot and rapidly urinates what he drinks. This illness of the kidneys and urinary bladder is comparable to lientery of the stomach and the intestines. *De locis affectis* 6.[206]

(95) If the stomach suffers harm from the biting effect of food that is not digested, together with the intestines it expels [this food] until it is completely discharged. This affliction is called "diarrhea." *De propriorum animi cuiuslibet affectuum dignotione [et curatione]*.[207]

(٩٢) إذا كانت الفضول المؤذية للطبيعة رطبة دفعتها القوة الدافعة بهذا الارتعاد الشديد العنيف الذي يكون في النافض أو في السعال فصارت إلى جميع المواضع التي من شأنها أن تقبلها. فبعضها يصير إلى البطن الأعلى وهي المعدة ويحصل فيها وبعضها يصير إلى البطن الأسفل وهي الأمعاء ويحصل فيها وبعضها يصير إلى خارج الجلد. خامسة العلل والأعراض.

(٩٣) إذا حدث في الأمعاء الدقاق ورم صلب أو سدّة عظيمة من ثفل حتّى يتقيّأ الإنسان رجيعه فتلك العلّة تسمّى ايلاوس فقلّ من يسلم منها. وإذا اعتلّت الأمعاء كلّها والمعدة ولا تقدر أن تضبط ما في جرمها ولو وقتا يسيرا أو لا تكون العلّة لذّاعة فتلك العلّة يقال لها زلق الأمعاء. وتسمّى أيضا علل البطن ويسمّى صاحبها مبطونا. سادسة التعرّف.

الذي يسمّى بالحقيقة إسهال الدم هو الذي يكون من قبل قرحة الأمعاء. سادسة التعرّف.

(٩٤) العلّة التي تسمّى استطلاق البول وقوم يسمّونها ديابيطس وقوم آخر العطش المبّرح وصاحب هذه العلّة يعطش عطشا شديدا فيشرب شربا كثيرا ويبول ما يشربه سريعا ومنزلة هذه العلّة من الكليتين والمثانة بمنزلة زلق الأمعاء من المعدة والأمعاء . سادسة التعرّف.

(٩٥) المعدة إذا تأذّت بما ينالها من اللذع الحادث عن الطعام الذي لا يستمرأ دفعته هو والأمعاء حتّى يخرج كلّه وهذا العارض يسمّى خلفة. في مقالته في تعرّف الإنسان عيوب نفسه.

---

١ إذا . . . والأعراض.] om. G || ٣ وهي . . . الأسفل] om. B || ٥ والأعراض] ومهما كان جوهر النفس فيشبه أن يكون هذا الباب لا ينفكّ عن أحد الأمرين] إمّا أن يكون هذا الجوهر يستعمل الروح والدم والحرارة التي في كلّ واحد منهما وفيهما جميعا في جميع أفعاله على جهة ما تستعمل الآلات وإمّا أن يكون إنّما هي في هذه العضوين add. B || ٩ علل] علّة L || ١١ يسمّونها] يسمّيها B || ١٥ تعرّف] عرف B

(96) The neck of the uterus and the cervix of the uterus are two synonyms for one and the same organ. The side of that cervix that is close to the uterus is called "os uteri," and this is the one that is hermetically closed during pregnancy. The side [of the cervix] that is close to the vulva and into which the penis penetrates is called the "mouth of the neck of the uterus." *In Hippocratis Aphorismos commentarius* 5.[208]

(97) The [illness called] *raḥā*[209] that develops in the uteri of women is the formless flesh that a woman produces. *De methodo medendi*, last treatise.[210]

The medicines that are taken internally are called "antidotes" by the physicians. *Mayāmir* 1.[211]

(98) The remedies that are called "useful for many purposes" are remedies that are beneficial for many illnesses and are, so to say, compounded from medicines that are opposite not only in their quality and first [degree of their] potency, but also in the second [degree of their] potency. *Qaṭājānas* 5.[212]

(99) "Thinning" and "rarefaction" are synonyms. For every medicine that heats without causing harm and that dries less than it heats and whose substance contains some fineness such as chamomile [*Matricaria chamomilla* and var., or *Anthemis nobilis* and var.] and marshmallow [*Althaea officinalis*], that medicine widens the pores and loosens the skin. A medicine that is hot and that has a thick substance is called "opening" because it opens the mouth of the vessels from below, such as garlic [*Allium sativum*], onion [*Alllium cepa*], cyclamen[213] [*Cyclamen purpurascens*], and bile of a bull. *De* [*simplicium*] *medicamentorum* [*temperamentis ac facultatibus*] 5.[214]

(100) A cleansing and clearing medicine uproots sordidness from the outer layer of the pores and openings, such as honey, white lupine [*Lupinus albus*] flour, barley, broad beans [*Vicia faba*], bitter vetch [*Vicia ervilia*], and a number of seeds. A medicine that purifies the pores and openings is any alkaline, fine medicine and is also called "opening." The difference between [this medicine] and a clearing [medicine] is only a quantitative one. *De* [*simplicium*] *medicamentorum* [*temperamentis ac facultatibus*] 5.[215]

(٩٦) عنق الرحم ورقبة الرحم اسمان مترادفان على عضو واحد بعينه. وطرف ذلك العنق الذي يلي الرحم يسمّى فم الرحم وهو الذي يتضمّم غاية الانضمام عند الحمل. وطرفه الذي يلي الفرج وفيه يلج الإحليل يسمّى فم رقبة الرحم. في شرحه لخامسة الفصول.

(٩٧) الرحا المتولّد في أرحام النساء وهو لحم تلده المرأة لا صورة له. آخرة الحيلة.

الأدوية التي ترد البدن من داخل يسمّونها الأطبّاء الأدوية المقابلة للأدواء. في أوّل الميامر.

(٩٨) الأدوية المسمّاة الكثيرة المنافع هي الأدوية التي تصلح لعلل كثيرة وكأنّها مؤلّفة من أدوية متضادّة لا في كيفيتها وقواها الأوّل فقط لكن وفي قواها الثانية أيضا. خامسة قاطاجانس.

(٩٩) التسخيف والتخلخل اسمان مترادفان وذلك أنّ كلّ دواء يسخّن تسخينا لا أذى معه وتجفيفه أقلّ من إسخانه وجوهره فيه لطافة ما بمنزلة البابونج والخطمي فإنّ ذلك الدواء يوسع المسامّ ويخلخل الجلد ولذلك تسمّى أدوية مسخّفة ومخلخلة. أمّا الدواء الحارّ الغليظ الجوهر فيسمّى مفتّح لأنّه يفتّح أفواه العروق من السفلة بمنزلة الثوم والبصل وشجرة مريم ومرارة الثور. خامسة الأدوية.

(١٠٠) الدواء الغسّال والجلّاء هو الذي يقلع الوسخ من الصفيخة الظاهرة من المسامّ والثقب كالعسل ودقيق الترمس والشعير والباقلّي والكرسنّة وعدّة من البزور. والدواء المنقّي للمسامّ والثقب هو كلّ دواء بورقي لطيف ويقال له أيضا مفتّح. والفرق بينه وبين الجلّاء في الزيادة والنقصان فقط. خامسة الأدوية.

---

٢ الذي . . . وطرفه] om. EL | يتضمّم . . . الذي] om. B || ٤ الرحا] الرجا SG || ١١ الدواء] om. ELBOU || ١٣ مفتّح] فتّاحا L

(101) Remedies that warm and moisten until they corrupt what they encounter are truly called "putrefying remedies." Similarly, all remedies that are hot and dry and whose substance is thick, if they bite or burn somewhat without causing pain, are called "putrefying" because they dissolve and corrode the flesh. They have the same effect on it as the truely putrefying remedies. These include the two types of arsenic, chrysocolla, stinging[216] or urticating caterpillar of the pinewoods, and aconite[217] [*Aconitum napellus*]. *De* [*simplicium*] *medicamentorum* [*temperamentis ac facultatibus*] 5.[218]

(102) The[219] king's nut is the edible[220] nut (i.e., walnut, *Juglans regia*). The[221] small nut is the hazelnut [*jillawz*], that is, *bunduq* [*Corylus avellana*]. Sorghum[222] [*Sorghum bicolor*] is called *shaylam*[223] by the ancients; millet[224] [*Panicum miliaceum*] is a type of sorghum. *De bonis* [*malisque*] *sucis*.

(103) Concentrated[225] grape juice is the must that has been extremely well cooked. *De victu attenuante*.[226]

(104) The difference between [soft][227] fat and suet (i.e., hard fat) lies in their moistness and dryness. For [soft] fat is moist, similar to olive oil that has become thick and dry because[228] of its age. Suet is very dry; therefore if you melt it and then leave it, it solidifies quickly. *De alimentorum facultatibus* 3.[229]

(105) Sour[230] milk is [the milk] from which only the buttery part has been removed and that was then left until it turned sour. An egg that has been boiled for a long time is called "hard [boiled]"; the one that reaches moderate thickness from boiling is called "moderately[231] boiled" and is the same as a soft-boiled egg.[232] The egg that is heated only by boiling is called "the[233] one that can be supped." *De alimentorum facultatibus* 3.[234]

(١٠١) الأدوية التي تسخن وترطّب حتّى تفسد ما تلقاه هي التي تسمّى بالحقيقة أدوية معفّنة. وكذلك أيضا يسمّى جميع الأدوية الحارّة اليابسة الغليظة الجوهر إذا كانت تلذع قليلا أو تحرق قليلا من غير أن تحدث وجعا تسمّى معفّنة لأنّها تذيب وتأكّل اللحم وتفعل فيه ما تفعل المعفّنة بالحقيقة وهي كالزرنيخين ولصاق الذهب ودود الصنوبر وقاتل الذئب. خامسة الأدوية.

(١٠٢) جوز الملك وهو الجوز المأكول والجوز الصغير هو الجلّوز وهو البندق. والدخن يسمّونه القدماء الشيلم والجاورس نوع من الدخن. في مقالته في جودة الكيموس.

(١٠٣) الميبختج هو العصير الذي قد طبخ طبخا كثيرا جدّا. في مقالته في التدبير الملطّف.

(١٠٤) الفرق بين السمن والشحم في الرطوبة واليبس وذلك أنّ السمن رطب بمنزلة الزيت الذي قد غلظ ويبس بسبب تقادمه. والشحم يابس كثيرا ولذلك إذا أذبته وتركته جمد سريعا. ثالثة الأغذية.

(١٠٥) اللبن المحمّض هو الذي أزيل زبده فقط وترك حتّى يحمض. البيض الكثير النضج يقال له المنعقد. والذي يبلغ من إنضاجه أن يغلظ غلظا معتدلا يقال له المترجّج وهو النيمبرشت والذي يبلغ من إنضاجه أن يسخن فقط يقال له المتحسّى. ثالثة الأغذية.

---

٣ لأنّها . . . المعفّنة] om. B || ٤ كالزرنيخين] كالزرنيخ O | ولصاق] ELOU لازق B || ٨ الميبختج . . . الملطّف] om. B || ١٣ المحمّض] المحيض S المحموض ELO || ١٤ يغلظ غلظا معتدلا] ينضج نضجا معتدلا B | المترجّج] المرجرج ELO المترجرج BU || ١٥ النيمبرشت] النيمرشت ELO النيرمشت B | والذي . . . المتحسّى] om. B

(106) The least nourishing of all types of wine is that whose color is white and whose consistency is thin and that is similar to water. Such[235] a kind of wine is [similar to water that is] suitable and fit for preparing honey water from it, which is called "hydromel." *De alimentorum facultatibus* 3.[236]

(107) Among the names of [different] types of milk are the following: if milk is churned and its butter removed, the rest is called "buttermilk." It is also called *dūgh.*[237] If buttermilk is boiled until it becomes thick and some salt is added to it, it is called *kashk.*[238] If it is then placed in the sun until it becomes dry and more sour, it is called *maṣl* [whey]. If the milk congeals completely either by rennet or by leaving it [standing] for days until it becomes thick, it is called *rāʾib*[239] [thick, coagulated]. It is also called *al-māst.*[240] If it is left [standing] for a long time until its sourness increases, it is called *al-ḥāzir.*[241] If [the milk called] *al-māst* is boiled until it is [completely] thick and dry, it is called *aqiṭ.*[242] From the *Ikhtiyārāt al-Ḥāwī,* by Ibn al-Tilmīḏ.[243]

(١٠٦) أقلّ أنواع الشراب كلّها غذاء ما كان لونه أبيض وقوامه رقيق وكان شبيها بالماء. وما كان من الشراب كذلك فهو <شبيه بماء> موافق صالح لأن يتّخذ منه ماء العسل المسمّى ادرومالي. ثالثة الأغذية.

(١٠٧) في أسماء أصناف اللبن اللبن إذا مخض وأزيل عنه زبده سمّي ما يبقى المخيض ويسمّى الدوغ. وإذا غلي الدوغ حتّى يغلظ وأضيف إليه ملح سمّي الكشك. وإن شمّس بعد ذلك حتّى يجفّ ويشتدّ حمضه سمّي المصل. وإذا جمد الحليب بجملته إمّا بإنفحة أو بتركه أيّاما حتّى يختر سمّي رائبا ويسمّى الماست. وإن طال لبثه حتّى تشتدّ حموضته سمّي الحازر. وإذا غلي الماست حتّى يغلظ وجفّف سمّي الأقط. من اختيارات الحاوي لابن التلميذ.

---

٢ لأن] لكلّ من LO لمن U لكلّ ما E لما B || ٣ ادرومالي] اضرومال L ابرومالي B ادروماليا E || ٥ ملح] من غير أن يوضع في الشمس add. B || ٧ الماست] وبالعربية سمّي ارائب اللبن إذا خثر add. B || ٨ اختيارات] اختيرة B || ٩ التلميذ] אמר המעתיק: מכל תשעה השמות האילו אשר זכר בפרק זה שהם יוצאים ונעשים מן החלב איני מוצא מהם בלשון העברי כי אם שנים בלבד והם החלב ומיץ החלב כי שם חמאה אינה בכלל אילו התשעה כי החלב הנקפא והחלב החמוץ הם שמות נגזרים הנקפא מההקפאה והחמוץ מהחימוץ על כן זכרתי כל אילו התשעה שמות בלשון ערבי והם החלב שהוא הסוג העליון ותחתיו השבעה מינים מהחלב שכל אחד ממנו אינו דומה לחברו ואם תרצה לקראם אישים ויהיה החלב שם המין תוכל לומר בו זה והתשעה שמות אשר בכללם שבעה מיני חלב אשר לא ידעתי להם שם עברי כי אם מיץ חלב הם תחלה תחלה זכר מכיץ והוא אשר יוסר ממנו החמאה והנשאר הוא מכיץ וקורין אותו דוג כמו כן והשלישי שזכר נקרא כשך והרביעי נקרא מצל והחמישי ראיב ונקרא כמו כן מאסית והששי נקרא חאריז והשביעי נקרא אלאקט add. Z

(108) If[244] the watery part of milk is boiled and the fatty parts that separate from it through the boiling are taken from it, it is called *al-lawr*.[245] Colostrum is that which is produced [by the mother's breasts] at the time of the delivery and for some days afterwards as long as it is thick. If salt is added to butter and boiled until the watery part vanishes, it is called "clarified butter." From the *Ikhtiyārāt al-Ḥāwī*.

(109) Ancient [physicians] call the alteration of a substance to another type of a different variety "putrefaction." Examples are the alteration of wine if it changes and turns into vinegar, or the corruption that develops in some [types of] wood until it crumbles and turns, as it were, into dust and ashes. However, modern physicians and people in general apply the name "putrefaction" to an alteration that destroys a substance completely and that is accompanied by a stench. This develops especially in substances that tend strongly towards fluidity and moisture. *In Timaeum commentarius* 2.[246]

*This is the end of the twenty-third treatise, by the grace of God, praise be to Him.*

(١٠٨) ماء الجبن إذا غلي والتقطت منه تلك الأجزاء الدسمة المنفصلة عنه بالغليان فإنّها تسمّى اللور. وأمّا اللبأ فهو ما احتلب عند الولادة وبعدها بأيّام طال ما هو خاثر. والزبد إذا ألقي فيه ملح وغلي حتّى تذهب مائيته سمّي السمن. من اختيارات الحاوي.

(١٠٩) القدماء يسمّون تغيّر الجوهر إلى نوع آخر غير نوعه عفونة كتغيّر الخمرة إذا استحالت فصارت خلّا. ومثل الفساد الذي يحدث لبعض الخشب حتّى يتفتّت ويصير كأنّه غبار ورماد. لكن الحدث من الأطبّاء وعامّة الناس إنّما يوقعون اسم العفونة على التغيّر المفسد للجوهر بأسره ومعه نتن. وهذه إنّما يحدث في الجواهر التي هي أميل إلى النداوة والرطوبة. في الثانية من شرحه لكتاب طيماوس.

تمّت المقالة ولله الحمد والمّنة.

---

٢ اللور] اللوز SG الزبدة L اللوغ L[1] الليد B || ٩ تمّت المقالة ولله الحمد والمّنة] ولله الحمد والمّنة G تمّت المقالة الثالثة والعشقون ولله الحمد والتوفيق والمنّة S تمّت المقالة الثالثة والعشرون الحمد لله وعدد فصولها مائة وثلاثة عشر فصلا L تمّت المقالة الثالثة والعشقون وعدد فصولها مائة وثلاثة عشر والحمد لله E كملت المقالة B تمّت المقالة الثالثة والعشقون والحمد لله على حسن عونه وعدد فصولها مائة وثلاثة عشر فصلا O تمّت المقالة الخامسة عشر U

*In the name of God,*
*the Merciful, the Compassionate.*
*O Lord, make [our task] easy.*

# The Twenty-Fourth Treatise

*Containing curiosities that figure in the medical books and unusual, rare occurrences*

(1) In the book *On Women's Diseases* composed by Hippocrates, translated by Ḥunayn, and commented[1] upon by Galen, I found an addition that is not part of Ḥunayn's translation nor of Galen's commentary. In that additional commentary there are strange things, among them that he says: Porphyry[2] has related that there was a great eclipse of the sun in Sicily [and that] in that year women gave birth to abnormally shaped babies that had two heads, and that some women menstruated from their mouth through vomiting.[3]

(2) In that additional commentary it is also [stated] that the uterus sends the menstrual blood through small vessels to the buttocks and that the vessels there open and that this [blood flow] is instead of menstruation.

بسم الله الرحمن الرحيم

ربّ يسّر

# المقالة الرابعة والعشرون

## تشتمل على نوادر جرت وحكيت في كتب الطبّ وعلى أمور شاذّة قليلة الوقوع

(١) كتاب أوجاع النساء لبقراط أخرجه حنين وشرحه جالينوس ووجدت زيادة في هذا الكتاب أخرجها غير حنين وشرحها غير جالينوس. ووجد في شرح تلك الزيادة أمور غريبة منها أنّه قال: حكى فرفوريوس أنّه كان للشمس كسوف عظيم في صقلية يعرض في تلك السنة أنّ النساء ولدن أولادا مشوّهي الصور لهم رأسان. وأنّ بعض النساء عرض لهنّ أن يطمثن من أفمامهنّ بالقيء.

(٢) وفي تلك الزيادة أيضا أنّ الرحم قد تبعث دم الطمث في عروق دقيقة إلى المقعدة فتنفتح العروق هناك ويكون ذلك بدل الطمث.

---

١ بسم الله الرحمن الرحيم ربّ يسّر] om. ELBU بسم الله الرحمن الرحيم O || ٣ الرابعة والعشرون] الخامسة عشر OU || ٤ على] فصول تتضمن add. ELO || ٦ لبقراط] لابقراط ELBOU || ٧ ووجد] ووجدت S ووجد في شرح تلك الزيادة أمور غريبة] om. B || ٨ فرفوريوس] فورفوريوس BO || ١٠ أفمامهنّ] أفواههنّ ESL

(3) A stone at this site grows no less than a plant. When something grows, it necessarily feeds itself. This is the wording of Galen['s statement] at the end of his treatise *De nominibus medicis*.[4]

(4) [Galen] promised a patient that a crisis would befall him, yet it did not befall him. He examined him and found the house [in which the patient was] to be cold. He heated the air [of the house] with fire, the patient began to sweat, and the crisis befell him. *De [optimo] medico cognoscendo*.[5]

(5) A young man [once] suffered from a wound in his breastbone. Then pus developed there, he was operated upon, but [subsequently] the bone there got corrupted [again]. [The corrupted bone] was removed, and his heart became visible and exposed beneath it. He became completely healed since the chest [itself] had not been perforated. *De anatomicis administrationibus* 7.[6]

(6) I [once] saw an astonishing thing, namely, that a young man suffered from a perforation in one of the two anterior ventricles of his brain, but God saved him and he escaped unharmed. If both anterior ventricles of his brain had been perforated at the same time, he would not have lived even for an instant. *De usu partium* 8.[7]

(7) The reason that I drew blood from [one of] the pulsatile veins was that I was twice told in my dream to bleed the pulsatile vein between the index finger and thumb of the right hand. I let the blood flow until it stopped by itself because I was told so in my dream. [The quantity] that flowed was less than a *raṭl*,[8] and immediately the pain that I had felt for a long time in the spot where the liver is connected to the diaphragm was alleviated. I was a young man when this pain occurred. *De venae sectione*.[9]

(8) As for the bodies that come out with the urine resembling bundles of hair, sometimes one of these is longer than a span of the hand. They originate from a thick, viscous humor that is heated and dries up in the vessels in the manner of the Guinea worms[10] [*Dracunculus medinensis*] that are formed in the thighs in certain places of Tihāma,[11] as they say. The substance of these worms resembles the sort of substance that a nerve has, and their [external] form is similar to that of intestinal worms in color. *De locis affectis* 6.[12]

(٣) إنّ الحجارة في هذا الموضع تنمو نماء ليس بدون النبات ومتى كان الشيء ينمو فهو لا محالة يغتذي. هذا نصّ جالينوس في آخر مقالته في الأسماء الطبّية.

(٤) وعد مريضا أن يجيء بحران فلم يجئه فافتقده فوجد البيت باردا فأسخن الهواء بالنار فعرق المريض وجاءه البحران. في مقالته في امتحان الطبيب.

(٥) غلام أصابته جراحة بقصّه ثمّ حصلت هناك مدّة وبطّ وفسد هناك عظم فقلع وظهر قلبه من تحت ذلك العظم وانكشف ثمّ برأ بروء تامّا إذ ولم ينثقب الصدر. في سابعة التشريح الكبير.

(٦) رأيت أمرا عجيبا وهو أنّ فتى انثقب أحد بطني دماغه فنجّاه اللّه وسلم. ولو كانا بطنا دماغه المقدّمان كلاهما انثقبا في وقت واحد لما عاش طرفة عين. في ثامنة منافع الأعضاء.

(٧) السبب الذي دعاني لفصد العروق الضوارب هو أنّي أمرت في منامي مرّتين بفصد العرق الضارب الذي بين السبّابة والإبهام من اليد اليمنى. وتركت الدم يجري إلى أن انقطع من تلقاء نفسه لأنّي بذلك أمرت في منامي. فكان ما جرى أقلّ من رطل فسكن عني على المكان وجع كنت أجده قديما في الموضع التي تتّصل فيه الكبد بالحجاب. وكنت في وقت ما عرض لي هذا الوجع غلاما. في مقالته في الفصد.

(٨) وأمّا ما يخرج في البول من الأجسام الشبيهة بطاقات الشعر ففي بعض الأوقات تطول الواحدة منها أكثر من شبر. وتحدث من خلط غليظ لزج يسخن ويجفّ في العروق على النحو الذي به يتولّد في الساقين في بعض بلاد التهامة على ما يقولون العروق المدنية التي جوهرها من جنس جوهر العصب وخلقتها شبيهة بخلقة الحيات التي تتولّد في البطن في ألوانها. في سادسة التعرّف.

---

١ نماء] نموء L || ٣ أن] بأن ELBOU || ١٠ أمرت] رأيت B || ١٢ بذلك] كذلك ELBOU || ١٧ يتولّد] تتمّ ELO

(9) There are other types of cleansing that are different from these and that are almost unknown, [as they occur only] exceptionally. An example is what I have seen, [namely], how an abscess in the lung was evacuated through the urine and an abscess in the chest through the stools. *Ibidem.*[13]

(10) A man once carried a pork liver with him from one village to another. When he had to relieve himself, he placed the liver on [some] herbs until he came back [to take it with him again]. When he came back he found that blood serum of the liver had dripped on the herbs. He then took from those herbs and gave it to [some] people to ingest. Whosoever took it did not stop suffering from bloody diarrhea until he died. With [these herbs] he killed many people. Then the ruler [of that country] had him captured and severely tortured until he told him who had informed him about [the effect of] that herb and from whom he had this information. He told him that he had not heard this from anyone and that he had not passed this information on to someone else, but told the story of what happened to him with the pork liver. He told him that it is a very common herb that grows anywhere. Then the ruler ordered to blindfold his eyes so that he would not be able to point that herb out [to someone else] so that this person would know about it. [Subsequently] he had him executed. *De purgantium medicamentorum* [*facultate*].[14]

(11) If abscesses are cut open, one finds different types [of things] in it. Sometimes one finds things similar to mud, urine, [clots[15] of] blood, a[16] honeylike mucous nasal discharge, stones, nails, and flesh. And sometimes one finds living creatures in it, similar to the living[17] creatures that originate from putrefaction. *De tumoribus* [*praeter naturam*].[18]

(12) Sometimes a superfluity descends from the head to the lungs and from the lungs to the testicles because of the natural connection between the organs in the chest and the reproductive organs. *In Hippocratis Epidemiarum librum* 1 *commentarius* 1.[19]

(13) He said in the fourth book of his *Commentary to Epidemics* 2: If blood flows outside the vessels beneath the skin, that site takes on the color of eggplant [*Solanum melongena*].[20]

(٩) وهاهنا ضروب آخر من النقاء خارجة عن هذه لا تكاد تعرف إلا في الندرة بمنزلة ما رأينا خراجا كان في الرئة فاستنقي بالبول وخراجا كان في الصدر تنقى بالغائط. في تلك المقالة.

(١٠) الرجل الذي كان يحمل كبد خنزير من قرية إلى قرية فاحتاج أن يغوط فوضعها على حشيش حتّى يرجع فرجع فوجد الكبد قد سال صديدها على الحشيش. فصار ذلك الرجل يأخذ من تلك الحشيشة ويسقي الناس فكلّ من شربها فلا يزال يسهل دما حتّى يموت. فقتل بها خلقا كثيرا فأخده السلطان وعذّبه عذابا شديدا حتّى يخبر من علّمه هذه الحشيشة ومن تعلّمها منه. فأخبر بأن لم يتعلّمها من أحد ولا علّمها لغيره بل حكى ما جرى له في كبد الخنزير وأخبر أنّها حشيشة كثيرة الوجود تنبت في كلّ مكان. فحينئذ أمر السلطان بتعصيب عينيه حتّى لا يشير إلى تلك الحشيشة فتعلّم وأخرجه للقتل. في مقالته في الأدوية المنقّية.

(١١) الخراجات إذا بطّت رئي فيها أنواع مختلفة. وقد توجد فيها أشياء شبيهة بالحمأة والبول والغبيط والعسل والمخاط والحجارة والأظفار واللحم. وقد يوجد فيها أيضا حيوان شبيه بالحيوان المتولّد عن العفونة. في مقالته في الأورام.

(١٢) قد ينحدر من الرأس فضل إلى الرئة وينحدر من الرئة إلى الأنثيين بسبب المشاركة الطبيعية التي بين آلات الصدر وأعضاء التوليد. في الأولى من شرحه للأولى من أبيديميا.

(١٣) قال في المقالة الرابعة من شرحه لثانية أبيديميا: انصباب الدم من خارج العروق تحت الجلد يصير منه لون الموضع لون الباذنجان.

---

٢ في تلك المقالة] سادسة التعرّف BU || ٥ حتّى يرجع فرجع فوجد] ثمّ يرجع ووجد ELB حتّى يرجع فرجع فوجد الكبد قد سال صديدها على الحشيش om. OU || ٧ يخبر] يخبره B || ٨ أحد] ولا أحد منه L | لغيره] لأحد B || ١٦ أبيديميا] أفيديميا ELO || ١٧ أبيديميا] أفيديميا ELO

(14) Ibn[21] Riḍwān drew the attention to this [statement] and said: This proves that the eggplant was known to Galen, but he only mentioned it in this place.

(15) Says Moses: It is my most firm [opinion] that Galen did not know [the eggplant] and that is why he did not mention it. Perhaps he described [a similar plant] whose color was between black and red and the translator identified it with the eggplant.[22]

(16) Only in a few cases do those suffering from tremor or dropsy or similar ailments benefit from bleeding; in most cases it is harmful to them. It is especially beneficial for someone whose illness started from a congestion of blood streaming from the openings of the vessels in the buttocks and [for a woman whose illness started] from a congestion of menstrual blood and for someone in whose body such a large quantity of blood has accumulated for whatever reason that there is no guarantee against the extinction of the innate heat. *In Hippocratis Epidemiarum librum* 2 *commentarius* 4.[23]

(17) There are bodies that are extremely emaciated and [yet] have much blood, and there are other bodies that are obese and fat and [yet] have little blood. Galen reports [the case] of a woman whose menstruation was retained for eight months and who was extremely emaciated. When he saw that the blood was flowing copiously in her vessels but that it had a livid color, he bled her and extracted on the first day a quantity of one and a half *raṭl* of dark blood resembling liquid tar. On the second day he extracted one *raṭl* and on the third day eight ounces.[24] And he said that she was cured and her body returned to its [normal] condition in a short time. *In Hippocratis Epidemiarum librum* 6 *commentarius* 3.[25]

(18) Examine a male at the time he reaches puberty. If his right testicle is larger [than the left], he will beget male offspring, but if the left testicle is larger [than the right one], he will beget female offspring. The same applies to the breasts of a girl at the time of her puberty. *In Hippocratis Epidemiarum librum* 6 *commentarius* 4.[26]

(١٤) ابن رضوان نبّه على هذا الموضع وقال: هذا يدلّ أنّ الباذنجان كان معروفا عند جالينوس وما ذكره في غير هذا الموضع.

(١٥) قال موسى: الأقوى عندي أنّ جالينوس لم يره ولذلك لم يذكره ولعلّ وصف لونا ما بين السواد والحمرة فقال المترجم عنه باذنجان.

(١٦) قد ينتفع بالفصد في الندرة أصحاب الرعشة وأصحاب الاستسقاء ومن يجري مجراهم وإن كان الفصد يضرّهم في أكثر الحالات. وإنّما ينفع خاصّة من ابتدأت به العلّة من احتقان دم يجري من أفواه العروق التي في المقعدة واحتقان الطمث ومن اجتمع في بدنه دم كثير بسبب من الأسباب وبلغ من كثرته أنّه لا يؤمن معه انطفاء الحرارة الغريزية. في الرابعة من شرحه لثانية أبيديميا.

(١٧) قد تكون أبدان في الغاية القصوى من الهزال وفيها دم كثير وأبدان آخر ضخمة سمينة والدم فيها قليل. وحكى جالينوس أنّ امرأة انعاق طمثها ثمانية أشهر وكانت في غاية الهزال ورأى عروقها دارّة وفيها كمودة ففصدها وأخرج لها في اليوم الأوّل رطل ونصف دما أسود بمنزلة الزفت السائل. وأخرج لها في اليوم الثاني رطل وفي اليوم الثالث ثمانية أواق قال فبرأت وعاد بدنها لحاله في مدّة يسيرة. في الثالثة من شرحه لسادسة أبيديميا.

(١٨) تفقد الذكر عند بلوغه فإن تزيّدت اليمنى من الأنثيين فهو يلد ذكرا وإن تزيّدت اليسرى فهو يلد إناثا. وهكذا الحال في ثديي المرأة عند البلوغ. في الرابعة من شرحه لسادسة أبيديميا.

---

٣ ولعلّ وصف] ولعلّه ELO | وصف لونا ما بين] ما وصف لونين B || ٩ أبيديميا] أفيديميا ELO || ١٤ أبيديميا] أفيديميا ELO || ١٥ ذكرا] ذكورا ELBOU || ١٦ المرأة] الجارية ELOU || ١٧ أبيديميا] أفيديميا ELO

(19) Itches, cough, hiccups, sneezing, and the like sometimes subside when a person endures and tolerates them, especially if they are few and weak. *In Hippocratis De humoribus commentarius* 1.[27]

(20) If someone sees someone else suffering from ophthalmia and he is not used to seeing such a thing, his eyes will initially fill with moisture, and if he looks for a long time, he will also suffer from ophthalmia.[28] Similarly, sometimes a person sees someone else urinating or defecating or yawning or stretching oneself and this prompts him to do exactly the same thing. *De motibus dubiis.*[29]

(21) Some people often fall asleep while sitting and walk while asleep. I used to hear this but did not believe it until I was obliged to walk while asleep [throughout[30] the whole night. I learned the truth by experience and had to believe it. I walked] nearly a sixth of a mile and, absorbed in a dream, did not wake up until I stumbled upon a stone. *De motu musculorum* 2.[31]

(22) A man [once] was delirious for thirteen days and thought that he was in the city of Athens while [in reality] he was in the city of Rome. He thought that he had just arrived from a [long] journey and wanted to go to the bathhouse to be treated. He knew [very well] all he had said and done except for the illusion of his arrival from a journey at Athens. After thirteen days had passed, a severe nosebleed overtook him, and [then] a sweat suddenly broke out and he recovered. But after his recovery he did not remember anything of what had happened to him. *De motu musculorum* 2.[32]

(23) A servant [once] became angry and threw himself on the ground. He held his breath for a long time, and then he[33] convulsed and died. He (i.e., Galen) says: Someone stayed silent for a year or more than a year by his own free will. *De motu musculorum* 2.[34]

(١٩) الحكاك والسعال والفواق والعطاس وما أشبهها قد تسكن متى احتملها الإنسان وصبر عليها وبخاصّة إذا كانت يسيرة ضعيفة. في الأولى من شرحه للأخلاط.

(٢٠) من رأى من به رمد وهو غير معتاد لرؤية ذلك فإنّ عينيه أوّلا تمتلئان رطوبة فإن أطال النظر فإنّه يرمد هو أيضا. وكذلك ربّما رأى الإنسان آخر يبول أو يتغوّط أو يتثاءب أو يتمطّى فيدعوه ذلك إلى أن يفعل ذلك الفعل بعينه. في مقالته في الحركات المعتاصة.

(٢١) كثيرا ما ينام بعض الناس في حال جلوسه ويكون ماشيا فينام ويمشي. وكنت أسمع هذا ولا صدّقته حتّى اضطررت أن سرت نائما قريبا من سدس ميل وأنا أرى حلما ولم أنتبه حتّى عثرت بحجر. الثانية من كتاب حركات العضل.

(٢٢) إنّ رجلا ذهب عقله ثلثة عشر يوما وكان يظنّ أنّه في مدينة أثينيا وكان في مدينة رومية ويظنّ أنّه الآن قدم من سفر ويريد يدخل الحمّام تطبّبا. وليس كان ينكر من أحواله كلّها لا في الأقوال ولا في الأفعال شيئا إلا ما يتعلّق بخيال قدمه من سفر إلى أثينيا. ولّما كان بعد ثلثة عشر يوم عرض له رعاف شديد وعرق بغتة فبرأ وما كان يذكر بعد البروء شيئا ممّا كان يأتي به. في الثانية من حركات العضل.

(٢٣) عبد غضب وألقى جسمه على الأرض وحبس نفسه مليّا ثمّ تضرّب ومات. قال: وقد مكث إنسان صامتا سنة وأكثر من سنة بإرادته. في تلك المقالة.

---

٤ يتغوّط] يتبرّز Arabic translation MS Ayasofya 3631, fol. 104b || ٥ المعتاصة] قال موسى كان بمصر ملوك الحمدان وكان الريس ناصر الدولة وكان يشكو وجع القولنج فأعيا الأطبّاء ولم يوجد له دواء. ثمّ أنّ السلطان دسّ على قتله فأرصد رجل معه خنجر. فلما جاء في بعض دهاليز القصر وثب عليه الرجل وضربه فجاءت الضربة أسفل خاصره. فأصاب طرف الخنجر المعاء الذي كان فيه القولنج فخرج ما فيه من الخلط. ثمّ عافاه اللّه فصحّ وبرأ لأحسن ما كان add. G[1] || ١١ بخيال] بحال SGB | قدمه] قدومه ESLBOU

(24) A woman who was pregnant[35] for some months at first saw blood, then thin, fetid blood serum. With the passing of time she miscarried. After this, every day part of the placenta was extruded because it had putrefied internally. When the remains of the placenta stopped [coming out], the midwives and all the attending physicians except me thought that she was completely cleansed. When I felt her pulse, I realized from its beat that something remained in her uterus that should be expelled. I informed the woman and her husband about it and that she needed to expel that which remained in the womb. On the sixteenth day after her miscarriage, [another] putrid fetus was aborted. *De [optico] medico cognoscendo.*[36]

(25) A woman suffered from an illness that was so harmful for her stomach that she lost her appetite and was close to death because of her extreme weakness and little intake of food. [Physicians] famous for their medical practice treated her but without success. I told them to prepare absinthe wine for her. Immediately after she had imbibed it, her stomach strengthened and she wanted to eat immediately. *De theriaca ad Pisonem.*[37]

(26) A boy suffered from an abscess that was ready to be incised, but[38] he was very fearful of an incision. [His father] took some theriac, made a salve from it, and put it on the [abscess]. It perforated the skin more rapidly than surgery and extracted the pus it contained. *De theriaca ad Pisonem.*[39]

(٢٤) امرأة حامل في بعض أشهر حملها رأت دما أوّلا ثمّ صديدا رقيقا منتنا. فلمّا تمادى بها الزمان أسقطت ثمّ من بعد ذلك يخرج من المشيمة في كلّ يوم شيء لأنّ المشيمة عفنت داخلا. فلمّا تقطّع بقايا المشيمة ظنّ القوابل وجميع من حضر من الأطبّاء غيري أنّ المرأة قد نقيت النقاء التامّ. فجسست أنا نبضها فتبيّن لي من نبضها أنّ في الرحم شيئا باقيا ينبغي أن يخرج. وأعلمت المرأة وزوجها بذلك وأنّها تحتاج إلى نفض الشيء الذي بقي في الرحم. فلمّا كان في اليوم السادس عشر من اليوم الذي أسقطت فيه سقط منها طفل قد عفن. في مقالته في محنة الطبيب.

(٢٥) امرأة مرضت مرضا أضرّ معدتها حتّى بطلت شهوتها للطعام وأشرفت على الموت من شدّة ضعفها وقلّة رزءها من الطعام. وطبّها مشاهير في أعمال الطبّ ولم ينجحوا فأمرتهم أن يتّخذوا لها شراب الأفسنتين فحين شربته قويت معدتها واشتهت الطعام من ساعتها. في مقالته في الدرياق إلى قيصر.

(٢٦) صبي أصابه ورم وصلح لأن يبطّ واستهال بطّه وأخذ من الدرياق وجعله بمنزلة المرهم ووضعه عليه فثقب الجلد أسرع من ثقب الحديد وأخرج ما كان هناك من المدّة. في تلك المقالة.

١ في بعض أشهر حملها] في الشهر الرابع من حملها *De optico medico cognoscendo*, ed. Iskandar, p. 130, line 13 || ٥ وزوجها] زوجها G || ٨ معدتها . . . (٤٧) ويحيي الشخص من ساعته] om. O || ٩ من الطعام] للطعام ELU | مشاهير] مشهور B | ينجحوا] تنجو B || ١١ الدرياق] الترياق ELBU || ١٢ الدرياق] الترياق ELBU

(26a) It is related that the queen of Egypt killed herself by letting a viper free on her breast.[40] [The viper bit her] and she died immediately. The reason she did so was because another king had defeated her and usurped the land that was in her possession. Says Galen: I saw with my own eyes in Alexandria how fast this viper kills [someone]. For when the judge in that city sentences a prominent person to death, they bring this viper and let her bite him in the chest and he dies immediately. *De theriaca ad Pisonem.*[41]

(26b) I was informed about an ancient [physician] that he wished to have a fair son born to him and that he painted a portrait on the wall of a boy as handsome as possible. When he had sexual intercourse with his wife, he ordered her to look at that portrait constantly and not to look away from it even for a short moment. She got a son who was as beautiful as that portrait but did not resemble his father. *Ibidem.*[42]

If vipers eat bread, the bread obstructs the passages of the teeth so that they bite without causing any damage. Someone who sees this is amazed, not knowing the wickedness and cunning of their hunters. *Ibidem.*[43]

(27) Once a plague erupted from the borders of Ethiopia to Greece. Hippocrates acted skillfully [against the plague] and saved the inhabitants of his city by instructing them to ignite a fire around the city and [to put onto it] large quantities of wood and other things, namely, blossoms and leaves of plants and fragrant trees. He also told them to put on the firebrand many spices and odiferous oils. When they did so, they were saved from the death they were so close to. *Ibidem.*[44]

(٢٦a) ذكر ملكة مصر التي قتلت نفسها بأن أرسلت على ثديها أفعى فماتت لحينها لمّا غلب عليها ملك آخر وأخذ البلاد منها وهم بأخذها. قال جالينوس: وقد شاهدت بالإسكندرية هذه الأفعى وسرعة قتلها. وذلك أنّ القاضي هناك إذا حكم على إنسان شريف بالقتل يجيئون بهذه الأفعى ثمّ ينهشون بها في صدره فيموت من ساعته. في مقالته في الدرياق إلى قيصر.

(٢٦b) بلغني عن بعض القدماء أنّه أحبّ أن يولد له غلام جميل فصوّر في حائط صورة الغلام من أحسن ما يصوّر وعندما واقع زوجته أمرها أن تطيل النظر إلى تلك الصورة ولا تصرّف نظرها عنها لحظة فجاء ولدها بحسن تلك الصورة ولم يشبه الأب. في تلك المقالة.

الأفاعي إذا أكلت الخبز يسدّ الخبز مجاري أسنانها حتّى أنّها تنهش ولا تضرّ شيئا. ويتعجّب من يرى ذلك ولا يعلم خبث صيّاديها وحيلتهم. في تلك المقالة.

(٢٧) عرض وبأ من حدّ بلاد الحبشة إلى بلاد اليونان فتحيّل أبقراط وخلّص أهل مدينته بأن أمرهم أن يوقدوا حوالي المدينة النار ويكثروا من الحطب وأشياء آخر من زهر النبات وورقه ومن الأشجار الطيّبة الروائح. وأمرهم أن يلقوا على ذلك الجمر طيبا كثيرا وأدهانا طيّبة الروائح. ولمّا فعلوا ذلك خلّصوا من الهلاك الذي كانوا أشرفوا عليه. في مقالته تلك.

---

١ ذكر . . . قيصر om. EL | ثديها] يدها GU يديها B || ٣ وسرعة] وسرع B || ٤ مقالته في الدرياق إلى قيصر] تلك المقالة BU || ٦ بلغني . . . في تلك المقالة] om. EL[1] || ٩ يسدّ] يفسد ESGLU | أسنانها] أنيابها B || ١١ وخلّص] وتخلّص SG || ١٤ خلّصوا] خلّصهم SG | تلك] תמת אלמקאלה י״ה בעון מאלך אלדוניה אלחכים עלא אל ספלייה ואלעלאויה וחאכים עלא עלאוייה ואל ספלייה צחיב אל דוניה אל מצ׳ייא. שנת ה׳ר׳צ׳ה add. U, fol. 106b

(28) Who is not amazed over the work of nature and what it does in the case of the female bear? It gives birth to an animal that is similar to a piece of meat in which none of its parts nor the shape of an animal is recognizable. But when she has given birth to it, she does not stop to lick it with her tongue until all the parts of this animal become apparent. *Ibidem.*[45]

(29) If you excise the testicles[46] of a female animal, she does not have [sexual] desire and does not admit the male to copulate with her and she loses her femininity. Thus[47] female swine are castrated by our countrymen in Athens but also by other nations. Then their bodies become fat and corpulent and their flesh becomes sweeter than that which is eaten of [other] female swine. If someone wants to castrate a female [swine], he is forced to[48] cut [around] both the flanks. For this reason the castration of the female is much more risky [than that of males]. *De semine* 1.[49]

(30) A female secretes sperm without a man approaching her, and this occurs during nocturnal pollution, which happens to her while she is asleep just as it happens to men. It also occurs during the accumulation of sperm as I described in the case of that woman [who was] a widow. *De semine* 2.[50] The woman he referred to there is the same whose story he related in the last [book] of *De locis affectis*.[51]

(31) He says in *De alimentorum* [*facultatibus*]: In the past people used to live only on acorns because it nourishes the body similar to many seeds and grains from which bread is prepared.[52]

(32) I know a man who ate lots of mushrooms that had not been properly cooked. As a result, he felt pressure and heaviness in the cardia of his stomach, his respiration was difficult, he fainted, and his sweat was cold. He was barely saved and rescued from death by taking [remedies] that disperse thick juices such as oxymel with[53] a decoction of thinning roots. *De alimentorum* [*facultatibus*] 2.[54]

(٢٨) من لا يعجب من فعل الطبيعة وما تفعله في الحيوان من الدبّ الأنثى؟ فإنّها تلد حيوانا كالبضعة لا يتبيّن فيه شيء من أعضائه ولا صورة حيوان. وإذا ولدته لا تزال تلحسه بلسانها حتّى تتبيّن أعضاء ذلك الحيوان كلّها. في تلك المقالة.

(٢٩) إن أنت قطعت من حيوان أنثى بيضتيها لم تشتهي ولم تطاوع الذكر على النزو وتبطل منها القوة الأنوثية. فإنّ إناث الخنازير قد تخصى عندنا في بلاد أثينية وعند أمم آخر غيرنا وتخصب أبدانها وتسمن ويكون لحمها ألذّ ما أكل من لحوم إناث الخنازير. ومتى أراد الإنسان أن يخصي الإناث اضطرّه الأمر إلى أن يشقّ الخاصرتين كلتيهما وبهذا السبب صار إخصاء الإناث أعظم خطرا. في الأولى من كتاب المنّي.

(٣٠) الأنثى ترمي بالمني من غير أن يقربها رجل عند الجنابة يصيبها في النوم كما يعرض ذلك للرجال وعند ما يكثر اجتماعه على ما وصفنا من أمر تلك المرأة الأرمل. في الثانية من كتاب المني. وهذه المرأة التي أشار إليها هي التي ذكر قصّتها في آخر التعرّف.

(٣١) قال في الأغذية: إنّ في ما سلف من الدهر كان الناس يعيشون ببلّوط وحده لأنّه يغذو البدن مثل كثير من البزور والحبوب الذي يتّخذ منها الخبز.

(٣٢) أنا أعرف رجلا أكل وأكثر من الفطير وكان لم يحكم طبخه فأحسّ منه في فم معدته بضغط وثقل وضاق عليه نفسه وأصابه غشي وعرق عرقا باردا وأفلت وتخلّص من الموت بعد جهد بأن استعمل أشياء تقطع الأخلاط الغليظة بمنزلة السكنجبين بطبيخ أصول ملطّفة. ثانية الأغذية.

---

١ لا] MS P starts here || ٥ آخر] om. G || ١٠ اجتماعه] اجتماعها B || ١٢ قال... الخبز] om. G

(33) He says: I know a small child whose first wet nurse died and was then nursed by another who had bad humors. As a result, his body was covered all over with many ulcers. This second wet nurse used to feed herself in the springtime with vegetables of poor quality because of a famine that had befallen the inhabitants of her land. Her body, too, became completely covered with ulcers, similar to the ulcers that covered the small child. *De alimentorum* [*facultatibus*] 3.[55]

(34) The intestines have been provided with two tunics, and both are alike to[56] strengthen their expulsive faculty and to minimize the occurrence of injuries. I have frequently seen in many persons such putrefaction of a large part of the intestines that in some of them the inner tunic of their intestines was completely destroyed, and [yet] they were saved and lived. If there had not been a second tunic to the intestines, besides the one that had putrefied and been destroyed, they could not have lived. *De usu partium* 4.[57]

(35) I have seen something amazing and unusual, namely, that a boy was hit on the pupil with[58] the end of a sharp iron instrument. Watery moisture flowed from the opening and his pupil became smaller and the hornlike tunic contracted completely. When he had been treated, he saw well again because that moisture that had suddenly flowed reaccumulated slowly. This is something that occurs only rarely. *De* [*morborum*] *causis et symptomatibus* 4.[59]

(36) Someone who was stung by a scorpion recently said that he thought that he was pelted and hit by hailstones. His entire body was cold, and he broke out in a cold sweat. He was barely saved after he was treated with remedies that are used for scorpion stings. *De locis affectis* 3.[60]

(٣٣) قال: إنّي أعرف طفلا توفّيت المرضعة الأولى فأرضعته أخرى رديئة الأخلاط فامتلأ بدنه كلّه قروحا كثيرة وكانت هذه المرضعة الثانية تغتذي وقت الربيع بالبقول الدنيئة بسبب مجاعة كانت أصابت أهل بلدها. فامتلأ بدنها هي أيضا قروحا كمثل القروح التي امتلأ بها بدن الطفل. ثالثة الأغذية.

(٣٤) إنّما جعل للأمعاء صفاقان وكلاهما بالسواء لتزيد قوتها الدافعة و وتبعد عن قبول الآفات. وقد رأينا مرارا كثيرة قوما كثيرين ممّن قد عفن جزء عظيم من أمعائهم حتّى أنّ بعضهم ذهب الصفاق الداخل من صفاقي أمعائهم كلّه وأفلتوا وعاشوا. ولو لم يكن للمعاء صفاق آخر غير الذي عفن وفسد لم يمكن أن يعيشوا. رابعة المنافع.

(٣٥) لقد رأيت أمرا عجيبا ليس من العادة أن يكون مثله وذلك أنّ غلاما أصابته ضربة بطرفة حديدة حادّة أمام الحدقة فجرت الرطوبة المائية وسالت من الثقب وصغرت حدقته وتكمّشت الطبقة القرنية بأجمعها. فلمّا عولج أبصر جيّدا لأنّ تلك الرطوبة التي سالت دفعة اجتمعت أوّلا أوّلا. وهذا أمر قلّ ما يعرض. في رابعة العلل والأعراض.

(٣٦) إنسان لسعته قريبا عقرب وكان يصف أنّه يظنّ أنّه يضرب و يرمى بحجارة الجمد والبرد وكان بدنه كلّه باردا وكان يعرق عرقا باردا وأفلت بعد كدّ عند ما عولج بالأشياء التي يعالج بها من لسعته عقرب. ثالثة لتعرّف.

---

١٠ فجرت] فخرجت $GS^2$ || ١٢ وهذا أمر قلّ ما يعرض] ههذا كلّ ما عرض B || ١٣ يصف أنّه يظنّ] يصيّره L

(37) He says: There are illnesses that I have only rarely seen. For instance, that a person suffered from a sudden cough and expectorated a moisture resembling thin bile and that he continued to expectorate this moisture, daily and constantly. Later on he expectorated sputum and after some months some blood. Then his body wasted away and his strength waned and he died. *De locis affectis* 4.[61]

I have seen someone cough and expectorate pieces of putrefied lung. I have also seen someone who had been coughing for a long time expectorate small pieces of matter. Then he expectorated something resembling small hailstones and continued to expectorate them until[62] his life span was completed. *Ibidem*.[63]

(38) One day a person famous for his medical practice met with me. I felt his pulse[64] and noticed therein all kinds of irregularities but without fever and without feeling anything at all during respiration. I told him that in my opinion this irregularity arose from a pressure and stenosis of the pulsatile vessels in his lungs [and that this was caused] either through an obstruction of thick, sticky humors or through the development of an abscess that was not ripe. He said to me: Then I should be suffering from an asthmatic orthopnea. I then said to him that orthopnea arises from the accumulation of a thick, viscous humor in the subdivisions of the trachea (i.e., bronchial tubes) but not from their accumulation in the pulsatile vessels. *Ibidem*.[65]

(39) Polyuria, also [called] "diabetes" or "severe thirst," is an illness that is only rarely found and that I until now have observed only twice. These are Galen's very words.[66]

(٣٧) قال: هاهنا علل رأيتها في الندرة وهو أنّ إنسانا سعل بغتة وقذف خلطا شبيها بالمرّة الرقيقة ولم يزل في كلّ يوم يقذف من ذلك الخلط دائما وفي آخر الأمر قذف قيحا وبعد أشهر قذف دما يسيرا وجعل بدنه بعد ذلك يذوب ثم ضعفت قوته ومات. رابعة التعرّف.

رأيت إنسانا يسعل أجزاء من الرئة قد عفنت. ورأيت أيضا إنسانا يسعل دهرا طويلا ويقذف شيئا يسيرا ثمّ أنّه قذف شيئا شبيها بحجر برد صغير ولم ينقطع عنه ما كان يرميه من حجارة البرد حتّى انقضت مدّة عمره. في تلك المقالة.

(٣٨) لقيني في بعض الأوقات رجل مشهور بأعمال الطبّ فجسست عرقه فوجدت فيه كلّ نوع من أنواع الاختلاف من غير حمّى ولا يحسّ في نفسه شيئا أصلا. فقلت له إنيّ أرى أنّ هذا الاختلاف يكون من ضغط وضيق يكون في العروق الضوارب التي في الرئة إمّا بسبب سدّة من أخلاط غليظة لزجة أو من تولّد خراج لم ينضج. فقال لي: وقد كان يجب أن يكون في التنفّس الانتصاب الربوي. فقلت له إنّ الانتصاب يكون عند اجتماع الخلط الغليظ اللزج في أقسام قصبة الرئة لا عند اجتماعه في العروق الضوارب. في تلك المقالة.

(٣٩) استطلاق البول وهو ديابيطس والعطش المبرّح هي علّة قلّ ما توجد إلا في الندرة فإنّي أنا إلى هذا الوقت لم أرها إلا مرّتين فقط. هذا نصّ كلام جالينوس.

---

١ سعل] أخذه سعال B || ٨ نفسه] تنفّس ELBP || ١٣ إلا] ولا B || ١٤ هذا نصّ كلام جالينوس] om. L

(40) Says[67] Moses: This illness has never passed by me in the Maghreb,[68] nor did any one of my elders tell me about it. But here in the land of Egypt, in a period of twenty[69] years I have seen about twenty men and[70] three women suffering from this illness. This prompts me to say: This illness only rarely occurs in cold countries but often in hot ones because it is caused by excessive heat prevailing over the kidneys, as can be deduced from what Galen says in *De locis affectis* 6.[71]

(41) I have seen several times that the movement of the pulsatile vessels subsided and abated, and then the patient recovered, regained his strength, lived, and was saved, especially a patient who was of the age of the elderly. *De pulsu* 14.[72]

(42) I once saw a man on one of my travels who had a vessel filled with honey and who stood before two men who were physicians in a shop and offered it to them for sale. He allowed them to lick some of the honey to try how good it was. They did so and started to bargain with him. He then said to them that he would not sell it to them for the price [they offered] and left them. Both men died shortly after his departure from them. For this reason and similar ones, no one should rely on whomever one happens to meet. *De [simplicium] medicamentorum [temperamentis ac facultatibus]* 10.[73]

(43) Pork resembles human meat. I have seen many innkeepers who are visited by travelers who sell human meat, once it had been cooked together[74] with some pork. Some honest persons told me that they had been eating in some inns what they were sure was pork until they found human fingers in their food. When the ruler was informed that they slaughter human beings and cook their meat, he had them executed. *De [simplicium] medicamentorum [temperamentis ac facultatibus]* 10.[75]

(٤٠) قال موسى: لم تمرّ بي قطّ هذه العلّة في بلاد الغرب ولا أخبرني عنها شيخ من شيوخي أمّا هنا في مدينة مصر فإنّي رأيت من أصحاب هذه العلّة في مدّة عشرين سنة نحو العشرين رجلا وثلاث نسوة. وهذا يدعوني إلى أن أقول إنّ هذه العلّة قلّ أن تحدث في البلاد الباردة وتكثر في البلاد الحارّة لأنّ سببها حرارة مفرطة تستولي على الكلى كما تبيّن من كلام جالينوس في سادسة التعرّف.

(٤١) قد رأيت مرارا شتّى حركة العروق الضوارب فترت وسكنت ثمّ عاد المريض وقوي وعاش ونجا ولا سيّما من كان من المرضى سنه سن الشيوخ. رابعة عشر النبض.

(٤٢) قد رأيت أنا رجلا مرّة في بعض تطوافي ومعه إناء فيه عسل وهو قائم بين يدي رجلين طبيبين في دكّان يعرضه عليهما للبيع. وأذن لهما أن يلعقا منه ليختبرا جودته ففعلا وأخذا في مماكسته وقال إنّه لا يبيع بهذه العطية وانصرف عنهما. ومات الرجلان بعد مفارقته لهما بمدّة يسيرة. فلهذا وأشباهه لا ينبغي لأحد أن يطمئنّ لكلّ من اتّفق. عاشرة الأدوية.

(٤٣) لحم الخنزير شبيه بلحوم الناس فقد رأينا كثيرا من أصحاب الخانات التي تمرّ بهم السابلة يبيعون لحوم الناس بعد أن يطبخونها في عدد لحوم الخنازير. وأخبرني عدّة من أهل الصدق أنّهم أكلوا في بعض الفنادق ما لم يشكّوا أنّه لحم خنزير حتّى وجدوا في الطعام إصبعا. ولمّا علم السلطان أنّهم يذبحون الناس ويطبخون لحومهم قتلهم. في تلك المقالة.

---

١ في بلاد الغرب] om. EL || ٢ شيوخي] في بلادنا add. EL | أمّا هنا في مدينة مصر] أمّا في مصر EL || ٣ أقول] أدّعي EL | إنّ هذه العلّة قلّ أن تحدث] قلّة حدوث هذه العلّة EL || ٤ وتكثر] وكثرة حدوثه EL | سببها] غلبة add. EL | تستولي] om. EL | كما تبيّن من كلام جالينوس في سادسة التعرّف] om. EL | تبيّن] يبدو BP || ٨ تطوافي] تطوفي EL || ١٤ في الطعام] om. EL في اللحم B

(44) Among all the medical works in our possession there is a treatise that bears the title "A[76] treatise by Galen on the prohibition of the burial [of the dead] within twenty-four hours," translated by al-Biṭrīq.[77] [The authorship of] this treatise is without doubt only for someone who is not familiar with the language of Galen. It seems to me that it refers to a man—a physician who was also a Greek and whose name was [also] Galen, but that he lived later than Galen the eminent physician—famous for his works. When this treatise fell into the hands of al-Biṭrīq, he translated it into Arabic and thought that it [was composed] by the famous Galen because he, I mean al-Biṭrīq, was of a much lower level than Ḥunayn in[78] his capacity of a translator.[79] But to put it briefly, since this treatise belongs to that which has been composed in the field of medicine, I thought it a good thing to mention some unusual aphorisms from it.

(45) He says in this treatise: A torpor may happen to a person that lasts for six or seven days, during which he does not use [the faculty of] reason and does not eat and does not drink, and his vessels are dry and his respiration is irregular. Then he mentions unusual methods of treating apoplexy patients.

(46) He further says in [this treatise]: Sometimes black bile increases in the heart and the blood thickens and so much wind is emitted into the vessels that life disappears. It can also happen that all the signs of life disappear from [such a patient], except for his complexion and the horripilation of the hair on his fingers. However, this indicates only that he is [still] alive, nothing else.

(47) He further says in [this treatise]: Sometimes an overfilling occurs that is such that the pulse ceases in the entire body and the heart does not move and the person [to whom this occurs] is as dead. But his large vessels are full and replete and of good appearance and warm to the touch. If you see this, whatever vessel you see replete, whether it is tortuous or not tortuous, hasten to make an incision lengthwise and let the blood flow out because then the pneuma will stream through the vessels and the person will be revived immediately.

(٤٤) من جملة كتب الطبّ الموجودة لدينا مقالة مكتوب عليها مقالة جالينوس في تحريم الدفن قبل أربعة وعشرين ساعة. إخراج البطريق. وهذه المقالة لا يشكل أمرها إلا على من لا أنسة له بكلام جالينوس. والذي يبدو إليّ أنّها لرجل طبيب مقصد أيضا يوناني كان اسمه جالينوس وكان بعد جالينوس الطبيب الفاضل المشهور كتبه. ولمّا وقعت هذه المقالة ليد البطريق أخرجها إلى اللسان العربي وظنّها لجالينوس المشهور لكونه أعني البطريق مقصرًا جدّا عن درجة حنين فيما أخرج. وبالجملة هي من جملة ما ألّف في الطبّ فلذلك رأيت أن أذكر فصولا مستغربة ممّا في تلك المقالة.

(٤٥) قال في تلك المقالة: يصيب الإنسان إغماء يمكث الستّة أيّام والسبعة لا يعقل ولا يأكل ولا يشرب وتكون عروقه يابسة ونفسه يتحرّك. ثمّ ذكر فيها أنواعا غريبة من طبّ المسكوتين.

(٤٦) وقال فيها: قد تكثر المرّة السوداء في القلب ويغلظ الدم ويبعث ريح في العروق حتّى تذهب الحياة. ويعرض أن يذهب منه دلائل الحياة كلّها إلا لونه وكون الشعر الذي على أصابعه يقشعرّ ويقوم وذلك يستدلّ على أنّه حيّ لا غير.

(٤٧) وقال فيها قد يحدث من الامتلاء أن يتعطّل النبض من البدن كلّه ولا يتحرّك القلب ويكون الشخص كالميّت. لكن عروقه الكبار تكون دارّة ممتلئة حسن السحنة سخن المجسّة. فإذا رأيت ذلك فأيّ عرق رأيته دارّا ملتويا كان أو غير ملتوي فبادر بشقّه شقّا طويلا واترك الدم يجري فإنّ الروح يجري في العروق ويحيى الشخص من ساعته.

٤ ليد] بيد G يبدو S || ٥ إلى اللسان العربي] للسان العربي EL للسان العرب BP || ٨ cf. MS Ayasofya 3724, fol. 143b | إغماء] om. B $L^1$ أنّه EL || ١١ cf. MS Ayasofya 3724, fol. 145b

(48) He further says in [this treatise]: It sometimes happens because of a fall from a high place or because of a very loud cry or because of a prolonged immersion in water that a person loses consciousness for forty-eight hours and becomes quasi-dead in that he assumes an ashy and dust-colored appearance and his nails become dust-colored [as well]. He then mentions indications of this person being still alive and gives information about how, in his opinion, one should treat him.

(49) He also says therein that if one buries a deceased person who died without fever and without a chronic illness within seventy-two hours following his death, one might kill him because it is possible that one buries him while he is still alive. He then gives indications of this person being still alive and gives information about the treatment of such a person.

(50) He also says therein: If someone has not eaten bread for a long time and then suddenly eats it, or if someone has not had intercourse for a [long] time and has intercourse, or if he stayed for a long time in a dark subterranean place and then suddenly emerges to the light of the sun, he may suffer from a condition similar to death and may really die. He then mentions the indications [of this person being still alive] and his therapy.

(51) He also says therein: Sometimes a condition similar to death occurs because of the consumption of poisons or stings or bites by vermin or by putting on a liniment of soporific ingredients. The same may occur because of immoderate consumption of moistening foods and drinks followed by a sleep on the left side in which he is completely immersed so that one thinks that he is dead. Then he mentions the indications [of this person being still alive] and his therapy.

(52) When Galen mentioned the ignorance of the physicians of his time and that he did not debate with them nor teach them anything when he met them at the [bedside of the] sick because they made themselves important and swelled over incorrect opinions, he expressed himself in the following words: Teaching[80] the followers of Moses and Christ is easier and faster than teaching these physicians and philosophers who are deluded by heretic tendencies. *De pulsu magno* 3.[81]

(53) Says Moses: It is known to you without any doubt that the Christian religion had appeared and had become well known and spread before Galen. However, it had not spread to Greece at the time of Galen.

(٤٨) وقال فيها: وقد يحدث من قبل سقطة من موضع عال أو من قبل صيحة شديدة أو طول غوص في الماء أن يغشى على الإنسان ثمانية وأربعين ساعة ويصير شبه الميّت تعلوه غبرة وخضرة وتخضرّ أظفاره. ثمّ ذكر هناك علامة كونه حيّ وعلاجه بزعمه.

(٤٩) وقال فيها من دفن ميّت مات من غير حمّى ولا علّة لازمة له من قبل اثنان وسبعون ساعة من بعد موته فقد قتله لأنّه يمكن أن دفنه حيّا. ثمّ أعطى هناك علامات كونه حيّا وعلاج الحيّ منهم.

(٥٠) وقال فيها: من فقد أكل الخبز زمانا طويلا ثمّ أكله دفعة أو فقد الجماع زمانا ثمّ جامع أو أقام في سرداب مظلم مدّة ثمّ خرج إلى ضوء الشمس دفعة فإنّه يعرض له حالة شبيهة بالموت وقد يموت حقيقة. ثمّ ذكر العلامات والعلاج.

(٥١) وقال فيها: قد يحدث من قبل تناول السموم أو لسع الهوامّ أو الطلاء بالأشياء المخدّرة حالة شبيهة بالموت. وكذلك من الإسراف في أكل الأغذية والأشربة المرطّبة والنوم بعقبها على اليسار فيستغرق ويظنّ به الموت. ثمّ ذكر هناك العلامات والعلاج.

(٥٢) لمّا ذكر جالينوس جهل أطبّاء عصره وكونه لا يجاوبهم ولا يعلّمهم شيئا عند اجتماعه بهم عند المرضى لكونهم قد كبروا وربوا على آراء غير صحيحة قال ما هذا نصّه: إنّ تعليم أدبة موسى والمسيح أهون وأسرع من تعليم هؤلاء الأطبّاء والفلاسفة المغترّين بالأهواء. ثالث النبض الكبير.

(٥٣) قال موسى: فقد تبيّن لك بيانا لا ريب فيه أنّ الملّة النصرانية كانت قد ظهرت واشتهرت وانتشرت قبل جالينوس لكنّها ما كانت عمّت بلاد اليونان في زمان جالينوس.

---

١ cf. MS Ayasofya 3724, fol. 146a || ٤ cf. MS Ayasofya 3724, fol. 146b || ١٤ إنّ] وذلك أنّ ELBOP || ١٥ أدبة (= أدباء) أدوية G || ١٨ واشتهرت] وشهرت P? ELBO

(54) He says: A deep wound that occurs in the lobes of the liver can be cured. Similarly, if one of the lobes of the liver is cut off. Sometimes we see that the neck of the bladder is healed from a cut made to extract a stone because the neck of the bladder is fleshy. But all these things happen only rarely. Some say that the wound occurring in the stomach can be cured. I have seen a man who suffered from a large deep wound in the brain and was cured, although such a thing happens only rarely. *In Hippocratis Aphorismos commentarius* 6.[82]

(55) In the first treatise of the book *On the Doctrines of Hippocrates and Plato*, Galen says: I once told someone who was with me during surgery to hold the heart with a smith's tongs since it jumped and slipped from his fingers when he tried to hold it. During this pressure on his heart, the animal did not lose any of its sensibility or voluntary movements, but screamed, moved,[83] and breathed. It was not lacking anything except for the movement of the pulsation of the vessels.

On another occasion, when I wanted to excise the[84] broken [fragments of a] bone of the cranium, I was forced to insert underneath that bone the instrument called "protector of the dura mater" as a precautionary measure. If we increase the contact and pressure on the brain with that instrument only a little bit, the [patient's] sensation and all voluntary movements are immediately abolished.[85]

(56) In the third treatise of *On the Doctrines of Hippocrates and Plato*, he says: With the Slavs[86] and non-Arabs[87] and barbarians anger is stronger than reason, but among us, the community of the Greeks, we find a similar matter only in the case of youngsters and those who have neither training nor education.[88]

(٥٤) قال: الجراحة الغائرة تقع في زوائد الكبد يمكن بروءها وكذلك إذا انبترت أحدى زوائد الكبد. وقد نرى رقبة المثانة تبرأ من القطع الذي يحدث فيها لاستخراج الحصى من قبل أنّ رقبة المثانة لحمية. وكلّ هذه الأمور إنّما تتّفق في الندرة. وقد قال قوم: إنّ الجراحة الواقعة بالمعدة يمكن بروءها. وقد رأيت رجلا أصابت دماغه جراحة عظيمة غائرة فبرأ إلا أنّ هذا من الأمور التي تحدث في الندرة. في شرحه لسادسة الفصول.

(٥٥) قال جالينوس في المقالة الأولى من كتابه في آراء أبقراط وأفلاطون: أمرت في بعض الأوقات إنسانا حضرني في وقت التشريح أن يضبط القلب بالكلبتين لأنّه كان يطفر و يفلت من الأصابع إذا مسك بها. ولم يفقد الحيوان في حال ضغط القلب شيئا من حسّه ولا حركاته الإرادية بل كان يصيح ويمشي و يتنفّس ولم يفقد شيئا إلا حركة نبض العروق.

و إضطرّنا الأمر مرّة عندما أردنا أن نخلّص العظام المكسورة من القحف أن ندخل تحت تلك العظام على جهة الاحتياط الآلة التي يقال لها حافظة غشاء الدماغ. إن نحن زدنا في غمزنا وضغطنا الدماغ بتلك الآلة فضل قليل فيعطّل حسّ الإنسان على المكان وبطلت جميع حركاته الإرادية.

(٥٦) وقال في المقالة الثالثة من آراء أبقراط وأفلاطون إنّ عند الصقالبة والأعجام والبربر الغضب أقوى من الفكر وعندنا نحن معشر اليونانين نجد الأمر كذلك في الصبيان وفي قوم لا دربة لهم ولا أدب.

---

١٠ مرّة] منه L || ١٤ الصقالبة] الصقلابة B | والأعجام] والأعاجم ELOP || ١٥ معشر] معاشر B

(57) At the end of the sixth treatise of *On the Doctrines of Hippocrates and Plato*, Galen states: People in their generation used to inflict punishment on that bodily part with which that crime was committed. They scarified and beat the legs of a runaway and did the same with the hands of a thief, and, similarly, they scarified and beat the belly and stomach of him in whom gluttony and gormandize became apparent. They did the same with the tongue of[89] prattlers. Therefore their poet (Homer) says: So-and-so[90] who had shown his passion to the wife of so-and-so and committed adultery with her, two kites[91] ate his liver, which is the source and origin of lust.[92]

(58) He states in the fourth treatise of his *Commentary on the book "Timaeus"*: I have seen [how] many people whose body was naturally strong but whose soul was weak hardly moved [or] did not carry out any activity [at all]. They were then afflicted by illnesses that were of the same type as sleeplessness, apoplexy, or paralysis, and illnesses like epilepsy. Women with a similar constitution were affected by hysterical suffocation, and after hysterical suffocation paralysis quickly [ensued]. But of people whose soul was naturally strong and the body weak, I have only seen a few. One of these was Aristides, who was from the people of Mysia. He was one of the best orators, and this happened to him because during his whole lifetime he[93] was so fond of conversation and talking that his body wasted away entirely. *In Timaeum commentarius* 2.[94]

(٥٧) قال جالينوس في آخر المقالة السادسة من آراء أبقراط وأفلاطون إنّ كان الناس في دهرهم يوقعون العقوبة وينزلونها من أعضاء البدن بالعضو الذي به فعل الإنسان ذلك الفعل الرديء. فالآبق يشرطون رجله ويضربونه عليها وكذلك يفعلون بيد السارق وكذلك من ظهر منه النهم والشره يشرطون معدته وبطنه ويضربونه عليها. وكذلك يفعلون بلسان من كثر هذيانه وفضوله في الكلام. ولذلك يقول شاعرهم إنّ فلانا الذي فضح عشيقته زوجة فلان ونال منها الفحشاء أكلت الحديان كبده التي فيه ينبوع الشهوة ومبدأها.

(٥٨) قال في المقالة الرابعة من شرحه لكتاب طيماوس: قد رأيت خلقا كثيرا البدن منهم قويا بالطبع والنفس ضعيفة قليلة الحركة عطلة فحدثت لهم أمراض من جنس السهر والسكتة والاسترخاء وأمراض من جنس الصرع. وعرض للنساء التي كذلك اختناق الرحم وعرض بعد اختناق الرحم الفالج بسرعة. وأمّا الذي أنفسهم قوية بالطبع وأبدانهم ضعيفة فلم أر منهم إلا اليسير. أحدهم أرسطيدس الذي من أهل موسيا. وهذا الرجل كان من أفضل الخطباء فعرض له بسبب أنّه كان مغرى دهره كلّه بالمفاوضة والكلام أن ذاب بدنه كلّه.

---

٣ فالآبق] فلايق G || ٤ يفعلون] كانوا يفعلون ELBOP || ٥ شاعرهم] شعراهم O || ٨ السهر] السهو B || ٩ وعرض] ويعرض ELBOP || ١٠ وعرض] ويعرض ELBOP || ١١ اليسير . . . قال إنّ (25.4)] om. O | أرسطيدس] أرسطيروس B || ١٢ بسبب] om. SG

(59)[95] In the third treatise of *De simplicium medicamentorum* [*temperamentis ac facultatibus*], in the translation by al-Biṭrīq, Galen says: If someone takes resin spurge[96] [*Euphorbia resinifera*] slowly and little by little, it does not harm him. We know this from an[97] old woman who lived in the land of Italy and who, as is related by all the ancients as well, used to take spurge[98] and it did not harm her at all. The reason for this was that the first time she only took a small dose thereof. And when she continued to take it in larger doses, it did not harm her at all. [For] when she continued to take it and got used to it, it became part of her nature.

(60) And in the ninth treatise of this book, in the translation by al-Biṭrīq, he says: There is nothing more suitable for the concoction of food by the stomach than to bring the body of another person nearby and to attach oneself to it. Some people approach young children [for this purpose] and put them on their abdomen during the night and derive great benefit therefrom because their heat is more suitable, better and more intense than the heat derived from a hot compress. There are other people who put a puppy on their abdomen if they want to sleep and find great relaxation in this.[99]

*This is the end of the twenty-fourth treatise, by the grace of God, praise be to Him.*

(٥٩) قال جالينوس في المقالة الثالثة من الأدوية المفردة إخراج البطريق إنّ الفربيون إن تناول الإنسان منه يسيرا يسيرا وقليلا قليلا لم يضرّه. وعلمنا ذلك من قبل عجوز كانت في بلاد اطيلية وذكرها أيضا الأوّلون كلّهم وأنّها كانت تأخذ الفربيون فلم يكن يضرّها شيئا. وذلك أنّها تناولت منه في أوّل ما أخذت منه قليلا. ولمّا داومت ذلك ازدادت وأكثرت منه فلم يضرّها شيئا. ولمّا داومت أكله واعتادت صار لها طبيعة.

(٦٠) وقال في المقالة التاسعة من هذا الكتاب إخراج البطريق: لا شيء من الأشياء أوفق لإنضاج البطن للطعام من أن يقرب إليه بدن إنسان آخر ويلزمه. ومن الناس من يعمد إلى صبيان صغار فيضعونهم على بطونهم بالليل فيجدون منفعة عظيمة لأنّ الحرارة أوفق وأفضل وأحمى للحرارة من الحرارة الكائنة من قبل الكماد. ومن الناس من إذا أراد النوم أخذ كلابا صغارا فيضعها على بطنه فيجد من ذلك راحة عظيمة.

تمّت المقالة الرابعة والعشرون ولله الحمد والمنّة.

---

١ الفربيون] القونيون U || ٢ يسيرا] om. LB || ٣ اطيلية] انطليا L ?E | وأنّها] وإنّما U | كانت] om. L || ٤ وذلك . . . شيئا] om. L | ذلك ازدادت وأكثرت منه فلم يضرّها شيئا. ولمّا داومت] om. EL || ٦ التاسعة] الخامسة ELP || ١٠ من ذلك] لذلك EL || ١١ تمّت المقالة الرابعة والعشرون ولله الحمد والمنّة] om. P | تمّت المقالة B تمّت المقالة والحمد لله ربّ العالمين E | والمنّة] وكان مكتوب في آخر هذه المقالة ما هذا مثاله: هذه ما وجدت من خطّه لأنّي لا أبيّض هذه المقالة إلا بعد وفاته رحمة الله عليه وكتب <ا> بو الزكات الطبيب حامدا لله تعالى add. G

*In the name of God,*
*the Merciful, the Compassionate.*
*O Lord, make [our task] easy.*

# The Twenty-Fifth Treatise

*Containing some doubts that befell me concerning Galen's words*

(1) Says Moses: [With] these doubts that I raise [in this treatise], I do not have the same intention as al-Rāzī, as will be clear to the attentive [reader], because al-Rāzī did not cast doubt [on Galen in medical matters] but [immediately] started to refute him in matters that have no relationship at all to the medical art. Even the matters that pertain to the medical art are only dubious for him in the arguments that [Galen] adduces for them and of which he seeks to establish that they are not logical arguments. Thus, he (i.e., al-Rāzī) tries, as it were, to establish his (i.e., Galen's) deficiency in the art of logic. Moreover, he (i.e., al-Rāzī) often blames him (i.e., Galen) and ascribes to him conclusions derived from the abstract and absolute sense of those words [in question], without regard to the sense in which he uses them in that context. Ibn Zuhr and Ibn Riḍwān have already tried to resolve those doubts.[1] I have not set my mind to [say] anything in this regard, and I am also not going to say anything about those things that he (i.e.,

بسم الله الرحمن الرحيم

ربّ يسّر

# المقالة الخامسة والعشرون

## تشتمل على فصول تتعلّق ببعض الشكوك الحادثة لي في كلام جالينوس

(١) قال موسى: هذه الشكوك التي أذكرها لم أقصد فيها قصد الرازي كما يبين للمتأمّل لأنّ الرازي لم يشكك بل أخذ أن يردّ عليه في أمور لا مدخل لها في صناعة الطبّ أصلا. وحتّى الأمور التي تتعلّق بصناعة الطبّ تشكل عليه في استدلالاته عليها ويتبيّن أنّ هذا ليس بدليل برهاني فكأنّه يبيّن قصوره في صناعة المنطق. وأيضا فإنّه يعيبه كثيرا ويلزمه بما يلزم مجرّد تلك الألفاظ مطلقا من غير اعتبار المعنى الذي فيه يتكلّم في ذلك الموضع. وقد عنى ابن زهر وابن رضوان بحلّ تلك الشكوك وأنا لم أتعرّض

---

١ بسم الله الرحمن الرحيم ربّ يسّر] om. ELBP || ٥ ببعض الشكوك] بشكوك L ببعض شكوك EB | الحادثة لي] حادثت لي EL | لي] G[1] | في كلام جالينوس] في مواضع من كلام جالينوس L || ٧ يشكك] يشك B | أن] om. ELBP || ٨ الطبّ] om. B | تشكل] يشكك EGBP لم يشكك S || ٩ ويتبيّن أنّ هذا ليس] om. B | يبيّن] بين] G || ١٠ يعيبه] يعانده LB | مجرّد] تجرد (?)G

al-Rāzī) pretends to be doubts or to be solutions of doubts, for all this is, in my opinion, a useless waste of time. It is, even more, a waste of time for the worse because every obstinacy means in most cases to follow preconceived ideas, and every following of preconceived ideas is a mere evil.[2] But I will mention those doubts that befell me concerning his (i.e., Galen's) words in matters related to the medical art, since he is the master of this art. It is in this [field] alone that he should be followed; his words should not be heeded in any other [field]. That these doubts befell me can only be from one of three causes: it[3] may come either from a mistake that befell the ones who translated [Galen's] works into Arabic, or it may come from unmindfulness that happened to Galen, as nobody is free from these things except for exalted[4] human beings, or the cause may be my bad understanding. In any case, it is certainly useful to present in a combined form both contradictory statements, so that the point of doubt may become evident and the attentive reader may direct his interest to that matter, and that the truth on which he can rely may become manifest to him and his notions may not be deranged and he may not become confused, if a similar doubt presents itself to him.[5]

لشيء من هذا الغرض ولا أقول أيضا شيئا فيما زعم أنّه شكّ ولا فيما زعم أنّه حلّ الشكّ إذ هذا كلّه عندي إتلاف زمان بلا فائدة بل إتلافه في الشرور لأنّ كلّ تعصّب تتبّع هوى في الأكثر وكلّ تتبّع هوى شّر محض. وإنّما أذكر أنا الشكوك الواقعة لي في كلامه في ما يتعلّق بصناعة الطبّ إذ هو إمام هذه الصناعة وهو الذي يقتدى به فيها ولا ينبغي أن يتبع أقواله إلا فيها لا فيما سوى ذلك. وهذه الشكوك الواقعة لي لا يخلو الأمر في سببها من أحد ثلاثة أوجه: إمّا أن يكون ذلك من غلط وقع للذي أخرج الكتب إلى لغة العرب أو يكون ذلك من سهو وقع لجالينوس إذا لا يعصم أحد من هذه إلا عند أرباب العلو أو يكون السبب في ذلك سوء فهمي. وعلى كلّ حال فإنّ الفائدة قد حصلت بما أورده من الجمع بين القولين الموقعين ويتبيّن موضع الشكّ فيصير ذلك المعنى عرضة للمتأمّل فيتبيّن له الحقّ الذي يعمد عليه ولا تتشوّش عليه محفوظاته ولا يتحيّر عند ورود الشكّ عليه من ذلك.

١ الشكّ] شكّ SG || ٢ لأنّ] إذ ELBP | تتبّع هوى في الأكثر وكلّ] om. EL || ٣ هوى شرّ] هولا شرا G || ٥ سوى ذلك.] سواها ELBP || ٧ إلا عند أرباب] الاعتذاريات Sch | أرباب] أصحاب EL | العلو] الغلط علوي L || ٩ المعنى] الموضع B | فيتبيّن] يبين B || ١٠ يعمد] يعتمد ELB

(2) In the fifth [book] of *De usu partium*, he says: Only[6] one extremely weak nerve is distributed through the whole liver because it does not need much sensation. These are his words in that place. Similarly,[7] he explained in this treatise that the spleen, gallbladder, and kidneys have little sensation. In the sixth chapter of this treatise, he says, and these are his words: As[8] for nerves, we do not find any distributed and spread through the heart substance, just as we do not find this in the liver, kidneys, and spleen. But a small nerve reaches the membrane that surrounds the heart (i.e., pericardium). But in those animals that have large bodies, something of a nerve that is perceptible sometimes attaches to the heart. These are his words. If he meant to say that the small nerve that he says is distributed in the liver, spleen, and gallbladder is [nothing else but] the nerve that is distributed through the membrane of each of these organs, then that should have been clear from his words, as it is in the case of the heart.

(3) In the second [book] of *De naturalibus facultatibus*, he says that the sour phlegm does not undergo any concoction in the liver.[9] In the fifth [book] of *De locis affectis*, he says that a cold dyscrasia of the liver makes the humor that ascends to it phlegmatic, crude, and semiconcocted.[10] According to him, then, the crude [humor] is more easily concocted than the sour phlegm because the crude [humor] undergoes some concoction in the liver, while the sour [phlegm] undergoes some concoction only in the stomach. This ought to be contemplated.

(4) In the ninth [book] of *De pulsu magno*, he says that there are three causes that alter the pulse, namely, need, strength, and [the constitution] of the organs themselves.[11] In the second [book] of *De sanitate tuenda*, he says that there are four causes for the alteration [of the pulse] and mentions the three that he also mentions in *De pulsu* [*magno*] and adds the[12] quantitative dissolution of the psychical pneuma.[13] It is possible that this [fourth cause] belongs to all that which falls under [the category of] need. This ought to be contemplated.

(٢) في خامسة منافع الأعضاء قال: تنقسم في الكبد كلّها عصبة واحدة ضعيفة جدّا لأنّها لم يكن بها حاجة إلى كثرة الحسّ. هذا نصّه هناك. وكذلك بيّن في هذه المقالة أنّ الطحال والمرار والكليتين لها حسّ قليل. وفي سادسة هذا الكتاب قال بهذا النصّ: أمّا العصب فلسنا نجد منه شيئا ينقسم وينبثّ في جرم القلب كما لا نجد ذلك في الكبد والكليتين والطحال. لكنّه يصل من العصب إلى الصفاق المحيط بالقلب عصبة دقيقة. وفي ما عظم بدنه من الحيوان قد يتّصل من العصب شيء بالقلب اتّصالا يظهر للحسّ. هذا نصّه. فإن كانت العصبة الدقيقة التي ذكر أنّها تنقسم في الكبد وكذلك في الطحال وكذلك في المرارة يريد بذلك تلك العصبة المنقسمة في غشاء كلّ واحد من هذه الأعضاء فقد كان يجب أن يتبيّن ذلك من كلامه كما بيّن في القلب.

(٣) في ثانية القوى الطبيعية قال إنّ البلغم الحامض لم يقبل شيئا من النضج في الكبد وقال في الخامسة من التعرّف إنّ سوء مزاج الكبد البارد يجعل الخلط الذي يصعد إليها بلغميا خاما نضجا نصف نضجة. فيكون عنده إذا الخام أنضج من البلغم الحامض لأنّ الخام قد قبل بعض النضج من الكبد والحامض إنّما قبل بعض النضج في المعدة فقط فيتأمّل.

(٤) في تاسعة النبض الكبير قال إنّ الأسباب المغيّرة للنبض ثلاثة وهي الحاجة والقوة والآلة. وهو يقول في الثانية من تدبير الصحّة إنّ أسباب التغيّر أربعة وذكر الثلاثة التي ذكر في النبض وزاد تحلّل الروح النفساني في الكمية. وقد يمكن أن يكون هذا من جملة ما يعدّ في الحاجة فيتأمّل.

---

٤ فلسنا] فليس SG | وينبثّ] وينبعث B || ٧ المرارة] المثانة SG || ٨ يتبيّن] يبين ELBP || ٩ بيّن] يبين B تبين LP || ١٢ خاما] حامضا B | نضجا] نضوجا BP || ١٣ في] من L || ١٦ تحلّل] تحليل B

(5) The putrid humor that produces fever within the vessels—I found Galen's discussion of this confused from my own point of view, for from his discourse in the book *De febrium differentiis,* it sometimes seems [to me] that this humor flows throughout the entire body. At other times it seems [to me] that that putrid humor is confined to one place.[14] Similarly, it is clear from his discussion in *De* [*morborum*] *causis et symptomatibus* that it is confined to one place.[15] This is the correct [opinion]. Were it not so, it would not follow that there could be two or three continuous fevers [in the body at the same time]. This ought to be contemplated.[16]

(6) In his *De temperamentis,* he says that the [body] heat of children and of adolescents is the same.[17] Yet in the first [book] of *De sanitate tuenda,* he says that moisture and [body] heat diminish from the time of birth of a living being until the end of his life.[18] This ought to be contemplated.[19]

(7) In the seventh [book] of *De methodo medendi,* he says that a transformation to heat or cold is easier to treat and more rapid to cure, whereas a transformation to moisture and dryness is harder to treat and harder to cure.[20] These are his words there. After this, in the very same book, when speaking about the stomach he says: A moist dyscrasia is easier to treat and faster to cure than the other types of dyscrasia. This holds true whether it is only [moisture] or it is mixed with heat or cold.[21] These are his words as well. One might excuse this contradiction by saying that the first statement is [meant] in general, while the last one is [meant] specifically for the stomach, and this seems [to be the case]. But if the matter [really] is like this, then the first statement is not a general one, and this is the point of doubt. This ought to be contemplated.

(8) He says in the fourth [book] of *Mayāmir*: The thin part of egg white washes and cleanses the moistures from the eye, and through its agglutinant quality it makes the roughness occurring in the eye soft and smooth.[22] These are his words, and later in the same book he says: Egg white has no cleansing [quality].[23] This ought to be contemplated.

(9) In the book *De alimentorum* [*facultatibus*], he regards the milk of camels as more excellent than that of donkeys.[24] Yet in the fifth [book] of *De sanitate tuenda,* he regards donkey's milk as more excellent and gives it preference over all [other] kinds of milk.[25]

(٥) الخلط العفن المولّد للحمّى الكائن داخل العروق رأيت كلام جالينوس فيه مضطربا بحسب نظري. وذلك أنّ في كتاب أصناف الحمّيات يبدو من كلامه تارة أنّ ذلك الخلط يجري في جميع البدن وتارة يبدو من كلامه أنّ ذلك الخلط العفن محصور في موضع واحد. وكذلك يبين من كلامه في العلل والأعراض أنّه محصور في موضع واحد وهذا هو الصحيح. ولولا ذلك لمّا لزم أن توجد حمّاتان دائمتان أو ثلاثة فيتأمّل.

(٦) في كتاب المزاج يسوّي بين حرارة الصبيان وحرارة الشباب وفي الأولى من تدبير الصّحة يقول إنّ الرطوبة والحرارة متناقصتين منذ تولّد الحيوان إلى آخر العمر فتأمّل.

(٧) في سابعة حيلة البرء يقول إنّ الاستحالة إلى الحرارة والبرودة أسهل مداواة وأسرع برء. أمّا الاستحالة إلى الرطوبة واليبوسة فهما أعسر مداواة وأنكد برء. هذا نصّه هناك. ثمّ قال بعد ذلك في المقالة بعينها عند كلامه في المعدة: فأمّا سوء المزاج الرطب فهو أسهل مداواة وأسرع برء من سائر أصناف سوء المزاج. والأمر فيه كذلك إن كان وحده وإن كان مركّبا مع حرارة أو برودة. هذا أيضا نصّه. فإن اعتذر عن هذا التناقض بأن يقال إنّ الكلام الأوّل عامّ وهذا الآخر خاصّ بالمعدة. وهكذا يبدو لكنّ إن كان الأمر كذلك فالقول الأوّل ليس يعامّ وهذا هو موضع الشكّ فتأمّل.

(٨) يقول في رابعة الميامر لطيف بياض البيض يغسل ويجلو الرطوبات من العين ويغرّي ويملّس ما يحدث في العين من الخشونة. هذا نصّه وبعد ذلك في تلك المقالة بعينها قال: بياض البيض عديم الجلاء بتّة فتأمّل.

(٩) في كتاب الأغذية يفضّل لبن الإبل على لبن الأتن وفي الخامسة من تدبير الصحّة فضّل لبن الأتن وقدّمه على الألبان كلّها.

---

١ الكائن] om. G || ٢ يبدو] لي add. B || ٣ يبدو] لي add. B || ٩ أمّا . . . برء] L[1] || ١٠ الرطب . . . المزاج] om. L || ١٣ وهذا الآخر] والكلام الأخير O | الآخر] الأمر SG | يبدو] لي add. B || ١٩ وقدّمه] وفضّله B

(10) In his treatise *De bonis malisque sucis*, he holds that pork excels any other [kind of] praiseworthy food. After that [in excellence] comes kid's meat and after that calf's meat and after that lamb's meat.[26]

(11) In a number of places Galen explains to us that [superfluous] matters in the beginning of their streaming, and also when inflammations get worse or reach their climax, should be attracted to the opposite side.[27] But if they have passed their climax and the humor is retained and settles in an organ and turns old or hard, the matter should be attracted from the filled organ itself, if possible, or from the organ that is closest to it. This is a fundamental rule that is repeatedly[28] mentioned in the writings of Galen and Hippocrates. It is a correct [rule] and fixed according to analogical reasoning. The entire medical practice is based on it, and its success is evident from experience. And because of this very beneficial fundamental rule, Galen instructs us to bleed the cephalic vein in the case of severe[29] illnesses of the eye, and angina[30] and the like. If the illness becomes prolonged and the inflammations become hard or adhere to an organ and become settled in it, then he tells us to bleed for illnesses of the eye [the vein alongside] the inner angle of the eye or a vein in the forehead or the veins behind the ears.[31] And for inflammations of the throat and uvula [he tells us] to bleed the veins under the tongue.[32] This is all correct and clear, and one should observe to draw [the matter] to the opposite side. In his commentary on the seventh [book] of [Hippocrates'] *Aphorisms*, he remarks: In the case of illnesses above the liver, one should bleed from the arms; and if [the illnesses] are below the liver, one should bleed from the legs.[33] This rule is repeated several times. However, in his *De venae sectione*, he says: If someone suffers from epilepsy, vertigo,[34] or dizziness, we should bleed him especially from the leg. Says Moses: This [rule] is the opposite of the rule established by him in his [previous] statement and the opposite of that demanded by analogical reasoning. I do not know any explanation of this [inconsistency], but it may be that the [last-mentioned] activity [of bleeding from the leg] has [special] conditions that have been omitted during the translation.[35]

(١٠) في مقالته في الخلط الجيّد والمذموم فضّل لحم الخنزير على كلّ غذاء محمود وبعده لحم الجدي وبعده لحم العجاجيل وبعده لحم الحملان.

(١١) قد بيّن لنا جالينوس في عدّة مواضع أنّ الموادّ في أوّل انصبابها وفي حال تزيّد الأورام الحارّة أيضا وعند منتهاها تجذب المادّة إلى خلاف الجهة. فأمّا إذا تمّ الانتهاء واحتقن الخلط ورسخ في العضو وقدم أو تحجّر فتجذب المادّة من نفس العضو الممتلئ إن أمكن أو من أقرب الأعضاء إليه. وهذا أصل تكرّر ذكره كثيرا في كلام جالينوس وأبقراط. وهذا صحيح ومقيّس وعليه عمل الطبّ كلّه ونجحه ظاهر بالتجربة. ومن أجل هذا الأصل العظيم النفع يأمرنا جالينوس بفصد القيفال في أمراض العين الشديدة وفي الخوانيق ونحوها. فإذا طالت العلّة وتحجّرت الأورام أو تشبّثت بالعضو وثبتت أمرنا حينئذ أن نفصد في أمراض العين المأق الأكبر أو عرق الجبهة أو العروق التي خلف الأذنين. ونفسد في أورام الحلق واللهاة العروق التي تحت اللسان. وهذا كلّه صحيح بيّن والمراعاة الجذب إلى خلاف الجهة. قال في شرحه لسابعة الفصول إنّ في العلل التي فوق الكبد ينبغي أن تفصد اليدين ومتى كانت تحت الكبد ينبغي أن تفصد الرجلين. وتكرّر له ذكر هذا القانون مرّات. لكنّه قال في مقالته في الفصد: من كانت علّته الصرع أو دوران أو سدر فينبغي أن نفصد خاصّة من الرجل. قال موسى: هذا خلاف ما تأصّل من كلامه وخلاف ما يقتضيه القياس. ولا أعلم لهذا تأويلا بوجه ولعلّ لهذا الفعل شرائط حذفت عند الإخراج.

---

٤ واحتقن EL وتتقن GP وتقن S وثبت B || ١٢ اليدين ... تفصد] om. G || ١٣ ذكر] om. ELOP || ١٤ سدر] سهر B || ١٦ أقول المفهوم من كلام جالينوس من كانت علّته الصرع أو الدوار أو السدد فينبغي أن يفصد خاصّة من الرجل يعني إذا كان سبب الصرع أو الدوار أو السدد احتباس ما اعتيد استفراغه من دفع الطبيعة كما إذا احتبس الباسور ويخاف من حدوث هذه الأمراض فإذن فصد الرجل من أوفق المعالجات لهذه الأعراض لجذبه إلى الخلاف البعيد ولتحريك الدم المتراقي إلى الدماغ نحو المحلّ المعتاد استفراغه بالطبع منه. هذا غاية ما يمكن فهمه بسبب الاحتباس وتأويله <... add. L?>

(12) In the first [book] of his commentary on *Epidemics* 1, he states that ardent fever does not originate from the burning of yellow bile in whatever organ this occurs. Rather, it develops if the yellow bile in the stomach has putrefied and especially in the cardia of the stomach or the concave side of the liver.[36] Then he says in the second book of his commentary to [*Epidemics* 1][37] that ardent fevers occurs if the yellow bile in the vessels—and especially in the vessels close to the liver, stomach, or lungs—putrefies.[38] This ought to be contemplated.

(13) In his treatise *De clysteribus*, he says: And detrimental foods such as cabbage [*Brassica oleracea*] and the like are among the cold and dry vegetables.[39] And in the seventh book of *De simplicium medicamentorum* [*temperamentis ac facultatibus*], he says that [cabbage] has no evident sharpness or acridity and that its taste contains bitterness.[40] He also says that its strength heals ulcers that have indurated. Everything that he mentions concerning its activity indicates that it contains some heat, although not strong. In this manner, Ibn Wāfid and others considered it as hot in the first [degree].[41]

(14) In his treatise *De bonis malisque sucis*, Galen says: One cannot find [any type of] cabbage that has a cooling effect, nor any type of onion [*Allium cepa*], garlic [*Allium sativum*], or leek [*Allium porrum* and var.] with such an effect.[42] Concerning a solution of the doubt [raised by these contradictory passages], it seems to me that it is the moisture in the [cabbage] that contains heat but that its very substance, if that moisture separates from it, is cold. But he (i.e., Galen) should have elucidated this, just as he elucidated such a matter in other cases. And in the first [book] of *De febrium* [*differentiis*, he says]: Hot foods, such as onion, garlic, leek, garden cress [*Lepidium sativum*], cabbage, and sweet basil [*Ocimum basilicum*].[43]

(15) If a hot humor ascends to the upper parts of the body, ulcers develop in the head by themselves. Then it is necessary to expel it from the nearest site through emesis and not through bleeding. Says Moses: Galen mentions this matter in the sixth [book] of his commentary on *Epidemics* 2. I have very grave doubts concerning this [statement], since it is contradictory to what is well known from the medical rules.[44]

(١٢) ذكر في الأولى من شرحه للأولى من أبيديميا أنّ الحمّى المحرقة لا تتولّد من احتراق الصفراء في أيّ عضو اتّفق و إنّما تتكوّن إذا كان عفن المرار الأصفر في المعدة وبالخاصّة فمها أو في مقعّر الكبد. ثمّ قال في المقالة الثانية من شرحه لهذه المقالة الأولى إنّ الحمّى المحرقة تحدث إذا عفنت المرّة الصفراء في العروق وبخاصّة في العروق التي تلي الكبد والمعدة والرئة فيتأمّل.

(١٣) في مقالته في الحقن قال: والأغذية الرديئة مثل الكرنب وأشباهه من البقول الباردة اليابسة وفي مقالته السابعة من الأدوية المفردة قال إنّه ليس بظاهر الحدّة والحرافة وفي طعمه مرارة. وقال إنّ قوته تشفي القروح التي قد صلبت. وكلّ ما ذكر من فعله يدلّ على أنّ فيه حرارة ليست بالقوية وهكذا جعله ابن وافد وغيره حارّ يابس في الأوّل.

(١٤) وقال جالينوس في مقالته في جودة الكيموس ورداءته قال: ولا تجد كرنبا يبرد ولا تجد أيضا في البصل والثوم والكرّاث جنسا يبرد. ويبدو إليّ في حلّ هذا الشكّ أنّ الرطوبة التي فيه هي التي فيها حرارة ونفس جرمه إذا فارقته تلك الرطوبة بارد. لكنّه كان ينبغي له أن يبيّن ذلك كما بيّن هذا المعنى في غيره. وفي الأولى من الحمّيات: الأطعمة الحارّة مثل البصل والثوم والكرّاث والحرف والكرنب والباذروج.

(١٥) إذا تعالى خلط حارّ إلى أعالي البدن حدثت قروح في الرأس من تلقاء نفسها فينبغي أن يستخرج من أقرب موضع بالقيء لا بالفصد. قال موسى: ذكر جالينوس هذا المعنى في المقالة السادسة من شرحه لثانية أبيديميا. وقد أشكل هذا عليّ غاية الإشكال فإنّه خلاف المشهور من قوانين الطبّ.

---

١ أبيديميا] أفيديميا ELO || ٧ السابعة] الثالثة L || ١٠ جالينوس] ببيان add. ELBOP | ولا. . . يبرد] om. B || ١١ والكرّاث] om. G | إليّ] لي ELBOP || ١٦ يستخرج] يستفرغ LPB | في المقالة السادسة من شرحه] في سابعة شرحه L || ١٧ أبيديميا] أفيديميا ELO

(16) In the fourth [book] of *De [morborum] causis et symptomatibus*, he makes the following statement, and these are his words: Any damage that occurs to any of the senses happens only because of an illness affecting the nerves by[45] which they (i.e., the senses) [are well supplied] when [the nerves] are healthy.[46]

(17) Says Moses: I wish I knew whether a cataract in the eye and a deep ulceration of the hornlike [tunic], if they are opposite the pupil and are joined together, are harmful for the sense of vision or not, and from what kind of damage the nerve through which the sense of vision is active suffers in these illnesses and similar ones. In the beginning of this treatise, Galen has informed us that a sense becomes impaired on account of the principal organ through which it functions, or on account of the faculty that impels this principal organ, or on account of the parts that were created for the benefit of this principal organ.[47] All this is correct. If one were to reverse this proposition (i.e., state the converse) and say that if the nerve of any sense whatsoever is harmed when the harm given to this sense is imparted to it (i.e., the nerve), then this proposition would be correct according to what we have [just] learned.[48] This ought to be contemplated.

(18) In his commentary on the second [book] of *De aeris aquis [locis]*, he says: No part of the body should be cauterized except for the hands, feet, and loins.[49] And in the seventh book of his commentary on *Epidemics* 6, he says: [In the case of] those who suffer from an ulcer in the lung, one should hurry to cauterize their chest.[50] These are his words, and [this statement] annuls the previous one. This ought to be contemplated.

(19) In the second [book] of *De locis affectis*, he says the following, and these are his words: Pulsation does not follow an[51] [inflammation in all parts of the body], as we said, but only in that part in which there are sensitive pulsatile vessels, if that part itself has sensory perception and the inflammation called "phlegmone"[52] is of noticeable size. For if these [things] occur together in that [bodily part], the patient feels a pulsatile pain, even if the affected part does not have a sensitive pulsatile vessel. These are his words.

(١٦) قال في رابعة العلل والأعراض كلاما هذا نصّه قال: كلّ مضرّة تنال حاسّة من الحواسّ أيّ حاسّة كانت إنّما تنالها من قبل آفة تحدث في العصب الذي منه تكون في وقت صحّتها.

(١٧) قال موسى: يا ليت شعري الماء النازل في العين وقرحة القرنية الغائرة إذا كانت مقابل الحدقة والتحمت تضرّ بحاسّة البصر أو لا تضرّ وأيّ آفة نالت العصبة التي بها تكون حاسّة البصر في هذه الأمراض ونحوها. وقد علّمنا جالينوس في أوّل هذه المقالة أنّ الحاسّة تنضرّ إمّا من قبل الآلة الأولى التي بها يكون الفعل أو من قبل القوة التي تأتي تلك الآلة الأولى أو من قبل الأعضاء التي خلقت لمنافع تلك الآلة الأولى. وهذا صحيح كلّه. ولو عكس هذه القضية وقال إنّ عصب كلّ حاسّة أيّ حاسّة كانت متى نالته آفة نالت تلك الحاسّة مضرّة لكانت القضية صادقة على ما علمناه فيتأمّل ذلك.

(١٨) في شرحه للمقالة الثانية من كتاب الأهوية والمياه قال: لا ينبغي أن يكوى عضو في البدن خلا اليدين والرجلين والحقوين. وفي المقالة السابعة من شرحه للمقالة السادسة من أبيديميا قال: أصحاب قرحة الرئة ينبغي أن يبادر بكيّ صدورهم. هذا نصّه فقد بطّل ما تقدّم فيتأمّل.

(١٩) في المقالة الثانية من التعرّف قال كلاما هذا نصّه قال: وأمّا الضربان فليس يتبعها كلّها على ما وصفنا بل إنّما يتبع منها ما فيه عروق ضاربة محسوسة إذا كان العضو في نفسه حسّاسا وكان الورم المسمّى فلغموني ذا قدر يعتدّ به في العظم. فإنّه إذا اجتمعت فيه هذه أحسّ المريض بوجع الضربان ولو لم يكن في العضو العليل عرق ضارب محسوس. هذا نصّه.

---

٨ أو . . . الأولى] om. B || ١١ ينبغي . . . والحقوين] ومنع أيضا من الكيّ للأعضاء التي لها غور سيّما إذا كان للعضو بطن غائر فإنّ للأعضاء كلّها بطونا ما خلا اليدين والرجلين والفخذين C, fol. 73r1sq. || ١٣ أبيديميا] أفيديميا ELO | بطّل] أبطل ELOP أبدل B

(20) Says Moses: If you consider this statement, it becomes clear to you that it is deficient since he mentions four conditions [for pulsatile pain], namely, that there is an inflammation, that it is of a large size, that it is in a sensible part, and that that part has sensitive pulsatile vessels. Then he says that when these conditions occur together, the patient feels pulsatile [pain]. Then he says [that this is the case] even if the affected part has no sensitive pulsatile vessel. With this last statement he canceled the specific condition necessary for pulsation [which he mentioned before], namely, the existence of a sensitive pulsatile vessel. The most probable solution [of this inconsistency], in my opinion, is that during the translation of this book from one language into another [some] words were omitted so that the meaning [of this text] was corrupted. [I also think] that the intention of Galen's statement is that the joined occurrence of these four conditions in the inflamed part necessarily leads to a pulsatile sensation, even if that sensitive pulsatile vessel is not in the inflamed [part] itself but in [a part] close to it. This ought to be contemplated.

(21) Others than us and many physicians have contemplated Galen's words on the causes of pain. We found that in a number of places he gives only one cause for it, namely, a[53] dissolution of continuity. He says about a hot cause of pain that it is comes with a loosening of a tight structure, and about a cold cause of pain that it comes with contraction and thickening.[54] It goes beyond doubt that if some parts of an organ become more tight, other parts become more loose. All of it goes back to a dissolution of continuity. On this fundamental principle he bases his statement in the fourth [book] of *De [morborum] causis et symptomatibus* in a number of places.[55] Then he explains in his treatise *De inequali intemperie* that a varying [kind of] dyscrasia is one of the causes of pain.[56] This is correct, and therefore every pain may have one of two causes: either a varying [kind of] dyscrasia or a dissolution of continuity. It is on this that he bases his assertion. There is no doubt that [initially] he had the first[57] opinion and that then it became clear to him that the matter is as he mentions it eventually, namely, that there are two causes of pain.[58]

(٢٠) قال موسى: إذا تأمّلت هذا الكلام بان لك اختلاله لأنّه ذكر أربعة شرائط وهي أن يكون الورم حارّا وأن يكون عظيم المقدار وأن يكون في عضو حسّاس وأن تكون في ذلك العضو عروق ضاربة محسوسة. وقال إنّ باجتماع هذه الشرائط يحسّ المريض بالضربان. ثمّ قال ولو لم يكن في العضو العليل عرق ضارب محسوس. وقد حذف في آخر كلامه الشرط الضروري الخاصّ بالضربان وهو وجود العرق الضارب المحسوس. والأقرب عندي أنّ في حال إخراج الكتاب من لغة إلى لغة سقطت كلمة أفسدت المعنى وأنّ الغرض كان من كلام جالينوس أنّ اجتماع هذه الأربعة شرائط في العضو الوارم يوجب إحساس الضربان ولو لم يكن ذلك العرق الضارب المحسوس في نفس الورم بل بالقرب منه فيتأمّل.

(٢١) قد تأمّل غيرنا وكثيرون من الأطبّاء كلام جالينوس في أسباب الوجع فوجدناه في عدّة مواضع يجعل سببه سببا واحدا وهو تفرّق الاتّصال فقط. ويقول في إيلام الحارّ إنّه بتفريقه الاتّصال وفي إيلام البارد إنّه بالجمع والتكثيف. وبلا شكّ أنّ إذا اجتمعت أجزاء من العضو فقد تفرّقت أجزاء آخر فيرجع الكلّ إلى تفرّق الاتّصال. وعلى هذا الأصل بنى كلامه في المقالة الرابعة من العلل والأعراض وفي عدّة مواضع. ثمّ بيّن في مقالته في سوء المزاج المختلف أنّ سوء المزاج المختلف سبب من أسباب الوجع. وهذا صحيح فيكون سبب كلّ وجع أحد سببين: إمّا سوء مزاج مختلف أو تفرّق اتّصال وعلى هذا بنى كلامه. ولا شكّ أن كان رأى الرأي الأوّل ثمّ تبيّن له أنّ الأمر كما ذكر أخيرا أنّ للوجع سببين.

١ بان] تبين ELBOP || ٦ كلمة] كل ما B || ٧ اجتماع] اجتمعت SG || ١٥ كلامه] في add. G

(22) In his treatise *Puero epileptico consilium*, he allows [an epileptic boy] the consumption of some common vegetables and some fruits because he is still young and is not capable of abstaining from food like a philosopher.[59] Then he mentions all the vegetables that he allows him and says, and these are his words: Also from these he should [only] take a moderate quantity.[60] Similarly, leek [*Allium porrum* and var.], garden celery [*Apium graveolens*], and mountain celery[61] [*Peucedanum oreoselinum*]. These are his very words. But when he continued his statement and started to speak about the things that he should abstain from entirely, he said the following, and these are his words: And among those things that are similar to those that I mentioned [to abstain from entirely] are all the things that ascend to the head through their heat and sharpness and fill it with vapors, such as wine, mustard, celery,[62] garlic,[63] and onions.[64] These are his words. It is dubious to me that [first] he permits two species of celery and then forbids it absolutely.[65] Also dubious to me is that he permits leek but forbids onion and garlic,[66] while all three of them equally fill the brain with vapors, just as he (i.e., Galen) treats them as equal in his *De alimentorum* [*facultatibus*].[67]

(23)[68] Says Moses: We do not know the causes of everything whose existence has been ascertained. The fevers that arise from the putrefaction of the humors belong to this class of things. That is, when Galen wanted to furnish the cause why some of them abate and others do not, and why some of the abating[69] [and attacking] ones adhere to one pattern and one cycle, while others of the abating [and attacking] ones follow no pattern, he started to present the causes of each of these four things whose existence is manifest. He said whatever he said in his [book] *De febrium* [*differentiis*]. He explained the difficulty of furnishing the cause for the regularity of the cycles. Moreover, he explained that he had shifted from one opinion to another but that later on he became confirmed in his final opinion. His explanation was quite lengthy. He claimed to have removed any difficulties and that what he stated was the most appropriate [thing] to be said about it. But when I contemplated his words thoroughly, I saw that there was [some] confusion in them. They became ever more dubious for me. The matter was not at all clear to me. I shall here quote his very words, and then I shall explain to you that which I found difficult. In book one of his treatise *De febrium* [*differentiis*], he stated the following, and these are his words:

(٢٢) في مقالته في تدبير صبي يصرع يسمح له لكونه صبيا في تناول بعض البقول المعتادة وبعض الفواكه لكونه صغيرا ولا يقدر يحتمي احتماء فيلسوف. وذكر جملة البقول التي أباح له وقال بهذا النصّ: وينبغي أن يكون ما يتناول من هذا أيضا بالمقدار القصد وكذلك من الكرّاث والكرفس البستاني والجبلي. هذا نصّ كلامه. ولمّا أمعن في القول وأخذ في ذكر الأشياء التي يمنع منعا كلّيا قال كلاما هذا نصّه: وممّا يجانس هذه التي ذكرت جميع الأشياء التي ترتفع إلى الرأس بحرارتها وحدّتها وتملأه بخارا كالشراب والخردل والكرفس والثوم والبصل. هذا نصّه. أشكل عليّ كون الكرفس أبيح نوعيه ثمّ منع مطلقا. وأشكل عليّ إباحة الكرّاث ومنع البصل والثوم وثلاثها في ملء الدماغ أبخرة سواء كما ساوى بينها في الأغذية.

(٢٣) قال موسى: ليس كلّ ما صحّ وجوده علمت أسبابه ومن جملة تلك الأشياء الحمّيات الكائنة من عفونة الأخلاط. وذلك أنّ جالينوس لمّا رام أن يعطي السبب في كون بعضها يقلع وبعضها لا يقلع وكون المفترة منها تلزم نظاما واحدا ودورا واحدا وبعض المفترة لا تلزم نظاما أخذ أن يعطي السبب في كلّ واحد من هذه الأربعة أشياء الظاهرة الوجود. فقال ما قال في ذلك في كتاب الحمّيات وصرّح بصعوبة إعطاء السبب في انتظام الأدوار وصرّح أيضا بانتقاله من رأي إلى رأي آخر ثمّ اعتمد على رأيه الأخير وطوّل في البيان وزعم أنّه قد رفع الإشكالات وأنّ الذي ذكره أولى ما يقال في ذلك. ولمّا تأمّلت كلامه تأمّلا جيّدا رأيت في الكلام اضطرابا وكثرت أشكالاته عليّ ولم يتخلّص لي المعنى في ذلك بوجه. وهاهنا أورد عليك نصوص كلامه وبعد ذلك أبيّن لك ما أشكل عليّ. قال في مقالته الأولى من كتابه في الحمّيات كلاما هذا نصّه قال:

---

١ يصرع ] MS O ends here | يسمح ] تسامح L تسمح B مسمح P || ٣ هذا... وكذلك ] om. B || ٥ التي... الأشياء ] om. L || ٧ الكرفس أبيح ] من الكرفس أباح L || ٨ ساوى ] سوى LBP || ١١ في كون ] فيكون B

As for the humors that putrefy in the viscera and in the major vessels—because these humors are always flowing, they cause to putrefy whatever they encounter. For[70] their putrefaction and the heat that originates from them are joined together and[71] result in [a putrefying heat that affects] one thing after another over a longer period. In sum, the determining factor of these things that happen inside the body is similar to [the determining factor] of that which happens at the outside to all the bodies that suffer from an unnatural heat, for whatever reason. For if that which becomes hot belongs to those things that do not putrefy, such as a stone or a piece of wood and other similar things, it keeps its warmth for some time until it [starts to] cool off slowly. But if it is one of those things that can putrefy, its heat spreads continuously from that part that is heated first to [the part] that is joined to it, like that which I once saw happening in some village to the dung of [some] animals and doves that had been collected in one place. One part of it became so heated by a very hot sun that a very large quantity of hot vapor started to arise from it, similar to smoke that has a strong biting effect and that is harmful for the eyes and nose of whoever gets close to it. Moreover, the heat of the dung was so strong when one touches it that if one put one's hand or foot into it and kept it there very well, it burned it. However, this symptom did not last forever, for the next day all the dung that had reached the highest degree of boiling heat on the previous day cooled off. And that part of the dung that was joined to the first part and that gradually absorbed the heat during the time that that first part was boiling hot started to become boiling hot as well when the heat of the first part began to diminish.

فأما الأخلاط التي تتعفّن في الأحشاء وفي العروق الكبار فمن قبل أنّ تلك الأخلاط تجري دائما وتعفن بعفونتها ما تلقاه. فإنّ عفونتها والحرارة المتولّدة عنها تتّصل ويحدث منها شيء بعد شيء في مدّة أطول. وبالجملة فإنّ الذي يعرض من هذا في البدن سببه ممّا يعرض من خارج بجميع الأجسام التي تسخن سخونة خارجة عن طبعها من أيّ سبب كان ذلك. فإنّ الشيء الذي يسخن إن كان ممّا لا يعفن مثل الحجر والخشبة أو غيرهما ممّا أشبههما فإنّه يبقى على حرارته مدّة ما إلى أن يبرد قليلا. وإن كان ممّا يمكن أن يعفن فإنّ حرارته تسعى دائما من الجزء الذي يسخن أوّلا إلى الذي يتّصل به مثل الذي رأيت مرّة في بعض القرى قد عرض في زبل دوابّ وحمام كان مجموعا في موضع فسخن جزء منه من شمس حارّة أصابته سخونة قوية حتّى جعل يرتفع منه بخار حارّ كثير جدّا جدّا بمنزلة الدخان يلذع تلذيعا قويا ويؤذي من دنى منه في عينيه ومنخريه. وكان أيضا قد بلغ من سخونة ذلك الزبل عند اللمس أنّه كان من أدخل فيه كفّه أو قدمه ولبث فيه أفضل لبث احرقه. إلا أنّ هذا العارض لم يكن يبقى دائما لكنّه كان من غدّ ذلك اليوم يبرد جميع ما كان من ذلك الزبل قد بلغت فيه الحرارة والغليان الأمس غاية منتهاها. ثمّ كان الجزء الذي يتّصل بذلك الجزء الأوّل التي كانت الحرارة لم تزال تتأدى إليه قليلا قليلا في وقت ما كان ذلك الجزء الأوّل في منتهى غليانه إذا بدأت حرارة ذلك الجزء الأوّل تنقص أخذ هذا الجزء الثاني أيضا في السخونة والغليان.

---

١ الأحشاء] الأغشية L الأحشاء L$^1$ || ٢ تلقاه] وتمامه L add. וכו P add. | فإنّ . . . ولا دور غيره] ثمّ تنقّل إلى قوله B ينقل إلى قوله LP || ١١ أفضل] أوصل S

Shortly afterwards [the second part] became extremely hot, while the first part [had cooled off].[72] Then the heat of that second part also began to diminish, and the part that was joined to it was gradually becoming hotter. And it did not take long before that third part became blazingly and extremely hot, while the second part [of the dung] cooled off. This cycle took about a day and a night so that it is an example of what is particular for quotidian fever. If this cycle would take two days and two nights, it would be an example of tertian fever. If it would take three days, it would be an example of quartan [fever], and if it would take five days, it would be an example of quintan fever, if there would be a fever that would attack on the fifth day. But I have not really seen such a cyclus nor another one beyond the cycle of quartan [fever].[73] This is his first formulation, in accordance with his first opinion.

Then, in the beginning of book two, he said, and these are his words: Intermittent fevers, that is, those that have a sensible abatement, occur only when the humor that produces the fever moves and flows throughout the entire body. But continuous fevers occur only when the humor that produces the fever is confined within the cavity of the vessels. This is the text of his second statement.[74] He then said [something else] in this book, namely, the statement in which he retracted his original opinion. These are his words: If you examine the matter closely, you will find that with some fevers paroxysms occur in cycles even more wondrous than these.

ثمّ أنّه بعد قليل يبلغ منتهاه من الحرارة فالجزء الأوّل قد <برد>. ثمّ أنّ حرارة ذلك الجزء الثاني أيضا كانت تبتدئ في الانحطاط فالجزء الذي يتّصل به يتزيّد قليلا قليلا حرارة. ثمّ لا يلبث ذلك الجزء الثالث أن يشعل ويبلغ منتهاه من الحرارة ويبرد الجزء الثاني منه. وكان هذا الدور يكون في قريب من يوم وليلة حتّى يكون مثالا خاصّة في الحمّى النائبة في كلّ يوم. ولو كان هذا الدور كان في يومين وليلتين لكان سيكون مثالا لحمّى الغبّ. ولو كان في ثلاثة أيّام لكان مثالا للربع ولو كان في أربعة أيّام كان مثالا للخمس إن كانت حمّى ينوب في الخامس. فإنّى أنا ما رأيت إلى هذه الغاية هذا الدور رؤية حقيقة ولا دور غيره من وراء دور الربع فهذا نصّه الأوّل على رأيه الأوّل.

ثمّ أنّه قال في أوّل المقالة الثانية كلاما هذا نصّه: إنّ الحمّيات المفارقة وهي التي تقلع إقلاعا محسوسا إنّما تكون متى كان الخلط المولّد للحمّى متحرّكا جاريا في البدن كلّه. وأمّا الحمّيات الدائمة فإنّما تكون إذا كان الخلط المولّد للحمّى محصورا في جوف العروق. هذا نصّ كلامه الثاني. ثمّ أنّه قال في هذه المقالة وهو القول الذي رجع فيه عن رأيه الأوّل كلاما هذا نصّه قال: على أنّك إن استقصيت النظر في الأمر وجدت أنّ حدوث النوائب في بعض الحمّيات على الأدوار أعجب من هذا.

٩ أنّه] om. B || ١٠ جاريا] جائرا P || ١٣ النظر في] om. ELP

For[75] the example of the dung that putrefies part after part and that I gave above, it is almost impossible that that would happen in the body of a living being, because it does not take long before the humors that putrefy get mixed with other humors that did not putrefy since the humors stream from every site in the body to every [other] site. If this is the case, then it is impossible that there is putrefaction in one part of the body but not in another and [only] at a certain moment but not at another, except when there is an [inflamed] tumor in some part that has bound the putrefied humor and retained it inside. If our words turned out to be opposite to the ones stated before and it is evidently more difficult to find the cause for fevers that attack in cycles than for continuous fevers, then we should attempt to discuss the situation with regard to both of them together.[76] This is the formulation of his third statement.

Later on in the same book, after he became confirmed in the second opinion, he said, when giving a cause for the cycles, that the organ expels its superfluities from one set time to the next and that it is those expelled superfluities that putrefy. He gave the cause for the length or brevity of the paroxysm in accordance with his last opinion. Then he said the following, and these are his words: Moreover, according to this reasoning it will not be difficult for you to know the cause whereby some bouts of fever abate, while others do not abate. The former are doubtless of such brevity that they terminate before the next bout begins. [The[77] putrefying humor] flows and moves through the entire body. Thus the entire period between the end of the first bout and the beginning of the second is a period of abatement and freedom from fever. However, when the second bout comes earlier, and it occurs before the first bout really ends, then no time at all remains between them during which the body is free from fever. This is his fourth formulation.[78]

فإنّ المثال الذي وصفناه في ما تقدّم من الزبل الذي يعفن شيء بعد شيء لا يكاد يمكن أن يكون في بدن الحيّ لأنّ الأخلاط التي تعفن لا تلبث أن تخلط بالأخلاط التي لم تعفن إذ كانت الأخلاط تجري من كلّ موضع من البدن كلّ موضع منه. فإذا كان الأمر كذلك فليس يمكن أن تكون العفونة في عضو من الأعضاء دون غيره وفي وقت من الأوقات دون غيره إلا أن يكون ورم في عضو من الأعضاء قد ربط الخلط الذي قد عفن وحصره فيه. فإذ كان الكلام قد آل إلى ضدّ ما كان نحا نحوه وبيّن أنّ وجود السبب في الحمّيات التي تنوب على أدوار أصعب من وجود السبب في الحمّيات المطبقة فقد ينبغي أن نروم نخبر عن الحال فيها جميعا. هذا نصّ كلامه الثالث.

ثمّ أنّه قال في هذه المقالة بعد اعتماده على هذا الرأي الثاني في إعطاء سبب الأدوار كون العضو يدفع فضلاته من الوقت إلى الوقت معلوم وتعفن تلك الفضلة المدفوعة. وأعطى السبب في طول النوبة وقصرها بحسب هذا الرأي الأخير. قال بعد ذلك كلاما هذا نصّه قال: وليس يعسر عليك أيضا على هذا القياس أن تعلم السبب الذي من أجله صارت بعض نوائب الحمّيات تقلع وبعضها لا تقلع وذلك أنّه متى كانت هذه النوبة الأولى من القصر بحال تنقضي معها قبل أن تبتدئ النوبة الثانية بلا شكّ ويكون جاريا متحرّكا في البدن كلّه صار ذلك الوقت كلّه الذي بين انقضاء النوبة الأولى وبين ابتداء النوبة الثانية وقت إقلاع ونقاء من الحمّى. ومتى سبقت النوبة الثانية فتحدث قبل أن تنقضي النوبة الأولى الانقضاء الصحيح لم يبق بينهما وقت أصلا ينقى فيه البدن من الحمّى. هذا نصّه الرابع.

١ الذي . . . الحمّيات المطبقة] وتمامه إلى قوله EL إلى قوله BP || ٧ نخبر] نذكر P? EL || ٩ كون] بأنّ ELBP || ١٠ فضلاته] فضلا G || ١٢ عليك] G[1] om. ELBP || ١٤ بلا شكّ ويكون جاريا متحرّكا في البدن كلّه] om. S || ١٧ يبق] يكن G

(24) Says Moses: The gist of his first statement is that the humor that putrefies gradually is within the vessels, and the period of abatement is that period between the putrefaction of a part of that thing and of that [part] that lies next to it, as he illustrated with [the example of] the dunghill. The fever attacks and the humor putrefies within the vessels, as he said. But the gist of his second statement is that there is no sensible abatement unless the putrefying humor is outside the vessels and moves and flows throughout the entire body. And[79] this is most astonishing, how it can be outside the vessels in one place, without any doubt, but [also] streaming and moving throughout the entire body. And the gist of his third statement—the one in which he became confirmed—is that the organ expels its superfluities outside of itself, and it then putrefies there, until that which is consumed is consumed and that which burns into ashes burns into ashes. This is a bout of fever. Later on it abates until it expels another superfluity to that place. The gist of his fourth statement is that continuous fever is the result of one paroxysm immediately following upon another. This ought to be contemplated.

(25) What I am going to say in this aphorism is not to express doubt regarding Galen but is something that those[80] engaged in speculation should consider and contemplate, [namely,] to which extremes the following of one's passion ultimately leads and how it blinds the perceptive faculties of the mind.[81] For this Galen was an earnest seeker of the truth, had a predilection for syllogistic demonstrations, composed a book [entitled] *De*[82] *demonstratione*, and questioned Aristotle's sayings about natural or supernatural matters when Aristotle did not demonstrate them logically, [by using,] for instance, mathematical demonstrations. But although he (i.e., Galen) had reached such a [high] level in seeking [logical] proof for everything, when he found out about the usefulness of the testicles and it became evident to him and [he held it for] the truth, while Aristotle had paid no attention to that usefulness and ignored it, he was very pleased with himself and, in a lengthy discussion, killed Aristotle off as an animal that is weakened [by hunger] kills its prey when it has found it. He then began to exalt the [usefulness of] the testicles and to magnify their importance until[83] he made them more eminent than the heart with his analogical reasoning. These are his words in the first book of the treatise *De semine*.[84]

(٢٤) قال موسى: المفهوم من كلامه الأوّل هو أنّ الخلط الذي يعفن أوّلا أوّلا يكون داخل العروق. وزمان الفترة هو الزمان الذي بين عفن جزء من ذلك الشيء وبين عفن ما يجاوره كما مثّل في المزبلة فتكون الحمّى تنوب والخلط يعفن داخل العروق كما قال. والمفهوم من كلامه الثاني أن لا يكون إقلاع محسوس إلا أن كان الخلط العفن خارج العروق ويكون متحرّكا جاريا في البدن كلّه. وهذا أعجب كيف يكون خارج العروق في موضع واحد بلا شكّ ويكون جاريا متحرّكا في البدن كلّه. والمفهوم من الكلام الثالث الذي اعتمد عليه أنّ العضو يدفع فضلاته خارجا عنه فيعفن هناك حتّى ينفد منها ما ينفد ويترمّد ما يترمّد وهي نوبة الحمّى ثمّ تقلع حتّى تدفع لذلك الموضع فضلا آخر. ومفهوم الكلام الرابع أنّ الحمّى الدائمة هي من أجل لحوق نوبة لنوبة. فيتأمّل هذا.

(٢٥) الذي أقوله في هذا الفصل ليس هو شكّ على جالينوس بل أمر ينبغي لأهل النظر أن يعتبرونه ويرون إلى أيّ غاية ينتهي تبع الهوى وكيف تعمى البصائر به. وذلك أنّ هذا الجالينوس رجل محقّق جدّا ويؤثر البراهين وألّف كتابا في البرهان ويشكّ في أشياء قالها أرسطو في أمور طبيعية أو إلاهية لمّا لم يأت عليها أرسطو ببرهان مثل البراهين التعليمية. ومع كونه في هذا الدرجة من طلب الأدلّة على كلّ شيء لمّا وجد منفعة الأنثيين وتبيّن له ذلك وهو حقّ وغفل أرسطو عن تلك المنفعة ولم يعلمها سرّ بنفسه وفرح وطوّل الكلام وافترس أرسطو افتراس الضعيف إذا وجد فريسته وأخذ في تعظيم الأنثيين وتشريف قدرها حتّى جعلها أشرف من القلب بقياس قاسه. وهذا نصّه في المقالة الأولى من كتاب المني.

---

١ أوّلا] om. B || ٣ في] ب- L || ٥ وهذا ... البدن كلّه] om. B وهذا ... موضع واحد om. BELP || ٧ منها] فيها B || ١٢ قالها] يقولها ELBP || ١٤ لمّا] لو B | عليها] عنها B || ١٦ الضعيف] الضعيفة ELBP | إذا وجد فريسته] om. EL | وجد] وجدت om. PB | فريسته] فريسة B فرسة P

(26) He says: Only the heart is the origin and root of living, but the testicles are the root and cause of living well. By as much as living well is better than plain living, by so much, among animals, are the testicles better than the heart.[85] These are the very words of this eminent, truth-seeking man, and this is his reasoning.[86]

Consider then, ye who possess insight, [whether this is correct], because if the heart would be excised from a living being, could he remain alive to live a good life? That is, could he have sexual intercourse and show his male sexual potency and not lack any vital function? But if his testicles are cut off, he remains alive as we see [in the case of] eunuchs. Are then the testicles more eminent than the heart? In short, this statement is so deficient that one does not have to refute it.

(27) In book five of *De [morborum] causis et symptomatibus*, he makes the following statement, and these are his very words: The afflictions that occur in [the case of] epilepsy are, in my opinion, caused by a surplus of phlegmatic superfluity that collects in the ventricles of the brain. Therefore, they appear suddenly and terminate suddenly. And this is something that can in no wise happen because of cold[87] of the body. These are his words there.[88]

(28) And in the third book of *De locis affectis*, he says: There are three types of epilepsy. One of these is that the illness [originates] in the brain itself, the second is that it originates from the cardia of the stomach [and ascends to the brain], and the third is that the illness ascends from any organ until it reaches the brain.[89] About the third type he states the following, and these are his words: That which arises is similar to a cold breeze. This cannot be [anything else] but a quality that arises and[90] is guided from organ to organ, or[91] some vaporous substance that comes with this quality, just as [is the case with] poison. These are his words. The point of doubt is clear: How can epilepsy be merely a dyscrasia without any substance whatsoever that happens in the brain? He himself has rejected this and said that it is not all possible.[92] This ought to be contemplated.

(٢٦) قال في القلب إنّما هو مبدأ وأصل للحياة فقط وأما الأنثيين فهما أصل وسبب لجودة الحياة. وبحسب فضل الحياة الجيّدة على الحياة المطلقة كذلك مقدار فضل البيضتين على القلب في الحيوان. هذا نصّ كلام هذا الفاضل المحقّق وهذا قياسه.

فاعتبروا يا أولو الأبصار لأنّه لو كان الحيوان يقطع قلبه فيبقى حيّا حياة جيّدة أعني أنّه يجامع وتظهر فيه قوة الذكور ولا ينقصه من أفعال الحياة شيء؟ فإذا قطعت أنثياه يبقى حيّا على ما نرى الخصيان لكانت الأنثيان أشرف من القلب؟ وبالجملة إنّ هذا الكلام من النقص في حيز لا ينبغي أن ينقض.

(٢٧) قال في المقالة الخامسة من العلل والأعراض كلاما هذا نصّه: والأعراض التي تعرض في الصرع أنا أرى أنّها إنّما تكون بسبب كثرة ما يجتمع في بطون الدماغ من الفضل البلغمي ولذلك صارت تحدث بغتة وتنقضي بغتة. وهذا شيء لا يمكن أن يكون أصلا من برودة الأجسام. هذا نصّه هناك.

(٢٨) وقال في المقالة الثالثة من التعرّف إنّ أنواع الصرع ثلاثة: أحدها أن يكون العلّة في نفس الدماغ والثاني أن يكون من أجل فم المعدة والثالث أن تكون العلّة يرتقي من عضو من الأعضاء إلى أن يصل إلى الدماغ. وقال في هذا النوع الثالث كلاما هذا نصّه: والشيء الذي يصعد شبيه بالريح الباردة وهذا لا يخلو إمّا أن يكون كيفية تصعد بالبذرقة من عضو إلى عضو وإمّا أن يكون مع الكيفية شيء من الريح على مثال ما عليه السمّ. هذا نصّه. وموضع الشكّ بيّن: كيف يكون الصرع بمجرّد سوء مزاج يحصل في الدماغ بلا مادّة أصلا وهو قد أنكر ذلك وقال أنّه لا يمكن أصلا. فيتأمّل.

---

٤ يا أولو] بأولى EL | حيّا حياة جيّدة] حيّا جيّدا L || ٥ أنّه يجامع] بأنثييه يجامع ELBP | أفعال] om. G || ٩ الفضل] الخلط LBP

(29)[93] In a number of places he says that males are warmer and drier than females, and in accordance to this [statement] he devised the fundamental principles of the entire [medical] art.[94] He adduced proof for this question and gave a lengthy explanation of it in the second book of *De semine*.[95] In his commentary on Hippocrates' book *On Women's Diseases*, he says that the rapid growth[96] of women indicates that they have extra heat that is matched by the moisture of their bodies. This is confirmed by the menstrual flow from their bodies every month, because where there is much blood, there is much heat.[97] These are his words.

If he means [with this] that the principal organs of a woman are colder and moister than those of men and that blood is more abundant in women, this is also problematic, because the vessels of men are wider. In addition, that first judgment [of his] in which he compares the female of every species with the male has a general character. Moreover, how can one conclude from a surplus of superfluities in a woman that there is [necessarily] a surplus of blood"? It seems to me that he (i.e., Galen) found this statement with another, earlier author, either with Hippocrates[98] or with one of the commentators of his books, and that he copied it once he found that commentary. He [must have] thought that it was correct, either because at that time he did not know about Aristotle's statement concerning this matter or because he had seen it but did not remember it when he commented upon this book (i.e., *On Women's Diseases*).

Listen to the wording of Aristotle's statement concerning this matter in the eighteenth book of his *De*[99] *animalibus*. He says: The heat found in female living beings is weak. However, some people assume the opposite, that is, that the blood in a female living being is more abundant than in a male one, and for this reason they think that a female living being is warmer than a male one, and this is so [according to them] because of the emission of menstrual blood—for blood is hot, and therefore that living being that has more blood has more heat. They imagine that this accident (i.e., menstruation) occurs only because of an excessive surplus of blood and heat. They also believe that all the blood can appear in this form (i.e., menstruation) and content themselves in this respect with the conclusion that it (i.e., the menstrual blood) is moist and that it has the color of blood. They do not know that pure blood that consists of good juices forms only a small part of [the menstrual blood], for menstrual blood, taken as a whole, is not pure. This is the wording of Aristotle's statement there, and it is correct, and Galen expresses himself in the same way in all his compositions.

(٢٩) قال في عدّة مواضع إنّ الذكور أسخن وأيبس من الإناث وعلى هذا مبنى الأمر في أصول الصناعة كلّها. وبرهن هذه المسألة وطوّل في بيانها في المقالة الثانية من كتاب المني. وقال في شرحه لكتاب بقراط في أوجاع النساء إنّ سرعة نشء النساء يدلّ على أنّ فيهنّ حرارة زائدة لحقتها رطوبة أبدانهنّ ويحقّق ذلك ما يجري من أبدانهنّ كلّ شهر من الطمث لأنّ حيث كثر الدم تكثر الحرارة. هذا نصّه.

فإن كان يريد أنّ أعضاء المرأة الأصلية أبرد وأرطب من أعضاء الرجال والدم في النساء أكثر فهذا أيضا مشكل إذ عروق الرجال أوسع. وأيضا فإنّ تلك القضية الأولى كلّية في مقايسة الأنثى كلّ نوع بالذكر. وأيضا كيف صار كثرة فضول النساء دليلا على كثرة الدم؟ والذي يبدو إليّ أنّ هذا الكلام وجده لغيره ممّن تقدّمه إمّا لأبقراط أو لأحد شارحي كتبه فنقله حين وجد هذا الشرح. وظنّه صحيحا إمّا بكونه لم يكن حينئذ وقف على كلام أرسطو في ذلك أو رآه ولم يذكره حين شرح هذا الكتاب.

واسمع نصّ كلام أرسطو في هذا المعنى في المقالة الثامنة عشر من كتابه في الحيوان قال: الحرارة الموجودة في الإناث ضعيفة وقد يتوهّم بعض الناس ما يضادّ ذلك أعني أنّ الدم في الأنثى أكثر منه في الذكر ولهذا السبب يظنّون أنّ الأنثى أشدّ حرارة من الذكر وذلك من قبل انبعاث دم الحيض. والدم حارّ والذي فيه دم أكثر فهو أشدّ حرارة. ويتوهّمون أنّ هذا العرض إنّما يكون من قبل إفراط زيادة الدم والحرارة ويظنّون أنّ الدم بأسره يمكن أن يكون بهذه الصورة ويكتفون في ذلك بأن يكون رطبا ويكون لونه لون الدم وليس يعلمون أنّ الدم النقي الجيّد الكيموس فيه قليل وذلك أنّه ليس دم الحيض بأسره نقيا. هذا نصّ كلام أرسطو هناك وهو الحقّ وعلى هذا جرى كلام جالينوس في جميع تآليفه.

---

١ وأيبس] كثيرا add. B || ١٠ فنقله] فنقل B | حين] حنين B حنين حين E | وجد] om. B || ١٣ ما يضادّ] ضدّ B || ١٧ ويكون لونه لون] ويكون له لون ELBP

(30) Whenever he mentions milk, in every place where he refers to it he says that it consists of three substances: the watery part, the cheesy part, and the fatty part. In *De bonis* [*malisque*] *sucis*, he makes the following statement, and these are his words: Watery moisture prevails more in the milk of camels and donkeys, cheesy [moisture prevails more] in sheep's milk, and fat in cow's milk. *De bonis* [*malisque*] *sucis*.[100] And likewise he explains in *De alimentorum* [*facultatibus*] that the fatty part—that is, the butter—prevails in cows' milk.[101] But in his treatise *De victu attenuante*, he says the following, and these are his words: And that milk in which the cheesy part greatly prevails such as cows' milk.[102] There is a point of doubt in that in the first statement he remarks that butter prevails more in cows' milk, while in the last statement he remarks that cheese dominates more in it. This ought to be contemplated.

(31) When he mentions the watery part of the milk in the tenth book of his treatise *De simplicium medicamentorum* [*temperamentis ac facultatibus*], he says the following, and these are his words: The strength of the watery part of this milk that is free from butter and cheese is that it purifies and cleanses the viscera and expels the putrefying superfluities from them, if it is imbibed or taken as an enema. It achieves this with no biting [effect]; on the contrary, it is also very effective in alleviating biting [pain]. These are his words there.[103] And in the third book of *De alimentorum* [*facultatibus*], he says the following about [the watery part of the milk], and these are his words: Do not be amazed that milk, once the watery part has been removed from it and water is again[104] added to it, has a sympathetic quality. For the physicians do this not because they shy away from the watery part of the milk but because they shy away from its sharpness, which causes the bowels to be relieved. These are his words.[105] The point of doubt is clear. In the first statement he says that it has no biting [effect] at all, but that on the contrary it alleviates [biting pain], while in the last statement he says that the watery part of milk has a sharpness that causes diarrhea. This ought to be contemplated.

(٣٠) لمّا ذكر اللبن في كلّ موضع ذكره وقال إنّ فيه ثلاثة جواهر: الجزء المائي والجزء الجبني والجزء الدسم. قال في مقالته في جودة الكيموس كلاما هذا نصّه: الأغلب على لبن اللقاح والأتن الرطوبة المائية وعلى لبن النعاج الجبنية وعلى لبن البقر الدسم. وكذلك بيّن في الأغذية أنّ الجزء الدسم وهو السمن في لبن البقر أغلب. وقال في مقالته في التدبير الملطّف كلاما هذا نصّه: وما غلب عليه من الألبان الجزء الجبني غلبة شديدة مثل لبن البقر. فموضع الشكّ كون لبن البقر يقول في الكلام الأوّل إنّ السمن أغلب عليه و يقول في الكلام الآخر إنّ الجبن أغلب فيه فيتأمّل.

(٣١) لمّا ذكر مائية اللبن في المقالة العاشرة من كتابه في الأدوية المفردة قال فيه كلاما هذا نصّه قال: فأما قوة ماء هذا اللبن الذي تخلّص من الزبد والجبن فإنّه منقّي غسّال يغسل الأحشاء و ينفي عنها الفضول العفنة إذا شرب أو احتقن به. و يفعل ذلك بغير لذع بل له أيضا في تسكين اللذع فعل جيّد. هذا نصّه هناك. وقال فيه في المقالة الثالثة من الأغذية كلاما هذا نصّه قال: ولا تعجب أنّ اللبن بعد أن يفنى ما فيه من الماء الذي هو له خاصّة يصبّ عليه من الرأس ماء آخر. وذلك أنّ الأطبّاء لم يهربوا في فعلهم هذا من رطوبة اللبن بل إنّما هربوا من حدّتها الذي بها يطلق البطن. هذا نصّه. وموضع الشكّ بيّن أنّ في كلامه الأوّل سلبه اللذع بالكلّية بل يسكن اللذع وفي الكلام الآخر قال إنّ في ماء اللبن حدّة بها يسهل. فيتأمّل.

---

٢ قال . . . الجزء الدسم ] om. EL || ٣ و كذلك بيّن في الأغذية أنّ الجزء الدسم ] om. G || ٤ السمن ] السمين EL || ٥ البقر ] هذا نصّه add B || ٦ فموضع الشكّ كون لبن البقر ] om. EL | عليه ] فيه ELBP || ١٣ يهربوا ] يتركوا L

(32) In the first book of *De naturalibus facultatibus*, he makes the following statement, and these are his words: All[106] the partly alterative faculties of the natural faculties produce the very substance of the two coats of the stomach, of the intestines, and of the uterus [and make them] what they are.[107] In the same book he also makes the following statement, and these are his words: The urinary bladder is an extremely thick and solid body, hard and consisting of two strong coats. These are his words.[108] And in the third book of this treatise he makes the following statement, and these are his words: For this reason any organ—even if it has only one coat, such as the urinary bladder, the gallbladder, the uterus, and the nonpulsatile vessels—necessarily has both kinds of fibers together, that is, those that stretch in the length (i.e., longitudinal) and those that stretch in the width (i.e., transverse).[109] The point of doubt is that whereas here he remarks that the uterus and the urinary bladder have one coat—and this is correct—in *De usu partium*, next to the earlier statement in the first book of *De [naturalibus] facultatibus*, he says they have two coats.[110] In my opinion there is no doubt that this is either an error by the translators or an error made during the copying (i.e., by the copyists).[111] If someone were to say that the urinary bladder really has only one coat, as mentioned by Galen, and that the upper coat is the membrane that covers every organ, this is problematic as well since every [organ] with two coats [also] has [this] membrane and he does not say that it has three coats. This ought to be contemplated.

(33) In the first book of *De [morborum] causis et symptomatibus*, he reviles those who sometimes call fever an illness and at other times—[namely,] when it is consequential upon a tumor—call it a symptom. He says that this is an error and that it is always an illness, and that sometimes illnesses come after other illnesses just as fever comes after a tumor.[112] And in the first book of *Ad Glauconem [de medendi methodo]*, he makes the following statement, and these are his words: Fevers that flare up from the putrefaction of the humors are especially known by this name, that is, that of fevers. They are not symptoms of other illnesses, but are illnesses themselves. These are his words.[113] One should contemplate how inconsistent he is in the terminology he uses.

(٣٢) قال في المقالة الأولى من القوى الطبيعية كلاما هذا نصّه قال: فأما جميع القوى المغيّرة الجزئية من القوى الطبيعية فهي المحدثة لنفس جوهر طبقتي المعدة وطبقتي الأمعاء وطبقتي الرحم على ما هي عليه. وقال أيضا في هذه المقالة كلاما هذا نصّه قال في المثانة إنّها جرم كثيف ملزّز بالغ الكثافة والتلزّز صلب مركّب من طبقتين قويتين. هذا نصّه. وقال في المقالة الثالثة من هذا الكتاب كلاما هذا نصّه قال: ويجب من هذا أن تكون الآلة وإن كانت إنّما لها طبقة واحدة مثل المثانة والمرارة والرحم والعروق غير الضوارب أن يكون لها الجنسان جميعا من الليف أعني الذي يمتدّ طولا والذي يمتدّ عرضا. موضع الشكّ كونه ذكر أنّ الرحم والمثانة ذات طبقة واحدة وهو الصحيح وكذلك بيّن في منافع الأعضاء وتقدّم ذكرهما هناك في أوّل القوى أنّ كلّ واحدة منهما ذات طبقتين. وهذا عندي من غلط المترجمين بلا شكّ أو من غلط النسخ. فإن قال قائل إنّ الطبقة الواحدة هي الخصيصة بالمثانة كما قد ذكر ذلك جالينوس والطبقة الفوقانية هي من الغشاء الذي يغشى كلّ عضو فهذا مشكل إذ كلّ ذي طبقتين عليه غشاء ولا يقال فيه إنّه ذو ثلاثة طبقات. فيتأمّل.

(٣٣) في المقالة الأولى من العلل والأعراض يشنّع على القوم الذي يسمّون الحمّى مرّة مرضا ويسمّونها إذا كانت تابعة لورم عرضا وقال إنّ هذا خطأ وإنّما هي أبدا مرض. وقد تتبع الأمراض أمراض آخر كما يتبع الحمّى الورم. وقال في المقالة الأولى من أغلوقن كلاما هذا نصّه قال: وأما الحمّيات التي تهيج عن عفونة الأخلاط فإنّها تعرف بهذا الاسم أعني اسم الحمّيات وليست هي بأعراض لأمراض آخر لكنّها هي أنفسها أمراض. هذا نصّه. فيتأمّل كيف ناقض أوضاعه في الأسميات.

---

٦ واحدة] om. G ‖ ٨ كونه] om. G ‖ ١٠ المترجمين] المخرجين ELBP | النسخ] الناسخ EL ‖ ١٦ تهيج ... هذا نصّه] تحدث من الأورام وكإنّما أعراض تابعة لتلك الأعضاء التي تحدث فيها الأورام EL

(34) In the second book of *De alimentorum* [*facultatibus*], he makes the following statement about citron [*Citrus medica*] peels, and these are his words: When used as a medicine, they are good for the digestion just as many other things that have a sharp, acrid quality.[114] And in the seventh book of *De simplicium medicamentorum* [*temperamentis ac facultatibus*], he says the following, and these are his words: Citron peels have no cooling [effect] but a moderate [effect] or a little less than moderate.[115] The point of doubt is that there he describes them as being among the sharp, acrid things, but here [he describes them as being] among the moderate things.

(35) When speaking about honey in the end of *De alimentorum* [*facultatibus*], he mentions the bile whose color is pale yellow and the bile whose color is yellow and remarks that there are other types of yellow bile besides these two. Then he says the following, and these are his words: We see with our own eyes how all these other types, except for the leek-green one, are evacuated from the body in the case of a severe and serious illness. Yellow bile, pale-yellow bile, and leek-green bile are often expelled through emesis and diarrhea while there is no illness.[116] This is a clearly defined formulation [as it can be found] in ancient writings. The point of doubt is how he [first] stipulated in the case of leek-green [bile] that it is only emitted in a severe, serious illness and then remarks that the leek-green [bile] is [often] emitted without any illness. If we try to explain [the contradiction by saying] that the meaning of his words is that in [the case] of a severe, serious illness there is no leek-green [bile] and therefore it does not emerge and is not seen, this is even more problematic in trying to provide a reason for this. To sum up, [it may be said that] it is a point that should be contemplated.

(٣٤) في المقالة الثانية من الأغذية قال في قشر الأترجّ كلاما هذا نصّه قال: فأما إن استعمل على طريق الدواء فهو ينفع في الاستمراء كما ينفع في ذلك أشياء آخر كثيرة ممّا له كيفية حادّة حرّيفة. وقال في المقالة السابعة من الأدوية المفردة كلاما هذا نصّه: فأما قشر الأترجّ فليس هو ببارد لكنّه إمّا معتدل وإمّا دون الاعتدال بشيء يسير. موضع الشكّ كونه وصفه هناك مع الأشياء الحادّة الحرّيفة وهنا مع المعتدلة.

(٣٥) قال في آخر الأغذية عند كلامه على العسل لمّا ذكر المرّة التي لونها أصفر والتي لونها أحمر وذكر أنّ للصفراء أنواع آخر غير هذين قال كلاما هذا نصّه قال: وهذه الأنواع الآخر كلّها نراها عيانا تستفرغ من البدن خلا المرّة الكرّاثية فكثيرا ما تخرج بالقيء والإسهال من غير مرض. هذا النصّ المحدّد من الكتب القديمة. موضع الشكّ كيف اشترط في الكرّاثية أنّها لا تخرج إلا في مرض صعب شديد ثمّ ذكر أنّ الكرّاثية تخرج من غير مرض. فإن تأوّلنا أنّ معنى قوله في المرض الصعب الشديد لا توجد الكرّاثية فلذلك لا تبرز ولا ترى كان هذا أيضا أشدّ إشكالا في إعطاء سبب ذلك وبالجملة هو موضع تأمّل.

---

٥ مع] مثل LEBP || ٩ تخرج] om. B || ١٠ مرض] موضع ELP || ١١ قوله] أنّ add. ELP

(36) In the sixteenth book of *De usu partium*, he says the following, and these are his words: No special, separate nerve was made to reach the skin, but it is reached by certain subdivisions of the nerves from the parts that lie beneath it. These subdivisions go to these parts in order that they are bonds between the skin and the parts beneath it and serve as sensory organs for them.[117] These are his words there. And in the end of book three of *De locis affectis*, he says the following, and these are his words: The physicians do not at all know that the nerves that are spread and distributed in the skin of the entire hand and provide it with sensation have special roots, and that the nerves for the movement of the muscles of the hand have other roots.[118] These are his words as well. The point of doubt is very clear in that in *De usu partium* he definitely states that the nerves of the skin are only [subdivisions] of the nerves that reach the muscles beneath the skin. And here in book three of *De locis affectis*, he says that the nerves that reach the skin of the hand are different from the nerves that reach the muscles that move the hand. I wish I knew whether this applies only to the hand among all the organs and [if this is the case] why he did not mention it.

(37) Says Moses: In my opinion, his statement in *De usu partium* is correct. The fact that the organ hidden beneath the skin can lose its sensation but not its motion is not caused by the nerves that are [inserted into] the muscle of that organ and that provide it with motion, but by the very nerves themselves (i.e., the part not inserted into the muscle), as he states in *De usu [partium]*. However, an affliction occurs in the ends of that fine nerve that is distributed in the skin, and therefore the sensation of the skin is abolished, but that affliction does not reach the root of that nerve—the root that is [inserted] in the muscle—and therefore motion is not abolished. This is in accordance with the principal rules that Galen taught us, namely, that the loss [of function] of a branch does not damage the root, but that the abolishment of the root necessarily causes loss [of function] of the branch.

(٣٦) قال في المقالة السادسة عشر من منافع الأعضاء كلاما هذا نصّه قال: لم يجعل للجلد عصبة تأتيه مفردة له خاصّة بل إنّما يأتيه من الأعضاء المستبطنة له أقسام من أقسام العصب التي يأتيها تكون رباطا للجلد بما يستبطنه من الأعضاء وتقوم له مقام آلة يحسّ بها. هذا نصّه هناك. وقال في آخر المقالة الثالثة من التعرّف كلاما هذا نصّه قال: والأطبّاء لا يعلمون بتّة أنّ العصب الذي ينبثّ ويتفرّق في جلدة اليد كلّها ويصل إليها منه الحسّ له أصول خاصّية به والعصب الذي يحرّك عضل اليد له أصول آخر غير تلك. هذا نصّه أيضا. وموضع الشكّ بيّن جدّا وهو أنّه أطلق القضية في منافع الأعضاء بأنّ عصب الجلد إنّما هو من العصب الذي يأتي العضل المستبطن للجلد. وهنا في ثالث التعرّف يقول إنّ عصبا يأتي الجلد من اليد غير العصب الذي يأتي العضل المحرّك لليد. ويا ليت شعري هل هذا شيء يخصّ اليد من بين سائر الأعضاء وكيف لم يذكر ذلك؟

(٣٧) قال موسى: الصحيح عندي هو ما ذكره في منافع الأعضاء وكون العضو المستور من الجلد يبطل حسّه ولا تبطل حركته ليس علّة ذلك كون العصبة المبثوثة في عضل ذلك العضو الذي يفيده الحركة بل هي العصبة بعينها كما ذكر في المنافع. لكنّ حلّت الآفة في أطراف تلك العصبة الدقيقة المبثوثة في الجلد ولذلك بطل حسّ الجلد ولم تصل الآفة إلى أصل العصبة المبثوث ذلك الأصل في العضل ولذلك لم تبطل الحركة. وهذا جار على الأصول التي علّمناها جالينوس وهو أنّ بطلان الفرع لا يضرّ بالأصل وبطلان الأصل يلزم عنه بطلان الفرع.

---

٥ اليد] الكف EL || ٨ المستبطن . . . العضل] om. B || ١١ المستور] المبطور (!)L || ١٢ من الجلد] بالجلد SG | عضل] om. L ?E || ١٦ وهو . . . (٤٠) محالة إلا] om. B

(38) In the first book of *De* [*morborum*] *causis et symptomatibus*, he says the following, and these are his words: These humors are mixed with one another, and one only rarely finds one of them that is pure not mixed with another one.[119] And in the second book of *De* [*morborum*] *causis et symptomatibus*, he says the following, and these are his words: Every singular one of these humors often streams to the organs while it is pure and unadulterated, not mixed with anything else. Sometimes, however, they stream [into them], mixed with one another.[120] These are his words there. The point of doubt is clear, namely, that in the first statement he considers the existence of one of the humors in a pure unadulterated form as a rare [phenomenon], but then he remarks in the second statement that more often [one finds one of them] streaming in an unadulterated form and that only occasionally one finds them mixed. What I observe constantly is [in agreement with] what he says in the first statement. This ought to be contemplated.

(39) In his treatise *De atra bile*, he makes the following statement, and these are his words: Black chymes are often excreted with vomiting or diarrhea, and this can in some cases be a good sign. But when black bile is excreted with vomiting or diarrhea, it indicates death because its development in the body is a fatal sign.[121] These are his words.[122] He makes it absolutely clear in that statement that the appearance of this humor is a sign of death and that ignorant[123] physicians think that the emission of this malicious humor is a good thing, but that this is not the case.[124] In his commentary on the fourth [book] of [Hippocrates'] *Aphorisms*, he states the following, and these are his words: Therefore black bile (and every other humor with a similar bad condition), if it appears at the end of the illness once signs of coction have become visible, it indicates that its evacuation has a wholesome [effect].[125] These are his words there as well. The point of doubt is clear, namely, that in this last statement he stipulates that the appearance of black bile after coction is a good sign, while in the first statement he states in a definite and absolute way that its excretion indicates death. It seems to me that the statement he makes in *De atra bile* is correct and that the statement he makes in his commentary on [the fourth book] of [Hippocrates'] *Aphorisms* is only correct for the other black humors but not for black bile. One should contemplate this matter very well.

(٣٨) في المقالة الأولى من العلل والأعراض قال كلاما هذا نصّه قال: هذه الأخلاط يخالط بعضها بعضا ولا يكاد تجد واحدا منها خالصا لا يخالطه غيره إلا في الندرة. وقال في ثانية العلل والأعراض كلاما هذا نصّه قال: وكلّ واحد من هذه الأخلاط كثيرا ما ينصبّ إلى الأعضاء محضا صرفا لا يخالطه شيء وربّما انصبّت مختلطة بعضها مع بعض. هذا نصّه هناك. وموضع الشكّ بيّن وهو كونه يجعل في القول الأوّل وجود واحد من الأخلاط خالصا محضا نادرا. ثمّ يقول في الثانية إنّ انصبابه محضا هو الأكثري وربّما وجد مختلطا. والذي نشاهده دائما هو ما قاله في الأوّلى. فيتأمّل.

(٣٩) في مقالته في المرّة السوداء قال كلاما هذا نصّه قال: كثيرا ما يخرج بالقيء والإسهال كيموسات سود وقد يدلّ خروجها على خير عدّة مرّات. وأما المرّة السوداء فهي إن خرجت بالقيء أو بالإسهال دلّت على الهلاك لأنّ تولّدها في البدن هو دليل الهلاك. هذا نصّه. وبيّن في ذلك الموضع غاية البيان أنّ ظهور هذا الخلط هي علامة الهلاك وأنّ جهّال الأطبّاء يظنون أنّ خروج هذا الخلط الرديء أمر نافع وليس الأمر كذلك. وقال جالينوس في شرحه لرابعة الفصول كلاما هذا نصّه قال: ولذلك صارت المرّة السوداء وكلّ خلط هو في الرداءة على مثل حالها إذا ظهر في آخر المرض بعد ظهور علامات النضج دلّ على أنّ استفراغه محمود. هذا نصّه هناك أيضا. موضع الشكّ بيّن وهو إشراطه في هذا الكلام الآخر بأنّ ظهور المرّة السوداء بعد النضج دليل محمود و إطلاقه القضية الكلّية في المرّة السوداء في الكلام الأوّل بأنّها متى خرجت دلّت على الهلاك. والذي يبدو إليّ هو أنّ كلامه الذي ذكر في مقالته في المرّة السوداء هو الصحيح وهذا الكلام الذي ذكره في شرح الفصول إنّما هو يصحّ في سائر الأخلاط السود لا في المرّة السوداء. فينبغي أن يتأمّل هذا جدّا.

٦ الأكثري] الابتداء E? L || ٩ فهي إن] فمتى BP || ١٦ بأنّها] فإنّها G

(40) In the second [book] of *De temperamentis*, he says the following, and these are his words: Of humors the most appropriate for the nature [of human beings] and the most beneficial is blood. Black bile is like a sediment and dregs of blood, and therefore it is colder and thicker than blood. Yellow bile is much hotter and drier than blood. Phlegm is colder and moister than all the [humors] in the body of a living being. The[126] instrument to measure this as well is the sense of touch.[127] These are his words. In [book] two of *De* [*morborum*] *causis et symptomatibus*, he says the following, and these are his words: That[128] which pours must inevitably and unavoidably be moist and fluid in its appearance, although it is not absolutely necessary that it is moist in its potency. Ancient physicians and philosophers speak about the potency of such humors. I too have commented upon [the matter of] this potency in the books[129] in which I describe the subject of medicines and in other books. But what I need for my present subject in this book is what I am going to say now, namely, that the potency of yellow bile is hot and dry, [that of] black bile is cold and dry, [that of] blood is hot and moist, and [that of] phlegm is cold and moist.[130] These are his words as well. The point of doubt is that in *De temperamentis* he explains that yellow [bile] is hot and dry as[131] it is measured with the sense [of touch], while here he says that it has [these qualities] potentially. The same is true for the other [three] humors: it is clear from his words in *De temperamentis* that these qualities are ascribed to them actually. But here he says that they are attributed [to them] potentially. This ought to be contemplated.

(41) In his commentary on [Hippocrates'] treatise *De natura hominis*, he says the following, and these are his words: I explained in my book *De temperamentis* that spring is moderate, while Hippocrates[132] says here that it is hot and moist.[133] The[134] matter is according to Hippocrates' statement. And in the first book of his commentary on Hippocrates' *De aeris aquis locis*, he says that spring is hot and moist with regard to its essence, [but] moderate in relation to the human body.[135]

(42) Says Moses: This last statement is correct. He did not formulate all his previous statements as accurately as he did this last statement.

(٤٠) قال في ثانية المزاج كلاما هذا نصّه قال: فأما الأخلاط فأطيبها وألأمها بالطبيعة الدم. وأما المرّة السوداء فهي كالثفل والدردي للدم ولذلك صارت أبرد وأغلظ من الدم. وأما المرّة الصفراء فهي أسخن كثيرا وأجفّ من الدم. وأما البلغم فهو أبرد وأرطب من جميع ما في بدن الحيوان والسبار في تعرّف هذا أيضا هو حسّ اللمس. هذا نصّه. وقال في ثانية العلل والأعراض كلاما هذا نصّه قال: الشيء المنصبّ لا بدّ من أن يكون في منظره رطبا جاريا لا محالة إلا أنّه ليس يجب أن يكون لا محالة رطبا في قوتة. وقد ذكر قوة الرطوبات التي حالها هذا الحال قدماء الأطبّاء والفلاسفة وبيّنّا نحن أيضا هذه القوة في الكتب التي وصفت فيها أمر الأدوية وفي كتب آخر. والذي يحتاج إليه من ذلك في هذا الكتاب الذي نحن فيه أنا ذاكره هاهنا وهو أنّ المرّة الصفراء قوتها حارّة يابسة والمرّة السوداء باردة يابسة والدم حارّ رطب والبلغم بارد رطب. هذا نصّه أيضا. وموضع الشكّ كونه بيّن في المزاج أنّ الصفراء حارّة يابسة بسبار الحسّ وهنا يقول إنّها بالقوة. وكذلك بقية الأخلاط الأربعة تبيّن من كلامه في المزاج أنّها توصّفت بتلك الكيفيات بالفعل وههنا يقول إنّها توصّفت كذلك بالقوة. فيتأمّل.

(٤١) قال جالينوس في شرحه لكتاب طبيعة الإنسان كلاما هذا نصّه قال: قد بيّنّا في كتاب المزاج أنّ الربيع معتدل وأبقراط يقول ههنا إنّه حارّ رطب. والأمر على ما يقول أبقراط فيه. وقال في شرحه لكتاب الأهوية والمياه والبلدان في المقالة الأولى إنّ الربيع حارّ رطب باعتبار ذاته معتدل بالإضافة لبدن الإنسان.

(٤٢) قال موسى: هذا الكلام الأخير هو الحقّ. وما تقدّم من قوليه جميعا فلم يحرّره كما حرّر في هذا الكلام الأخير.

---

٨ نحن فيه] om. EL | أنا] اذا (!)B || ١٥ الربيع . . . الإنسان] الربيع حارّ رطب وليس هو على هذا إن استقصى مستقص استقصاء شافيا .C, fol. 30v 12sq || ١٦ بالإضافة ل-] باضافته إلى ELBP || ١٧ الكلام الأخير] om. ELBP | وما . . . الأخير] om. L | يحرّره] يحرسه B

(43) When he describes in the seventh book of *De methodo medendi* the case of the man whose stomach was dried by the physicians [to a degree] that he suffered from marasmus, he says the following, and these are his words: Then, when they finally saw that his stomach could not digest any food at all, they prompted him to drink tanner's sumac[136] [*Rhus coriaria*] juice and put all[137] those medications on the outside of his stomach, which I mentioned before. By doing this they[138] made him like someone whose body was wasted away and depleted of moisture until he was as if he were dead. When I was charged with the treatment of this man, I started to moisten him in any possible way.[139] These are his words.

When he started to mention the treatment of that man, he made the following statement, and these are his words: Just as I treated that man whom the physicians had dried out [and] who in terms of heat and cold was healthy since none of these prevailed over him, neither in his body in general nor in his stomach, but he suffered from extreme dryness, emaciation, and leanness of the body.[140] These too are his words concerning this man. The point of doubt is very clear. How can a person whose body has become so utterly dry that he is like dead—as he says—have a moderate [constitution] between heat and cold? Rather, his body should be cold since the substance of the innate heat has dissipated.

In his discussion of this very same man in this treatise, he says the following, and these are his words: It is impossible that dryness remain on its own and by itself while heat and cold are counterbalanced without any blemish,[141] for organs, if not nourished, become cold very rapidly.[142] These too are his words there, and this is correct. But when he remarked in his earlier statement about this man that he was healthy in terms of heat and cold in his body, he started to correct this with the following words: But in this case I only treated, as I said, from the beginning of the matter the dryness that prevailed on its own and by itself and that persisted for a long time without being followed by cold of a perceptible size.[143] This is the end of his statement there in his own words.

(٤٣) المقالة السابعة من كتاب حيلة البرء لمّا ذكر فيها حال الرجل الذي جفّف الأطبّاء معدته حتّى ذبل قال فيها كلاما هذا نصّه قال: ثمّ أنّهم بآخره لمّا رأوا أنّ معدته ليس تستمرئ طعاما بتّة حملوه على شرب عصارة السمّاق ووضعوا على معدته من خارج جميع الأدوية التي ذكرتها قبل فصيّروه بذلك في حدّ من قد بلي وفنيت رطوبة بدنه حتّى صار كأنّه ميّت. فلمّا تولّيت أنا مداواة هذا الرجل جعلت أرطّبه بكلّ ضرب. هذا نصّه.

ولمّا أخذ في ذكر تدبير هذا الرجل قال أيضا كلاما هذا نصّه قال: على مثال ما دوينا نحن هذا الرجل الذي كان الأطبّاء قد يبّسوه فإنّه كان من طريق الحرّ والبرد سليما ليس يغلب عليه ولا واحد منهما لا في جملة بدنه ولا في معدته إلا أنّه كان من اليبس ونحافة البدن وقضفه في الغاية. هذا أيضا نصّه في هذا الرجل. وموضع الشكّ بيّن جدّا كيف يكون شخص جفّ في الغاية حتّى صار كالميّت كما ذكر ويكون معتدلا بين الحرّ والبرد؟ بل يبرد جسمه ضرورة لأنّ مادّة الحرارة الغريزية قد ذهبت.

وقد قال في هذه المقالة في حديثه في هذا الرجل بعينه هذا النصّ قال: ليس يمكن أن يبقى اليبس على حدته مفردا وتكون الحرارة والبرد متكافيتين لا يذمّ من أمرهما شيء لأنّ الأعضاء إذا لم تغتذ بردت في أسرع الأوقات. هذا نصّه أيضا هناك وهذا هو الحقّ. ولمّا تذكّر ما تقدّم له من قوله في هذا الرجل أنّه كان من الحرّ والبرد سليما أخذ أن يستدرك ذلك بهذا النصّ قال: ولكنّ نحن على ما قلنا منذ أوّل الأمر داوينا ههنا يبسا غلب وحده مفردا ولبث مدّة صالحة من غير أن تتبعه برودة ذات قدر يعتدّ به. هذا آخر كلامه هناك بنصّه.

---

٥ جعلت] رجعت B || ٧ فإنّه] om. G || ٨ بدنه] جسمه B || ١٥ أنّه] om. G | من] بين ELBP || ١٦ نحن] يجب GS نحن $S^2$ | داوينا] نحن add. S | ههنا] om. EL del. G نحن $G^1$ | مفردا] مفرطا B

I am [even] more doubtful [now]. I wish I knew [the answer to the following]: If in the case of someone whose [body] has become so dry that it is as if he is dead, there is no cold discernible in him, what is then the case of dryness that is necessarily followed by [perceptible] cold? Would you consider it to occur once he has died—being old and decayed? Even more amazing is his statement about him that he became utterly emaciated because of lack of food, while he says here that the organs, if they are not nourished, become cold very quickly. In general, this last statement is correct; there is no doubt about it.

(44) In the treatise *De pulsu parva*, he says the following, and these are his words: When the affliction is minor, it makes the pulse regularly unequal, and when the affliction is major, it makes the pulse [have] an irregular inequality.[144] These are his words there. In the fourteenth book of *De pulsu magno*, he makes the following statement, and these are his words: An irregularly unequal pulse indicates that the cause of the inequality shifts [from organ to organ] and is not stable. The illness may shift to an inferior organ and the patient is spared. But it may also shift to a noble organ and he dies. Therefore, one cannot use the irregularity [of the unequal pulse] as a genuine prognostic [sign].[145] This is his formulation, and the point of doubt is clear and evident. For in the first statement he declares positively that irregularity [of the unequal pulse] indicates that the affliction is a major one, and in this last statement he says that it is neither a good nor a bad sign. The doubt can be solved by saying: Irregularity [of an unequal pulse] indicates that the current affliction is severe but that one cannot know what will really be in the end. This too ought to be contemplated.

(45) In his treatise *De morborum temporibus*, he starts to explain that every illness from which one can be healed has four stages—beginning, increase, climax, and decline—and that in the case of some illnesses one thinks because of their short beginning that they do not have a beginning, while they do have a beginning without any doubt, but only a very short one. He then says the following, and these are his words: We find [that in the case of] an illness that is extremely detrimental—namely, apoplexy—its beginning and increase take place in a short time. The same holds true for epilepsy.[146] These are his words, and this statement is true without any doubt.

وقد زاد الشكّ يا ليت شعري إذا كان الذي يبس حتّى صار كأنّه ميّت لم يتبيّن فيه البرد فما هو اليبس الذي يتبعه البرد ضرورة أتراه بعد أن صار ميّتا رميما. وأعجب من هذا قوله فيه أنّه صار في غاية النحافة لعدم الغذاء وهو القائل هنا إنّ الأعضاء إذ لم تغتذي بردت في أسرع الأوقات. وبالجملة فإنّ هذا الكلام الأخير حقّا لا ريب فيه.

(٤٤) في كتاب النبض الصغير قال كلاما هذا نصّه: متى كانت الآفة يسيرة جعلت النبض مختلفا منتظما ومتى كانت الآفة عظيمة جعلت النبض مختلفا غير منتظم. هذا نصّه هناك. وقال في رابعة عشر النبض الكبير كلاما هذا نصّه: النبض المختلف اختلافا غير منتظم يدلّ على أنّ سبب الاختلاف منتقل غير ثابت. فقد تنتقل العلّة إلى عضو خسيس فيتخلّص المريض أو ينتقل إلى عضو شريف فيهلك المريض. فليس يستدلّ إذا من خلاف النظام على شيء حقيقي. هذا نصّه وموضع الشكّ بيّن واضح لأنّ في الكلام الأوّل قطع بأنّ خلاف المنتظم يدلّ على عظم الآفة وفي هذا الكلام الأخير قال إنّه لا يدلّ على خير ولا شرّ. وقد يحلّ الشكّ بأن يقال إنّ اختلاف النظام يدلّ على أنّ الآفة الموجودة الآن عظيمة ما يعلم مآلها الحقيقي لأيّ شيء يؤول. فيتأمّل أيضا.

(٤٥) في مقالته في أوقات الأمراض أخذ أن يبيّن أنّ كلّ مرض يبرأ منه له الأربعة الأوقات ابتداء وتزيّد وانتهاء وانحطاط وأنّ بعض الأمراض لقصر زمان الابتداء فيها يظنّ فيها أنّها لا ابتداء لها وهي بلا شكّ لها ابتداء وإنّما هو قصير جدّا. وقال كلاما هذا نصّه قال: نجد المرض الذي يكون في غاية الشدّة وهو السكتة ابتداؤه وصعوده في مدّة قصيرة وكذلك الصرع. هذا نصّه وهو كلام صحيح لا شكّ فيه.

---

٢ صار] يصير ELBP | ميّتا] om. ELBP | رميما] ذميما ELBP || ١٥ وانتهاء] ومنتهى EL

In the first book of the treatise *De crisibus*, when he began to explain that from the nature of an illness one can draw conclusions about its length or brevity, he makes the following statement, and these are his words: In the same way, in the case of the other illnesses, one can draw conclusions about their duration. Hectic fever, pleurisy, and pneumonia have a short beginning, but epilepsy, sciatica, arthritis, and nephritis have a long beginning. These are his words there.[147]

The point of doubt is that [in this last statement] he makes the beginning of epilepsy long. What does he mean with this statement? If he means the beginning of an epileptic fit, it is impossible that the time is shorter than that, for then it would be imperceptible, as he explained in the beginning of his statement in that treatise (i.e., *De morborum temporibus*). And if he means the beginning of the cause that produces epilepsy, [the question arises] as to what the observation of this matter has to do with the definition of the stages of an illness. The most probable [solution] in my opinion is that the epilepsy mentioned in *De crisibus* is originally a mistake by the copyist.[148]

(46) In the fourth book of *De simplicium medicamentorum [temperamentis ac facultatibus]*, he says the following, and these are his words: A similar [effect] as iron and a stone heated in the fire and the like is achieved by the drugs that kill through the corrosion they cause when they are brought to [the same degree of] heat as the body has. Examples are yellow[149] vitriol, green[150] vitriol, red[151] vitriol, and quicksilver, for all such drugs that are coarse and have a hot potency burn the stomach and the adjoining parts of the abdomen.[152] These are his words there.

And in the ninth book [of the same treatise], when speaking about quicksilver, he says: I [do not know from] testing or experience if it is fatal when it is ingested nor what effect it has if it is applied externally to the body. These, too, are his words concerning quicksilver. I wish I knew who is the [authority] he relies on for the judgment he passes on quicksilver in the fourth [book], namely, that it kills by burning just like the [different] types of vitriol.

وقال في المقالة الأولى من كتاب البحران لمّا أخذ أن يبيّن أنّ من طبيعة الأمراض يستدلّ على طول أوقات المرض أو قصرها قال كلاما هذا نصّه قال: وعلى هذا المثال يمكنك أن تستدلّ في سائر الأمراض على أوقاتها. فإنّ الحمّى المحرقة وذات الجنب وذات الرئة ابتداؤها قصير. وأما الصرع ووجع النساء ووجع المفاصل ووجع الكلى فإنّ ابتداؤها طويل. هذا نصّه هناك.

وموضع الشكّ كونه يجعل ابتداء الصرع طويلا أيّ شيء يريد بهذا القول؟ إن كان يريد به ابتداء نوبة الصرع فلا يمكن أن يكون زمان أقصر منه وهو غير محسوس كما بيّن في كلامه الأوّل في تلك المقالة. وإن كان يريد به ابتداء السبب المولّد للصرع فما هذا المعنى الملحوظ في تحديد أوقات الأمراض. والأقرب عندي أنّ هذا الصرع المقول في البحران غلط ناسخه في الأصل.

(٤٦) في الرابعة من كتاب الأدوية المفردة قال كلاما هذا نصّه قال: ونظير الحديد والحجر المحمّى بالنار وشبههما الأدوية التي تقتل بما تحدثه من التأكّل عندما تخرجها إلى تلك الحرارة التي في البدن بمنزلة القلقطار والزاج الأخضر والأحمر والزيبق لأنّ كلّ ما هذا سبيله من الأدوية التي هي غليظة وقوتها قوة حارّة تحرق المعدة وما يليها من البطن. هذا نصّه هناك.

وقال في التاسعة من هذا الكتاب عند كلامه على الزيبق: ليس عندي فيه محنة ولا تجربة هل يقتل إن شرب ولا ما الذي يفعل إن وضع من خارج البدن. هذا أيضا نصّه في الزيبق. فيا ليت شعري ذلك الحكم الذي حكم على الزيبق في الرابعة أنّه يقتل بالحرق كأنواع الزاج إلى من يستند فيه.

١ يستدلّ] تشتدّ G || ١٢ التي] لا add. G || ١٨ إلى] الذي G

(47) He says the following in the eleventh book of *De methodo* [*medendi*], and these are his words: It is most beneficial, as I have stated, to apply venesection not only in continuous fevers but in all fevers that arise from putrefaction of the humors.[153]

(48) Says Moses: One may doubt [Galen's] approval of venesection in [the case of] all putrid fevers. In his treatise *De venae sectione* and other places, he [himself] forbids venesection in pure phlegmatic fever because the humors are raw and crude.[154] He also forbids bloodletting in pure quartan fever, unless there is a clear indication for excess of blood.[155] To solve this doubt, it seems to me that when he speaks about all fevers that arise from putrefaction of the humors, he means that the putrefying substance consists of many humors and not one unadulterated humor. Thus, the meaning [of his words] is that [in the case of] every fever that arises from putrefaction of the blood, although that putrefying blood is mixed with an [even] larger quantity of phlegm or black [bile], venesection is beneficial. But if only the phlegm or the black [bile] putrefies, one should not apply venesection. But he would still be inconsistent [in his statements] if he used the following words: However, all fevers arising from putrefaction of one single putrid humor, whatever humor it may be.

(49) In the sixth book of *De simplicium medicamentorum* [*temperamentis ac facultatibus*], while discussing the plant [called] Roman nettle [*Urtica pilulifera* and var.] when he mentions the benefits of its seed and leaves, Galen says the following, and these are his words: Moreover, they both have flatulent strength, and for this reason they stimulate the sexual lust, especially when the seed of this plant is ingested with concentrated grape juice.[156] These are his words. When he describes the effects of this plant in more detail, he makes the following statement, and these are his words: The flatulence that I said is produced develops only from the plant when it is digested in the stomach. The reason for this is that [this plant] is not flatulent actually but only potentially.[157] These are his words.

(٤٧) قال في المقالة الحادية عشر من الحيلة كلاما هذا نصّه قال: الأجود على ما قلت أن يفصد العرق ليس في الحمّيات المطبقة فقط ولكنّ في جميع الحمّيات الحادثة عن عفونة الأخلاط.

(٤٨) قال موسى: قد يتشكّك الإنسان في استحسانه الفصد في جميع الحمّيات العفنية وقد نهى في مقالته في الفصد وفي مواضع آخر عن الفصد في الحمّى البلغمية المحضة إذ والأخلاط نيئة فجّة. وكذلك ينهى عن الفصد في حمّى الربع المحضة إلا أن تظهر علامة كثرة الدم. ويبدو لي في حلّ هذا الشكّ أنّه أراد بقوله في جميع الحمّيات الحادثة عن عفونة الأخلاط أن يكون الشيء العفن أخلاطا كثيرة لا خلط واحد محض. فيكون المعنى أنّ كلّ حمّى حادثة عن عفن الدم وإن كان البلغم هو الأكثر في ذلك الدم العفن أو السوداء فإنّه ينفع الفصد. أما إذا عفن البلغم وحده أو السوداء وحدها فلا يفصد. وإنّما كان يلزمه التناقض لو قال بهذا النصّ: ولكنّ جميع الحمّيات الحادثة عن عفونة أيّ خلط عفن من أحد الأخلاط.

(٤٩) قال جالينوس في المقالة السادسة من الأدوية المفردة عند كلامه على نبات الأنجرة لمّا ذكر منافع بزره وورقه قال كلاما هذا نصّه: وفيهما مع هذا قوة نافخة بسببها صارا يهيّجان شهوة الجماع وخاصّة متى شرب البزر من هذا النبات مع عقيد العنب. هذا نصّه. ولمّا أمعن في وصف أفعال هذا النبات قال كلاما هذا نصّه: وأما النفخة التي قلنا إنّه يولّدها فإنّما تتولّد منه عندما ينهضم في المعدة وذلك لأنّه ليس هو نافخا بالفعل بل نافخ بالقوة. هذا نصّه.

---

٩ وإن... الدم العفن] om. B | هو الأكثر] والأكثر EL أو الأكثر P || ١٠ وإنّما] والا B || ١٦ وذلك] وكذلك SG | هو] هذا G

(50) Says Moses: I can in no way understand what he said about this matter or what he is trying to say, and the way he expresses himself is confusing for the translator. The point of doubt is his statement that it is flatulent potentially but not actually; that is to say that any [substance] is flatulent only potentially but not actually, neither this plant nor any other flatulent one. But how does he conceive that a drug can actually be flatulent? He himself explained for us in a previous chapter of this book that any property that is ascribed to a drug—as when we say that it is hot or cold—refers only to its potential [effect], [but] not to the sensation of that drug as hot or cold. However, the heat of our body actualizes what is potentially in it. This ought to be contemplated.

(51) In the third book of his *In Timaeum commentarius*, Galen explains that only the liver transforms the food into blood and that the body of the vessels that contain the blood do not convert it into something bloodlike. He says with the following words: We find that every bodily organ that feeds itself with blood transforms its nourishment and makes it similar to its substance so that, if it is completely without blood like bones, cartilage, nerves, ligaments, tendons, and membranes, it transforms the blood into its [own] nature. How is it then possible that the body of a vessel produces blood, since it is white and a type of membrane, so that it nourishes only itself by altering and transforming the food into its own nature? These words are sufficient [to conclude] that it is the liver that transforms the food into blood.[158] Thus far his words.[159]

(52) In the third book of *De locis affectis*, when speaking about the pain of migraine, Galen states the following: If the pain is caused by wind, the patient feels a tension; if it originates from a surplus of superfluities, the patient also feels heaviness.[160] In his treatise *De venae sectione*, he says the following, and these are his words: A special sign for the kind of overfilling that is commensurate to strength is weight, and [a special sign] for the kind of overfilling that is commensurate to the vessels is tension.[161]

(٥٠) قال موسى: لم أقدر أن أعلم بوجه أيّ شيء قال في هذا المعنى أو أيّ شيء أراد أن يقول فتشوّشت العبارة على المترجم. وموضع الشكّ قوله نافخ بالقوة لا نافخ بالفعل وذلك أنّ كلّ نافخ إنّما هو نافخ بالقوة لا بالفعل لا هذا النبات ولا غيره ممّا ينفخ. وكيف يتصوّر أن يكون دواء نافخا بالفعل وهو قد بيّن لنا في ما تقدّم من مقالات هذا الكتاب أنّ كلّ صفة يوصف بها الدواء مثل قولنا حارّ وبارد إنّما ذلك بالقوة لا أنّ مجسّة الدواء حارّة أو باردة. وإنّما حرارة أبدانا تخرج ما فيه بالقوة الى الفعل. فيتأمّل.

(٥١) بيّن جالينوس في المقالة الثالثة من تفسيره لكتاب طيماوس أنّ الكبد وحدها هي التي تحيل الغذاء دما وأنّ جرم العروق الحاوية للدم لا تحيله للدموية. قال بهذا النصّ: نجد كلّ واحد من أعضاء البدن وهو يغتذي من الدم يحيل غذاءه فيشبهه بجرمه حتّى أنّه إن كان عديما للدم أصلا على مثال العظم والغضروف والعصبة والرباط والوترة والغشاء يحيل الدم إلى طبيعته. فكيف يمكن إذا أن يولّد بدن العرق دما وهو أبيض من جنس الأغشية على أنّه إنّما يغتذي بأن يحيل الغذاء ويغيّره إلى طبيعته؟ فهذا القول يكتفى به في أنّ الكبد هي التي تحيله إلى الدم. إلى هنا نصّ كلامه.

(٥٢) ذكر جالينوس في ثالثة التعرّف عند كلامه على وجع الشقيقة قال إنّه إن كان سببه ريح أحسّ صاحبه بتمدّد وإن كان عن كثرة الأخلاط فيحسّ معه بثقل. وقال في مقالته في الفصد كلاما هذا نصّه قال: الدليل الخاصّي بالصنف من الامتلاء الذي يكون بحسب القوة الثقل وأما الصنف من الامتلاء الذي يكون بحسب الأوعية فالتمدّد.

---

٥ مثل قولنا] لو قلنا LP لا قلنا (!)B | لا] بالفعل add. B لا أنّ] لان SG || ٩ فيشبهه] فيتشبه B || ١٠ والغشاء] om. SG || ١٣ كلامه] في الأصل [...] شطر أبيض بلا كلام كأنّه [...] على أن يذكر فيها تمام الكلام والله أعلم add. G1 وقال يبحث ههنا بعض ذكر أنه لا يوجد تمام الكلام في المصورة والأصل add. B והנה יבוקש הנה קצת זכרון שהוא לא יהיה נמצא השלמת המאמר בכתוב ובשורש add. Z Et verba sua propria sana sunt usque nunc, et cum in particula illa dictum suum exquisivi non invenitur complementum dictorum verborum in suo originali add. Bo || ١٦ بحسب . . . يكون] om. B

The point of doubt is that [in the first statement] he says that the sensation of heaviness that comes with the pain of migraine indicates a surplus of humors, while in the [second] statement he says that tension indicates overfilling that is commensurate to the vessels. And this overfilling originates without any doubt from a surplus of humors. It seems to me that the proof adduced in *De venae sectione* for two kinds of overfilling is [valid] only if the patient feels that heaviness or tension without pain, regardless of whether that [sensation] is [only] in one part or in the entire body. But if he feels a severe pain like migraine in a bodily part and next to the pain he feels heaviness, it indicates a surplus of humors and not only malignancy of humors. For overfilling commensurate to strength is only caused by malignancy of humors, and this is harmful for the strength of the organ so that he has a sensation of heaviness, while it is not severe. Some people say that this applies to the head especially. This is confirmed by what Galen says in the second book of *Mayāmir*, and these are his words: A surplus of humors in the head produces heaviness but not a headache unless an obstruction results from it. These are his words.[162] It is very difficult to provide a reason why only a surplus of humors, that is, overfilling commensurate to the vessels, causes heaviness in the head and tension in any other part of the body or in the entire body. This ought to be contemplated.

(53) In the fifth book of *De methodo medendi*, when he begins to describe how someone suffering from hemoptysis from the lungs should be treated, he says the following, and these are his words: Tell the patient not to take deep breaths and always to remain quiet, and immediately phlebotomize him from the[163] vein at the inner side [of the arm].[164] These are his words there. And in his commentary on the first book of *De humoribus*, he makes the following statement, and these are his words: It is not proper for someone who emits blood from the larynx, lungs, chest, or windpipe to raise his voice or breathe deeply. But to move his arms is not bad for him, and it is [even] more appropriate in this regard to move his legs moderately so that his pulse does not become spasmodic.[165] These are his words as well. The point of doubt is that in the first statement he instructs the patient to adhere to [a regimen] of rest and repose, while in the second statement he allows moderate movement. This ought to be contemplated.

موضع الإشكال كونه قال في حسّ الثقل مع وجع الشقيقة إنّه دالّ على كثرة الأخلاط وفي هذا الكلام الآخر يقول إنّ التمدّد دلّ على الامتلاء الذي بحسب الأوعية وهذا الامتلاء هو الكائن من كثرة الأخلاط بلا شكّ. والذي يبدو لي هو أنّ ذلك الاستدلال المذكور في مقالة الفصد على صنفي الامتلاء هو إذا أحسّ الإنسان بذلك الثقل والتمدّد دون وجع سوى كان ذلك في عضو واحد أو في البدن كلّه. أما العضو الذي يحسّ فيه وجع شديد كالشقيقة فإنّه إن أحسّ مع ذلك الوجع بثقل فهو دليل على كثرة الأخلاط لا على رداتها فقط لأنّ الامتلاء الذي بحسب القوة فقط إنّما سببه رداءة الأخلاط وذلك هو الذي أنكى قوة العضو حتّى استثقل ما ليس بكثير. ولقائل يقول إنّ هذا خصيصا بالرأس خاصّة. وممّا يؤكّد ذلك قول جالينوس في ثانية الميامر كلاما هذا نصّه: وأمّا كثرة الأخلاط في الرأس فتحدث ثقلا لا صداعا إلا أن حدثت عنها سدد. هذا نصّه. فيصعب جدّا إعطاء السبب في كون كثرة الأخلاط فقط الذي هو الامتلاء بحسب الأوعية يحدث ثقلا في الرأس ويحدث في كلّ عضو سواه أو في البدن كلّه تمدّدا لا ثقلا. فيتأمّل.

(٥٣) في المقالة الخامسة من حيلة البرء قال عندما أخذ أن يصف كيف يعالج من نفث الدم من رئته قال كلاما هذا نصّه: تأمر المريض أن لا يتنفّس تنفّسا عظيما وأن يلزم القرار والهدوء دائما وتفصد له من ساعته عرقا من مأبضه. هذا نصّه هناك. وقال في شرحه للمقالة الأولى من كتاب الأخلاط كلاما هذا نصّه: ليس ينبغي لمن ينبعث منه دم من حنجرته أو من رئته أو من صدره أو من قصبة رئته أن يكون له صوت ولا تنفّس عظيم. وأمّا تحريك اليدين فليس برديء له وأحرى بذلك تحريك الرجلين حركة اعتدال حتّى لا يحدث تواتر في نبض. هذا نصّه أيضا. وموضع الشكّ كونه يأمر المريض في الكلام الأوّل بالهدوء والسكون وفي الكلام الثاني أباح الحركة المعتدلة. فيتأمّل.

---

١ الإشكال] الشكّ EL || ٦ إنّ . . . فقط] om. B || ٧ أنكى] أرخى EL || ١١ يحدث . . . (?) ٦٥ ] om. S || ١٧ أو من رئته] om. G || ٢٠ أباح] يوجبه (?) في G

(54) When he mentions fleawort [*Plantago psyllium*] seed in the eighth book of *De simplicium medicamentorum* [*temperamentis ac facultatibus*], he makes the following statement, and these are his words: The most beneficial [part] of this plant is its seed; it is cold in the second degree and is in the middle between moisture and dryness, balanced.[166] These are his words there. In the second book of his treatise *Ad Glauconem* [*de medendi methodo*], when speaking about corrosive shingles he says the following, and these are his words: In this illness be careful not to use lettuce [*Lactuca sativa*], common knotgrass [*Polygonum aviculare*], common duckweed [*Lemna minor*], water lily [*Nymphaea alba* and var., or *Nuphar lutea*], fleawort seed, common purslane [*Portulaca oleracea*], tree aeonium [*Sempervivum arboreum*], or similar [ingredients] with cooling, moistening properties.[167] These are his words in this place. The point of doubt is that in this last statement he explains that fleawort seed is cold and moist and counts it with lettuce, purslane, duckweed, and water lily and says that all these have cooling and moistening properties, while in the first statement he says that [fleawort seed] is intermediate between dryness and moisture. This ought to be contemplated.

(55) In the thirteenth book of *De methodo* [*medendi*], when speaking about the treatment of tumors of the liver and spleen and comparing their remedies, he says the following, and these are his words: That is that both these organs require remedies that, although of a similar kind, differ in strength and weakness. For the spleen needs stronger remedies because of the greater amount of thickness of its nourishment over the nourishment of the liver.[168] These are his words there. And in the fourth book of *De usu* [*partium*], he makes the following statement, and these are his words: Note the [following] summary of my words to you concerning the nourishment of these three organs: the liver is nourished by thick, red blood; the spleen is nourished by thin, dark blood; and the lung is nourished by blood that is extremely well concocted, bright red, thin, and spirituous.[169] These too are his words.

(٥٤) لمّا ذكر البزر قطونا في المقالة الثامنة من الأدوية المفردة قال فيه كلاما هذا نصّه: أنفع ما في هذا النبات بزره وهو بارد في الدرجة الثانية ووسط في ما بين رطوبة واليبس معتدل. هذا نصّه هناك. أمّا في المقالة الثانية من كتابه إلى أغلوقن في كلامه على النملة المتأكّلة فقال كلاما هذا نصّه: واحذر أن يستعمل في هذه العلّة الخسّ أو عصا الراعي أو الطحلب أو النيلوفر أو البزرقطونا أو البقلة الحمقاء أو حيّ العالم أو غير ذلك ممّا شأنه التبريد والترطيب. هذا نصّه في هذا الموضع. وموضع الشكّ كونه صرّح في هذا الكلام الأخير بأنّ البزرقطونا بارد رطب وعدّه مع الخسّ والرجلة والطحلب والنيلوفر وقال إنّ هذه كلّها شأنها التبريد والترطيب وهو قال في الكلام الأوّل إنّه معتدل بين اليبس والرطوبة. فيأمّل

(٥٥) قال في ثالثة عشر الحيلة عندما تكلّم في مداواة أورام الكبد والطحال والمقايسة بين أدويتهما قال كلاما هذا نصّه: وذلك أنّ هذين العضوين كليهما يحتاجان إلى أدوية شبيهة بعضها ببعض في جنسها إلا أنّها تختلف بطريق الزيادة والنقصان أنّ الطحال تحتاج إلى أدوية أقوى بمقدار فضل غلظ غذائه على غذاء الكبد. هذا نصّه هناك. وقال في رابعة المنافع كلاما هذا نصّه: وافهم عني جملة أقولها لك في غذاء هذه ثلاثة الأعضاء وهي أنّ الكبد تغتذي بدم أحمر غليظ والطحال يغتذي بدم لطيف أسود والرئة تغتذي بدم قد نضج غاية النضج وهو مشرق الحمرة لطيف قريب من طبيعة الروح. هذا نصّه أيضا.

١ الثامنة] الثانية B || ٣ النملة المتأكّلة] الحملة الثالثة G(!) || ٥ شأنه] شأبه B(!)

The point of doubt is that in *De methodo medendi*, he explains that the nourishment of the spleen is thicker than that of the liver, whereas in *De usu partium* he explains that the nourishment of the spleen is thinner than that of the liver. His explanation in *De usu partium* is correct; there he compares the [degree] of thinness of the nourishment of the liver, spleen, and lung and says that the nourishment of the liver is thick according to its substance, the nourishment of the lung thin, and that of the spleen intermediate between these two, namely, thinner than the nourishment of the liver and thicker than that of the lung. Once he has compared the thinness of the blood, as we have [just] described, he compares the color of the blood of these three organs and says that the blood with which the lung nourishes itself is bright red, and that with which the spleen nourishes itself is dark, and that with which the liver nourishes itself is intermediate between these two, that is, less red than the blood of the lung and less dark than that of the spleen.

It seems to me that Galen did not forget all this, nor did he disregard it. But he expressed himself very carelessly in his statement in *De methodo* [*medendi*] and took [the term] *nutrition* in its most general sense, that is, something that has the property to turn into nutrition, just as one says of bread and beet that they are nutrition. There is no question that the [substance] that the spleen attracts before it transforms it and nourishes itself with it is thicker than that which is attracted by the body of the liver for nourishment. This is the matter he looked at in his statement in *De methodo* [*medendi*]. This ought to be contemplated.

موضع الشكّ كونه صرّح في حيلة البرء بأنّ غذاء الطحال أغلظ من غذاء الكبد وبيّن في منافع الأعضاء أنّ غذاء الطحال ألطف من غذاء الكبد. والذي بيّن لنا في منافع الأعضاء هو الصحيح وهناك قايس بين لطافة غذاء الكبد والطحال والرئة وقال إنّ غذاء الكبد غليظ بحسب جوهرها وغذاء الرئة لطيف وغذاء الطحال وسط بينهما هو ألطف من غذاء الكبد وأغلظ من غذاء الرئة. ثمّ قايس بين ألوان دم الثلاثة أعضاء بعد أن قايس بين لطف ذلك الدم كما ذكرنا فقال إنّ الدم الذي تغتذي منه الرئة أحمر مشرق والدم الذي يغتذي منه الطحال أسود والدم الذي تغتذي منه الكبد وسط بينهما وهو أقلّ حمرة من دم الرئة وأقلّ سوادا من دم الطحال.

ويبدو لي أنّ هذا كلّه لم ينسه جالينوس ولا غفل عنه. وإنّما تسامح جدّا في كلامه هذا الذي في الحيلة وأخذ الغذاء على الوجه الأعمّ أعني على ما شأنه أن يصير منه الغذاء كما يقال في الخبز والسلق إنّهما غذاء. ولا شكّ أنّ الشيء الذي يجتذبه الطحال قبل أن يحيله ويغتذي منه بما يغتذي هو أغلظ ممّا يجتذبه جرم الكبد لتغتذي به. وهذا المعنى هو الذي لحظ عند كلامه في الحيلة. فيتأمّل هذا.

---

١١ يجتذبه] يغتذي به EL يجذبه B || ١٢ يجتذبه] يغتذي به EL يجذبه B | وهذا المعنى هو الذي لحظ عند كلامه] وهذا هو المعنى في كلامه B

(56) In the second book of *De pulsu magno*, [Galen] makes the following statement, and these are his words: The[170] language of the Greek is the most pleasant of all languages and the most universal for all people [endowed] with logic, the most eloquent and most human. For if you pay attention to the pronunciation of the words in the languages of other peoples, you will certainly discern that some of them are very much like the grunting of pigs, others resemble the croaking of frogs, and yet others resemble the sound produced by the green[171] woodpecker. Then you will also find that [these words] originate in an ugly way in the movements of the tongue, lips, and entire mouth. For some people bring forth sounds mostly from deep within the throat as if they were snoring, others twist their mouth and whistle,[172] others roar and scream at the top of their voice, others make no perceptible or discernible sound at all. Some of them open their mouth widely and stick out their tongue, and others do not stick out their tongue at all; it seems to be idle and difficult to move as it is heavy and tied.[173]

(57) Says Moses: Al-Rāzī and others have cast doubt on these words of Galen.[174] The thrust of their objection is that he makes the Greek language into a unique one [among the languages] spoken by men and regards all the other languages as ugly ones. It is well known that the languages are conventional[175] and that every language is ugly, hard, and obscure for someone who does not know it and who has not been raised with it. This is the [basic] meaning [of the words] of every one who doubts this statement [by Galen]. It seems to me that what Galen said in this statement is correct—that is, that the difference in the pronunciation of the letters and the difference in the movement of the organs of speech during speaking are consequential upon the difference in climates, that is, the difference of the temperaments of their inhabitants and the difference of the shapes of their organs and their external and internal sizes.[176]

(٥٦) قال في المقالة الثانية من النبض الكبير كلاما هذا نصّه قال إنّ لغة يونان أعذب اللغات وأعمّها لذوي المنطق كلّهم وأطلقها وأشبهها بالإنس فإنّك إذا تفطّنت في ألفاظ لغات الأمم الآخر علمت علما يقينا أنّ بعضها أشبه شيء بصياح الخنازير وبعضها يشبه بصوت الضفادع وبعضها يشبه بصوت الشقرّاق. ثمّ تجدها مع ذلك سمجة المخارج في حركات اللسان والشفتين والفم كلّه. وذلك أنّ بعضهم يخرج الصوت أكثر ذلك من داخل من جوف الحلق بمنزلة من ينخر وبعضهم يعوّج فاه ويصفر وبعضهم ينعر ويصرخ بصوته كلّه وبعضهم لا يظهر صوته البتّة ولا يتبيّن منه شيء. ومنهم من يفتح فاه فتحا كثيرا ويخرج لسانه ومنهم من لا يخرج لسانه البتّة وترى لسانه عطلا عسر الحركة كأنّه مثقل مربوط.

(٥٧) قال موسى: قد شكّك الرازي وغيره على جالينوس هذا الكلام ومعنى الشكّ كونه جعل لغة يونان خاصّية بالإنسان واستسماجه لكلّ ما سواها من اللغات. ومعلوم أنّ اللغات اصطلاحية وأنّ كلّ لغة عند من لا يعلمها ولا ربّي عليها سمجة مستثقلة معجمة. هذا هو غرض كلّ من شكّك على هذا القول. وأنا يبدو لي أنّ الذي قاله جالينوس في هذا القول هو الصحيح. وذلك أنّ اختلاف مخارج الحروف واختلاف تحريك آلات الكلام عند الكلام تابع لاختلاف الأقاليم أعني اختلاف أمزجة أهلها واختلاف أشكال أعضائهم ومقاديرها الظاهرة والباطنة.

---

١ لغة ] لغات ELB || ٢ وأعمّها ] أشكلها Ra, p. 87, line 4 | المنطق ] النطق Ra, p. 87, line 5 | بالإنس ] باللسان B بالإنسان ?L بالنفس E الاسن Ra, p. 87, line 4 بالناس Ka || ٦ جوف ] حوق Ka | بمنزلة ] كمثل Ka || ١٠ بالإنسان ] الإنسان Ka || ١١ عليها ] G فيها G²

(58) This was mentioned by Abū Naṣr al-Fārābī in the *Kitāb al-ḥurūf* [*Book of Letters*].[177] For as, in general, people living in the temperate climatic zones have more perfect intellects and better forms (i.e., their shape and outline is more regular), their organs are better proportioned, and their temperament is more balanced than that of the inhabitants of the distant climatic zones in the extreme north and south, so the pronunciation of the letters by the inhabitants of the temperate climatic zones and the movement of their speech organs during speaking are more balanced and are closer to human articulated speech than the pronunciation of the letters and the movement of the speech organs of those [people], I mean, the inhabitants of the distant climatic zones in the extreme [north and south] and their language, as Galen remarks. Galen does not mean the Greek language only, but it and similar ones, namely, the Greek language, Arabic, Hebrew, Syriac, and Persian since these are the languages of the inhabitants of these moderate climatic zones, and they are natural to them according to the difference of the places [they live in], which are close to one another.

Regarding the Arabic and Hebrew language, everyone who knows these two languages agrees that they are undoubtedly a single language and Syriac is somewhat close to them and Greek is close to Syriac. The pronunciation of the letters in these four languages is the same, except for a few letters, perhaps three or four. Persian is more remote from these, and the pronunciation of its letters is very different. One should not be deluded by the fact that the current inhabitants of the[178] climatic zone that is in the middle [of the earth] speak in a very bad language. For they are immigrants to that place from remote places, just as one finds a Hebrew- or Arabic-[speaking person] in the extreme north or south who there speaks in the language he was raised with in his homeland.

(٥٨) وقد ذكر ذلك أبو نصر الفارابي في كتاب الحروف. فكما أنّ أهل الأقاليم المتوسّطة أكمل عقلا وأحسن صورة على العموم أعني أنظم شكلا وتخطيطا وأحسن تناسب أعضاء وأعدل مزاجا من أهل تلك الأقاليم المتباعدة في أقصى الشمال والجنوب كذلك مخارج أحرف أهل الأقاليم المتوسّطة وحركة آلات الكلام منهم عند الكلام أعدل وأقرب لنطق الإنسان من مخارج أحرف أولائك وحركة آلات الكلام منهم أعني أهل الأقاليم المتباعدة في الأقاصي ولغاتهم كما ذكر جالينوس. وليس يعني جالينوس لغة يونان خاصّة بل هي وما ماثلها وهي لغة يونان والعرب والعبرانيين والسريانيين والفرس إذ هذه هي لغات أهل هذه الأقاليم المتوسّطة الطبيعية لهم بحسب اختلاف مواعضهم المتقاربة.

أمّا اللغة العربية والعبرانية فقد اتّفق كلّ من علم اللغتين أنهّما لغة واحدة بلا شكّ واللغة السريانية قريبة منهما بعض القرب واليوناني قريب من السرياني. ومخارج أحرف هذه اللغات الأربعة واحدة إلا أحرف قليلة لعلّها ثلاثة أحرف أو أربع. أمّا الفارسية فأبعد من هذه وفي مخارج حروفها أيضا اختلاف كثير ولا يغلطك كون أهل الإقليم الوسط اليوم يتكلّمون بلغة رديئة جدّا لأنهّم ناقلة لذلك الموضع من مواضع قاصية كما تجد شخصا عربيا أو عبرانيا في أقصى الشمال أو الجنوب وهو يتكلّم هناك باللغة التي ربي عليها في بلاده.

٣ كذلك ] لذلك GKa || ٤ لنطق ] من نطق B || ٥ أولائك ] الحيك G || ٧ ماثلها ] من اللغات EL || ٩ اتّفق ] أيقن ELP || ١٠ بعض القرب ] om. Ka G[1] || ١٢ كثير ] أكثر ELBP || ١٣ اليوم ] بعضها B | ناقلة ] ناقلون EL || ١٥ بلاده ] MS S ends here

(59)[179] Says Moses: It[180] is a well-known saying of the philosophers that the soul can be healthy or ill just as the body can be healthy or ill. These healthy and ill [conditions] of the soul they allude to belong to [the field] of opinions and ethical qualities [of human beings] and are characteristic of them, without any doubt. Therefore, I call untrue opinions and bad ethical qualities with their many varieties "human"[181] diseases. Among all the human[182] diseases there is one disease that is so common that almost no one can escape from it, except for a few individuals in long periods. This disease varies among human beings in the greater or lesser degree [of its severity] just like the other physical and mental diseases. This illness that I mean is that every person imagines himself to be more perfect than he is and that he desires and wishes that all his opinions [that he acquired] without any effort and exertion pass as perfect.

Because of this common illness, we find that individuals who possess cleverness and alertness and have learned one of the[183] philosophical, theoretical, or speculative sciences, or one of the conventional[184] sciences, and have become proficient in that science, that such a person expresses his opinion not only in that science that he has mastered but also in other sciences that he does not know at all or only knows deficiently and speaks about those sciences [with the same authority] as about the science in which he has specialized. This is especially the case if that person happens to achieve one of the alleged felicities of being regarded as someone with authority and preeminence and has become one of the great masters who only has to speak in order to make his words accepted. No one refutes his words or objects to them. And as that alleged felicity becomes more established and stronger, that disease becomes more severe and stronger [as well], and that person begins, in due course, to talk nonsense and to speak whatever comes

(٥٩) قال موسى: من المعلوم قول الفلاسفة إنّ للنفس صحّة ومرض كما للجسم صحة ومرض. وتلك أمراض النفس وصحتها التي يشيرون إليها هي في الآراء والأخلاق وهذه خصيصة بالإنسان بلا شكّ. ولذلك أسمّي أنا الآراء الغير صحيحة والأخلاق الرديئة على كثرة اختلاف أنواعها الأمراض الإنسانية. ومن جملة الأمراض الإنسانية مرض عامّ ويكاد أن لا يسلم منه إلا آحاد في أزمنة متباعدة ويختلف ذلك المرض في الناس بالزيادة والنقصان كسائر الأمراض الجسمية والنفسية. وهذا المرض الذي أشير إليه هو تخيّل كلّ شخص نفسه أكمل ممّا هو عليه وكونه يريد ويشتهي أن يجوز كلّ ما يعتقده كمالا من غير تعب ولا نصب.

ومن أجل هذا المرض العامّ نجد أشخاصا من الناس ذوي حذق ونباهة قد علموا أحدى العلوم الفلسفية النظرية أو العلمية أو علم من العلوم الوضعية ومهروا في ذلك العلم فيتكلّم ذلك الشخص في ذلك العلم الذي أحكمه وفي علوم أخرى لا علم له بها أصلا أو يكون مقصّرا فيها ويجعل كلامه في تلك العلوم ككلامه في ذلك العلم الذي مهر فيه ولا سيّما إن كان ذلك الشخص قد اتّفقت له سعادة من السعادات المظنونة ولحظ بعين الرئاسة والتقدّم وصار من أرباب الصدور يقول ويتلقّى قوله بالقبول ولا يردّ عليه قول ولا يعترض فيه. فإنّ كلّما تمكّنت هذه السعادة المظنونة وقويت تمكّن ذلك المرض واستعضل وصار ذلك الشخص يهذي مع الزمان ويقول ما عنّ له أن يقول بحسب خيلاته أو بحسب

---

٢ هي] وهي GB | وهذه خصيصة بالإنسان] om. LP || ٤ الإنسانية] النفسانية EL | الإنسانية] النفسانية EL || ٦ الجسمية والنفسية] الجسمانية والنفسانية BP | إليه] هنا add. BP || ٧ يريد] يزيد Sch | يجوز] يجري (!)B || ٩ حذق] حدّة P || ١٠ النظرية] أو add. ELP | أو العلمية ELBP أو العملية correction Sch || ١٤ يقول] تقوول Ka || ١٤ يعترض] يعرض Ka || ١٦ عنّ] عزّ Ka

to his mind according to his fantasies or his dispositions, or according to the questions addressed to him. He answers whatever comes to his mind because he does not want to say that there is something he does not know. In some persons this illness becomes so inveterate that they are not content with all this, but begin to argue and explain that those sciences that they do not know are useless and needless and that there is no science worthy of a lifelong attention, except for that science that they know, be it a philosophical or conventional [science]. Many have composed refutations of sciences that they have not mastered. To sum up, this disease is very widespread, and if you look at the words of a person with an impartial eye, the degree [of severity] of this disease will be clear to you and whether this person is close to health or ruin.

And this [man] Galen, the physician, was attacked by this disease in the same degree as others who were equal to him in science. That is, this man[185] was very, very proficient in medicine, more than anybody we have heard about or whose words we have seen; he has achieved great things in [the field of] anatomy, and things became clear to him—and[186] to others in his time as well—about the functions of the organs, their usefulness and structure, and about the [different] conditions of the pulse, which were not clear in Aristotle's time. He, I mean Galen, has undoubtedly trained himself in mathematics and has studied logic and the books of Aristotle on the natural and divine sciences, but he is defective in all that. His excellent intellect and acumen that he directed towards medicine, and[187] his discoveries of some of the conditions of the pulse, anatomy, and the usefulness and functions [of organs]—which are undoubtedly more correct than what Aristotle mentions in his books, if one looks at them impartially—have induced him to speak about things in which he is very deficient and about which the experts have contradictory opinions.

السؤالات التي تردّ عليه فيجاوب بما عنّ له إذ لا يريد أن يقول إنّ ثمّ ما لا يدريه. وقد وصل استحكام هذا المرض في بعض الناس أن لم يقنع بهذا القدر بل أن يأخذ أن يحتجّ ويبيّن أنّ تلك العلوم التي لا يحسنها غير مفيدة ولا حاجة إليها وأنّ ليس ثمّ علم ينبغي أن يفنى فيه العمر إلا ذلك العلم الذي يحسنه هو لا غير كان ذلك علما فلسفيا أو وضعيا وكثيرون ألّفوا ردودا على علوم لا يحسنونها. وبالجملة فإنّ هذا المرض له عرض واسع جدّا وعند تأمّلك كلام الشخص بعين الإنصاف يتبيّن لك قدر مرضه هذا وهل ذلك الشخص قريب من الصحّة أو قريب من العطب.

وهذا جالينوس الطبيب لحقه من هذا المرض ما يلحق القوم الذين هم من قبيله في العلم. وذلك أنّ هذا الرجل مهر في الطبّ جدّا جدّا أكثر من كلّ من سمعنا خبره أو رأينا كلامه وكذلك أصاب في التشريح إصابة عظيمة وتبيّن له وفي زمانه لغيره أيضا من أفعال الأعضاء ومنافعها وخلقتها ومن أحوال النبض أشياء ما كانت تبيّنت في زمان أرسطو. وهو بلا شكّ أعني جالينوس ارتاض في رياضيات وقرأ منطق وقرأ كتب أرسطو في الطبيعيات والإلاهيات لكنّه مقصّر في جميع ذلك. ولجودة ذهنه وذكائه الذي صرفه إلى الطبّ وكونه وجد ما عرفه هو من بعض أحوال النبض والتشريح والمنافع والأفعال أصحّ ممّا ذكره أرسطو في كتبه بلا شكّ عند من ينصف فدعاه ذلك إلى الكلام في أمور هو مقصّر فيها جدّا وتضارب المهرة فيها.

١ يدريه ] يدركه B || ٢ بل أن ] ثمّ B || ٨ من ($G^1$) ] om. Ka || ٩ العلم ] العلوم Ka || ١٠ وفي ] في BP وتبيّن في EL | زمانه ] ما لا يتبيّن add. B ما لم يتبيّن add. Ka || ١٤ بعض ] om. Ka

So he refutes, as you know, Aristotle in logic and speaks about the natural and divine sciences, as he does [in] *On*[188] *My Own Opinions*, and [in] *On*[189] *the Doctrines of Hippocrates and Plato*, and [in] the book *On*[190] *Sperm*, which contain refutations of Aristotle. Likewise he composed a[191] book on motion, time, the possible, and the first mover, and about all these things he comes with opinions that are well known to the people of that branch. This led to the point where he composed his famous book *De demonstratione* and maintained that the physician is not perfect in medicine unless he knows [this book] and that it is very useful for the physician. He limited himself to those syllogisms that are necessary for demonstration, maintaining that those syllogisms are useful in medicine and in other [branches], and omitted the other [syllogisms]. But the syllogisms that he mentioned are not at all the demonstrative syllogisms, and he omitted those syllogisms that are very useful in the medical art and claimed that they are not at all useful and that Aristotle's and other people's study of them is a waste of time.

All this was explained by Abū Naṣr al-Fārābī[192]—that is, that he [Galen] omitted the hypothetical and the mixed syllogisms and confined himself to the absolute syllogisms (i.e., the hyparctic)[193] and did not pay attention to the fact that demonstrative syllogisms are necessary ones and not hyparctic ones and that that which is useful in medicine and in most arts is the hypothetical and mixed syllogisms. Hear the words of Abū Naṣr on this matter in his great commentary on the *Analytica* when he begins to explain the preliminary exposition that he (i.e., Aristotle) has made on the possible and the hypothetical syllogisms.[194] Abū Naṣr says: The question here is not as Galen the physician thinks, because in his book called *De Demonstratione* he mentions that the study of the possible and of the [hypothetical] syllogisms that are derived therefrom is superfluous. Galen the physician is one of the people for whom it would have been most proper to study the hypothetical syllogisms; even more so, he should have directed most of his attention in his book called *De Demonstratione* to the hypothetical syllogisms; for he pretends that he composed his book *De Demonstratione* in order that it might be useful in medicine. And the syllogisms that the physician uses for extracting the [different] parts of the medical art and the syllogisms that he employs for recognizing the internal diseases and their causes in every one of his [patients] whom he wants to cure, all these are hypothetical syllogisms, and there is no necessary [syllogism] among them, except for exceptional cases that are practically outside

فيردّ على أرسطو كما علمت في المنطق ويتكلّم في الإلاهيات وطبيعيات ككلامه في ما يعتقده رأيا لنفسه وككلامه في آراء أبقراط وأفلاطون وكتاب المني المضمّنة ما تضمّنته من الردود على أرسطو وكذلك ألّف كتابا في الحركة وفي الزمان وفي الممكن وفي المحرّك الأوّل ويأتي في جميع ذلك بما هو معلوم عند أهل هذا الشأن وانتهى به ذلك إلى أن ألّف كتابه المشهور في البرهان وزعم أنّه لا يكمل الطبيب في الطبّ إلا بمعرفته وأنّه نافع للطبيب جدّا. واقتصر من المقاييس على ما يحتاج إليه في البرهان بزعمه أنّ تلك المقاييس هي النافعة في الطبّ وغيره وحذف ما سوى ذلك. فكانت مقاييسه تلك التي ذكر ليست هي مقاييس البرهان أصلا وحذف المقاييس النافعة جدّا في صناعة الطبّ وزعم أنّها لا حاجة إليها أصلا وأنّ اشتغال أرسطو وغيره بها إتلاف للزمان

كلّ ذلك بيّنه أبو نصر الفارابي وذلك أنّه حذف المقاييس الممكنة والمقاييس المختلطة واقتصر على المقاييس المطلقة وهي الوجودية ولم يأبه إلى أنّ المقاييس البرهانية هي ضرورية لا وجودية وأنّ الشيء النافع في الطبّ وفي أكثر الصنائع هي المقاييس الممكنة والمختلطة واسمع نصوص أبي نصر في ذلك. قال في شرحه للقياس الكبير لمّا أخذ أن يشرح تلك التوطئة وطّأها للممكن وللمقاييس الممكنة. قال أبو نصر: وليس الأمر في ذلك على ما ظنّه جالينوس المتطبّب لأنّه ذكر في كتابه الذي سمّاه كتاب البرهان أنّ النظر في الممكن وفي القياسات الكائنة عنه فضل. وأولى الناس بالنظر في القياسات الممكنة جالينوس المتطبّب بل يلزمه

١ فيردّ] فردّ Sch | ككلامه] ككلام G بكلام Ka || ٢ في آراء أبقراط وأفلاطون وكتاب المني المضمّنة ما تضمّنته من الردود على أرسطو وكذلك ألّف كتابا] om. Ka Sch G | المني] الميز Ka || ٣ الممكن] المكان الأماكين Ka Sch $G^2L$ || ٥ المشهور] في آراء أبقراط وأفلاطون وكتاب المني المضمّنة ما تضمّنته من الردود على أرسطو وكذلك ألّف كتابه add. Ka Sch G || ٦ أن] conj. editor وأنّ MSS || ٩ للزمان] الزمان Ka

the medical art. Therefore, he should have spoken in his book called *De Demonstratione* about the kinds[195] of the hypothetical syllogisms only and not about those of the hyparctic [syllogisms], and if he has confined himself in his book to the hyparctic kinds in order to restrict himself to those syllogisms that are useful for demonstrations, then [one has to say that] the kinds relating to existence are not destined for demonstrations, because demonstrations are not made from this matter but are made from the necessary kinds only. End of the quotation from Abū Naṣr.[196]

(60) When Aristotle begins to explain the syllogisms that are mixed from hypothetical and absolute ones,[197] Abū Naṣr says the following in his commentary to this statement, and these are his words: This chapter is extremely useful and more useful than [the chapter on] the plain hypothetical ones because all the practical arts make use of this chapter, especially in finding out whether the individual phenomena that are in the future will occur or not, in medicine, agriculture, navigation, politics, rhetorics, general[198] premises, and in all the activities in which one needs prognostics; all that which can be found in the book of Hippocrates the physician on prognostics and in similar books resolves itself into these syllogisms. End of the quotation from Abū Naṣr. This ought to be contemplated.

أن يكون قد صرّف أكثر عنايته في كتابه الذي قد سمّاه كتاب البرهان إلى المقاييس الممكنة فإنّه زعم أنّه صنف كتابه في البرهان لينتفع به في الطبّ. والقياسات التي يستعملها الطبيب في استنباط أجزاء صناعة الطبّ والقياسات التي يستعملها في تعرّف الأمراض الباطنة وأسبابها في واحد واحد من الذين يقصدون علاجهم فكلّها قياسات ممكنة وليس في شيء منها ضروري إلا أن يكون الشاذّ الذي يكاد أن يكون خارجا عن صناعة الطبّ. فلذلك يلزمه أن لا يكون يتكلّم في كتابه الذي سمّاه كتاب البرهان إلا في أشكال المقاييس الممكنة فقط دون الوجودية وعلى أنّه إن كان إنّما اقتصر في كتابه على الأشكال الوجودية ليكون قد اقتصر من المقاييس على ما ينتفع به في البراهين فإنّ الأشكال الوجودية ليست هي معدّة نحو البراهين لأنّ البراهين ليست تعمل من هذه المادّة بل إنّما تعمل من الأشكال الاضطرارية فقط. انتهى كلام أبي نصر.

(٦٠) ولمّا أخذ أرسطو في تبيين المقاييس المختلطة من ممكنة ومطلقة قال أبو نصر في شرح ذلك الكلام ما هذا نصّه قال: هذا الباب عظيم النفع جدّا أعظم نفعا من الممكنة الصرف من قبل أنّ الصنائع العملية كلّها تستعمل هذا الباب ولا سيّما في استنباط الأمور الجزئية المستقبلة هل تكون أو لا تكون في الطبّ وفي الفلاحة والملاحة وفي تدبير المدن والخطابة والمشهورات وفي كلّ ما يتصرّف فيه ممّا يحتاج فيه إلى تقدمة المعرفة وما في كتاب أبقراط الطبيب في تقدمة المعرفة وما شاكله من الكتب فكلّه ينحلّ إلى هذه القياسات. انتهى كلام أبي نصر. فيتأمّل.

---

١ الذي] التي G || ٢ أنّه] إنّما add. ELP | والقياسات التي يستعملها الطبيب] om. B || ٣ أجزاء] om. Ka Sch أجز (?) del. G || ٤ يقصدون] يقصد EL || ٧ الوجودية] الوجودي ELP || ٨ البراهين] البرهان Sch || ٩ تعمل] تعمد Ka | تعمل] تعمد Ka || ١٣ أنّ] om. G || ١٥ والمشهورات] والمشاورات EL والمشورات KaBP | يتصرّف] ينعرف Ka | وما في] وأمّا EL وما... المعرفة] om. B | في] om. P || ١٦ ينحلّ] يحيل Ka

(61) One should be astonished by the words of this [man] Galen, of the fact that he exaggerates in his praise of logic in all his books and says that the affliction that has affected contemporary physicians, and the cause of their deficiency, is simply their lack of knowledge of logic, and that the cause of his skill lies in the fact that he was well trained in logic and that he always endeavors to show that the physician has need of logic. But when he composed this book, he not only did not mention one single kind of syllogism of the [different] kinds of hypothetical and mixed syllogisms that alone are useful in medicine, but rebuked him who studies them and said that there is no need for them at all. No one doubts that Galen studied Aristotle's books on logic and understood them better than others who are inferior to him. But because of that common illness we are speaking about, he imagined that the understanding of the art of logic and the other theoretical sciences is like the understanding of the medical art and that his skill in all those sciences is like his skill in medicine. Therefore he exposed himself to all [these errors].

He did not stop at this limit, but because of the excessive pleasure he took in what became evident to him about some of the uses of organs, he pretended to be a prophet and said that an angel came to him from God and taught him such and such and ordered him such and such.[199] If only he had stopped at this [point] and had arranged himself among the majority of the prophets—peace be upon them—and had not burst out against them. However, he did not do [so]; on the contrary, a wrong evaluation of his own value led him to eventually compare himself with Moses—peace be upon him—and to attribute to himself perfection and to Moses—peace be upon him—ignorance. God is exalted above the sayings of the ignorant.

(٦١) واعجب من كلام هذا جالينوس وكونه يطنب في مدح المنطق في جميع كتبه ويذكر أنّ آفة أهل عصره من الأطبّاء وعلّة تقصيرهم إنّما هو قلّة خبرتهم بالمنطق وأنّ علّة مهارته هو كونه تأدّب بالمنطق ويروم دائما أن يظهر حاجة الطبيب إلى المنطق. ولمّا ألّف ذلك الكتاب ما كفى أنّه لم يذكر ولا صنفا واحدا من أصناف المقاييس الممكنة والمختلطة التي هي فقط النافعة في الطبّ إلا عنّف المشتغل بها وقال إنّها لا يحتاج إليها أصلا. ولا يشكّ أحد أنّ جالينوس قرأ كتب أرسطو في المنطق وفهمها أكثر من فهم غيره ممّن هو دونه. لكنّ من أجل ذلك المرض العامّ الذي نحن نتكلّم فيه تخيّل أنّ فهم صناعة المنطق وسائر الصنائع النظرية كفهم صناعة الطبّ وأنّ مهارته في تلك العلوم كلّها كمهارته في الطبّ فتعرّض لكلّ ما تعرّض له.

وما وقف عند هذا الحدّ بل من شدّة التذاذه بما ظهر له من بعض منافع الأعضاء ادّعى النبوة وقال إنّ جاءه ملك من عند الله وعلّمه كذا وأمره بكذا. فيا ليته وقف عند هذا وكان ينظّم نفسه في جملة النبيّين عليهم السلام ولا يتهافت إليهم. لكنّه ما فعل بل انتهى به جهله بمقدار نفسه أن قايس بين نفسه وبين موسى عليه السلام ونسب لنفسه الكمال ونسب الجهل لموسى عليه السلام. تعالى الله من أقاويل الجاهلين.

---

١ كلام] حديث ELBP || ٥ عنّف] عن (...) G أنّه اعرف EL عند Ka Sch || ٩ فتعرّض] يعرض G Ka Sch || ٩ فتعرّض] يعرض Sch G || ١١ ليته] لو add. ELBP | هذا] الحدّ add. EL || ١٢ يتهافت] تهافت Ka | إليهم] عليهم ELP

Therefore, it seems to me a good thing to let you know the text of his own words—he who quotes the words of an unbeliever is not an unbeliever [himself]—and to refute him, although it is not a refutation of someone who committed an enormity like this, for Moses—peace be upon him—is not to him what he is to us, the community of followers of Divine Laws. Rather, in this my refutation I will explain that the ignorance that he attributes to our prophet Moses—peace be upon him—does not pertain to him, but that Galen is, in reality, the ignorant one. I will make my own [judgment] of both of them as if I am [judging] between two learned men, one of whom is more perfect than the other, and not as if I were deciding between the words of a great prophet and [those of] a medical practitioner, because this is the correct procedure if the matter is looked into.

(62)[200] I say that when Galen began to explain, in the eleventh book of *De usu partium*, the usefulness of the fact that the hair of the eyebrows does not grow long and hang down like the hair of the head, and the usefulness of the fact that the hair of the eyelids is rigid and does not grow long, he says the following, and these are his words: Do you say, then, that the Creator has commanded this hair to remain at all times at one and the same length and not to grow longer and that the hair has accepted that order, obeyed, and remained [at the same length], without deviating from what it had been ordered either out of fear and apprehension to offend against the command of God or because of politeness and awe before God who gave this command, or that the hair itself knows that it is more appropriate and better to do so? This is the opinion of Moses about the natural things, and I think that this opinion is better and more appropriate to be adopted than that of Epicurus, even though the best thing is to refrain from both and to maintain that God, may He be exalted, is the principle of the creation of all created things as Moses—peace be upon him—has said, but to add to this the material principle from which they were created.[201]

ولذلك حسن عندي أسمعك كلامه بنصّه إنّ حاكي الكفر ليس بكافر وأردّ عليه ليس ردّ على من تعرّض لهذه العظيمة إذ ليس موسى عليه السلام عنده كما هو عندنا نحن معشر المتشرّعين بل أبيّن في ردّي هذا أنّ الجهالة التي نسبها لنبيّنا موسى عليه السلام لا يلزمه وأنّ جالينوس هو الجاهل بالحقيقة. وأجعل كلامي بينهما كأنّي أتكلّم بين شخصين عالمين أحدهما أكمل من الآخر لا كمن يرجح بين كلام نبي عظيم وبين رجل متطبّب إذ هكذا هو الإنصاف في معرض النظر.

(٦٢) فأقول إنّ جالينوس لما أخذ أن يبيّن في المقالة الحادية عشر من منافع الأعضاء منفعة كون شعر الحاجبين لا يطول وينسبل كشعر الرأس ومنفعة كون شعر الجفنين منتصبا ولا يطول قال كلاما هذا نصّه قال: أتقول إنّ الخالق أمر هذا الشعر أن يبقى على مقدار واحد لا يطول أكثر منه في جميع الأوقات وإنّ الشعر قبل ذلك الأمر وأطاع فبقي لا يخالف ما أمر به إمّا للفزع والخوف من المخالفة لأمر اللّه وإمّا للمجاملة والاستحياء من اللّه الذي أمره بهذا الأمر وإمّا أنّ الشعر نفسه يعلم أنّ هذا أولى به وأجمل بفعله؟ أمّا موسى فهذا رأيه في الأشياء الطبيعية وهذا الرأي عندي أحمد وأولى بأن يتمسّك به من رأي أفيقورس إلا أنّ الأجود الضرب عنهما جميعا والاحتفاظ بأنّ اللّه تعالى هو مبدأ خلق كلّ مخلوق كما قال موسى عليه السلام وزيادة المبدأ الذي من قبل المادّة التي منها خلق.

٢ تعرّض] يعرض Ka Sch || ٣ أبيّن] ليس Ka | نسبها] ينسبها Ka || ٥ أكمل] الأكمل Sch | كمن] كما من L || ٨ شعر الجفنين] الجبين Ka || ٩ أتقول] نقولB || ١١ يخالف] مخالفKa | والاستحياء] وإما مستحيا Ka || ١٢ أنّ] om. Sch GB | يعلم] علم EL || ١٤ أفيقورس] أفيقوروس BP | الضرب] الهرب B || ١٥ عليه السلام] om. ELBP

Our Creator has made the eyelashes and eyebrows feel the necessity of remaining at one and the same length since this was more appropriate and better. And since He knew that it was necessary to make them so, he placed under the eyelashes a hard body similar to cartilage that extends along the eyelid, and spread under the eyebrows a hard skin adherent to the cartilage (i.e., the superficial fascia) of the eyebrows. And this because it would not have been sufficient, in order to retain this hair in one and the same length, that the Creator would have wished it to be so. In the same way, if he would wish to turn a stone into a man all of a sudden, without making the stone undergo the appropriate alteration, this would not be possible.

The difference between the belief of Moses—peace be upon him—and our belief and that of Plato and the other Greeks is the following: Moses claims that it is sufficient that God wishes to give shape and form to the matter in order to let it take shape and form instantly. This is because he thinks that all things are possible with God, and that if He wishes to create a horse or an ox from ashes instantly, He can do so. But we do not approve of this, but say that there are some things that are impossible in themselves and these God never wishes to occur, but he wishes only possible things to occur, and from the possible [things] he only chooses the best, most appropriate, and excellent. For this reason, as it is most appropriate and proper for the eyelashes and eyebrows to be always and forever of the same length and number, we do not say about this hair that God wished it to be so, and that straightaway it became as He wished it to be. For, if He had wished the hair to be so a[202] million times, it would never have been so, once He had let it grow from soft skin; if he had not planted the roots of the hair in a hard body, they would—while[203] greatly changing from their [initial] condition—not have remained erect and rigid.

وإنّ خالقنا إنّما جعل الأشفار وشعر الحاجبين تحتاج أن تبقى على مقدار واحد من الطول لأنّ هذا كان أوفق وأصلح. ولمّا علم أنّ هذا الشعر كان ينبغي أن يجعل على هذا جعل تحت الأشفار جرما صلبا شبيها بالغضروف يمتدّ في طول الجفن وفرش تحت الحاجبين جلدة صلبة ملصقة بغضروف الحاجبين وذلك أنّه لم يكن يكتفي في بقاء هذا الشعر على مقدار واحد من الطول بأن يشاء الخالق أن يكون هكذا كما أنّه لو شاء أن يجعل الحجر دفعة أنسانا دون أن يغيّر الحجر التغيير الموافق لذلك لم يكن ذلك بممكن.

والفرق فيما بين إيمان موسى عليه السلام وإيماننا وإيمان أفلاطون وسائر اليونانين هو هذا: موسى يزعم أنّه يكتفي بأن يشاء الله أن يزيّن المادّة ويهيّئها ليس إلا فتتزيّن وتتهيّأ على المكان. وذلك أنّه يظنّ أنّ الأشياء كلّها ممكنة عند الله وأنّه لو شاء أن يخلق من الرماد فرسا أو ثورا دفعة خلق. وأمّا نحن فلا نعرف هذا ولكنّا نقول إنّ من الأشياء أشياء في أنفسها غير ممكنة وهذه الأشياء لا يشاء الله أصلا أن تكون وإنّما يشاء أن تكون الأشياء الممكنة ومن الممكنة لا يختار إلا أجودها وأوفقها وأفضلها. ولهذا لمّا كان الأوفق والأصلح للأشفار وشعر الحاجبين أن تبقى على مقدارها في الطول وعلى عدده الذي هو عليه دائما أبدا لسنا نقول في هذا الشعر إنّ الله إنّما شاء أن يكون على ما هو عليه فصار من ساعته على ما شاء الله. وذلك أنّه لو شاء الله ألف ألف مرّة أن يكون الشعر على هذا لم يكن ذلك أبدا بعد أن يجعل منشأه من جلدة رطبة إلا أنّه لو لم يغرس أصول الشعر في جرم صلب لكان مع ما يتغيّر كثيرا ممّا هو عليه لا يبقى أيضا قائما منتصبا.

---

٣ شبيها] يشبه Ka || ٤ ملصقة] ملزقة BP | لم يكن يكتفي] ما كان يكفي Ka || ٦ التغيير] التغير G | بممكن] ممكن Ka || ٧ وسائر] وأرسطو Ka || ٨ يكتفي] يكفي Ka | الله] البارئ Ka || ٩ المكان] الحال Ka | الأشياء] الأعضاء B || ١٣ عدده] عددها ELB || ١٥ هذا] الحال add. B | يكن] يكون Ka || ١٦ يتغيّر] يتخيّر SchG || ١٧ أيضا] أبدا B

And since this is the case, we say that God has accomplished two things: firstly, the choice of the best, most suitable, and most appropriate condition for what he was going to do; and secondly, the selection of the appropriate material. Therefore, since it was most proper and good that the eyelashes be erect and rigid and that they remain always of the same length and number, he made the planting ground and center of the hair in a hard body. If he had planted them in a soft body, He would have been more ignorant than Moses and more ignorant than a foolish[204] army commander who laid the foundations of the walls of his town or fortress in soft ground that is submerged by water. Similarly, [the fact] that the hair of the eyebrows remains always in the same condition only comes from His choice of the [right] material. End of the quotation from Galen.[205]

(63) Says Moses: If a man, a philosopher, who is familiar with the basic rules of the Divine Laws known in our times, looks into these words, the confusion of this man becomes evident to him. For his words on the whole are neither congruous with the opinion of the followers of Divine Laws nor with that of the philosophers, because the rules of both opinions are neither well established nor accurately defined with Galen. Rather, he speaks about things the premises of which he does not understand, as I am going to explain [to you] now. For he ascribed to Moses—peace be upon him—in that statement [by Moses] that he refers to, four opinions; one opinion of the four is [really] the opinion of Moses—peace be upon him—but the remaining three opinions are not those of Moses. But Galen, through his lack of an established and accurate knowledge of all things about which he is talking, except medicine, thought that the four opinions that he mentioned are [only] one. I also [want to] say that that one opinion that is the opinion of Moses—peace be upon him—as mentioned by Galen is a[206] necessary consequence of the principle and basic rule of his Divine Law and that of his ancestor Abraham—peace be upon them. Therefore his words are neither confused nor contradictory, but follow the premises and consequences [of his Divine Law]. But all the assertions that Galen has

وإذا كان هذا هكذا فإنّا نقول إنّ اللّه جعل هذين الأمرين أحدهما اختيار أجود الحالات وأصلحها وأوفقها لما يفعل والثاني اختيار المادّة الموافقة. ومن ذلك أنّه لمّا كان الأصلح والأجود أن يكون شعر الأشفار قائما منتصبا وأن يدوم بقاؤه على حالة واحدة في مقدار طوله وفي عدده جعل مغرس الشعر ومركزه في جسم صلب ولو أنّه غرسه في جسم رخو لكان أجهل من موسى وأجهل من قائد جيش سخيف يضع أساس سور مدينته أو حصنه على أرض رخوة غارقة بالماء وكذلك بقاء شعر الحاجبين ودوامه على حال واحدة إنّما جاء من قبل اختياره للمادّة. انتهى كلام جالينوس.

(٦٣) قال موسى: إذا نظر في هذا الكلام رجل متفلسف عارف بقواعد الشرائع المشهورة في زماننا تبيّن له اختلاط هذا الرجل. فإنّ هذا الكلام لا ينتظم كلّه على رأي المتشرّعين ولا على رأي المتفلسفين لأنّ قواعد الرأيين عند جالينوس غير محصّلة ولا محرّرة. وإنّما يتكلّم في أمور يجهل أصولها كما أبيّن الآن. وذلك أنّه نسب لموسى عليه السلام في هذا الكلام الذي ذكره أربعة آراء، أمّا الرأي الواحد من الأربعة فهو رأي موسى عليه السلام وأمّا الثلاثة آراء الباقية فليست من رأي موسى وإنّما جالينوس بقلّة تحصيله وتحريره لكلّ ما يتكلّم فيه خارجا عن الطبّ ظنّ أنّ الآراء الأربعة التي ذكرها رأي واحد. وأقول أيضا إنّ ذلك الرأي الواحد الذي هو رأي موسى عليه السلام كما ذكر جالينوس هو فرع تابع لأصل شريعته وقاعدتها وشريعة جدّه إبراهيم عليهما السلام فلم تضطرب أقواله ولا تناقضت بل

---

١ نقول] القول Sch || ٢ والثاني] الثاني G | ومن] وفي Ka || ٣ حالة] حال ELBP || ٤ جسم] جرم ELBP || ٥ جسم] جرم ELBP | سخيف] ضعيف Ka Sch G | سور] صور Ka G || ٦ بقاء] om. Ka || ٩ اختلاط] اخلاط Ka | المتشرّعين] الشرعين Sch || ١٠ وإنّما] ولما Ka || ١١ يتكلّم] تكلّم Ka | نسب] ينسب Ka || ١٣ وإنّما] وأمّا B || ١٤ خارجا] خارج G || ١٦ شريعته وقاعدتها] شريعتنا وقاعدتنا P شريعتنا وقاعدتها EL

made for himself and claims to be his faith are not the consequence of his [own] fundamental belief, but what he says is the consequence of the belief of others. Therefore, his words are confused and his conclusions do not conform to his principles.

(64) I will now begin to explain those four opinions that he ascribes to Moses—peace be upon him—in that statement [quoted above]. The first one is his saying that God commanded the hair of the eyebrows not to grow long, and that it obeyed him; he says that this is the opinion of Moses regarding natural things. But [in reality] this is not the opinion of Moses, for according to Moses, God only gives orders and prohibitions to intelligent beings. The second opinion is his saying that Moses believes that all things are possible with God; this, too, is not the opinion of Moses, but his opinion is that the power to do impossible things cannot be ascribed to God. Galen, because of his distortion [of the facts], did not notice the point where opinions differ. For there are things of which Moses says that they are possible and of which others say that they are impossible. This difference of opinion concerning these things is a[207] necessary consequence of the difference in the principles. But Galen did not pay attention to this and did not know it, since he only proceeds at random.

The third opinion is his saying that Moses believes that God, if He wished to instantly create a horse or ox from ashes, could do so. It is true that this is the opinion of Moses, and it is a necessary consequence of one of his principles, as we are going to explain.

The fourth opinion is his saying that Moses believes that God does not choose the proper material for that which He wishes to come into existence in a certain manner, as, for instance, what he said about His choice of a cartilaginous body beneath the eyelashes. But Moses—peace be upon him—does not have a different opinion in this. One of the things that Moses—peace be upon him—clearly stated is that God does nothing in vain and by chance, but that He creates very well with justice and equity all that He creates, as I explained in my exposition of the principles of religion.[208]

تبعت أصولها وفروعها. و إنّ هذا الكلام كلّه الذي ذكره جالينوس هنا عن نفسه وقال إنّ هذا إيمانه لا يلزم أصل اعتقاده بل هذا الذي قاله لازم لاعتقاد غيره فاضطربت أقواله ولا اطّردت فروعه على أصوله.

(٦٤) والآن أبتدئ بشرح تلك الآراء الأربعة التي نسبها إلى موسى عليه السلام في هذا الكلام. أحدها وهو أوّلها قوله إنّ اللّه أمر شعر الحاجبين أن لا يطول فقبل منه وقال إنّ هذا رأي موسى في الأشياء الطبيعية. و إنّ هذا ليس رأي موسى ولا يأمر الله و ينهى عند موسى إلا ذا عقل. ورأيه الثاني قوله إنّ موسى يعتقد أنّ الأشياء كلّها ممكنة عند اللّه وهذا أيضا ليس هو رأي موسى بل رأيه أنّ لا يوصف اللّه بالقدرة على الممتنعات. و إنّما جالينوس بتحريفه لم ينتبه لموضع الاختلاف وذلك أنّ ثم أشياء يقول موسى هي من قبل الممكن وغيره يقول هي من قبل الممتنع. وهذا الاختلاف في تلك الأشياء فرع لازم لاختلاف وقع في الأصول. وجالينوس لا يأبه لهذا ولا يعرفه لكنّه يخبط فقط.

والرأي الثالث قوله إنّ موسى يعتقد أنّ اللّه لو شاء أن يخلق من الرماد فرسا أو ثورا دفعة خلق. هذا صحيح أنّه رأي موسى وهو فرع لازم لأصل أصله كما سنبيّن.

ورأيه الرابع هو قوله إنّ موسى يعتقد أنّ اللّه لا يختار المادّة الموافقة لكلّ ما يريد وجوده على صفة ما مثل ما ذكر من اختيار جسم غضرو في تحت الأشفار. وموسى عليه السلام لا يخالف في هذا ومما صرّح موسى عليه السلام أنّ اللّه لا يفعل شيئا عبثا ولا كيف اتّفق بل كلّ ما خلق حسنا جدّا خلقه وبعدل وتقسيط كما بيّنت فيما تكلّمت به في أصول الدين.

---

١ تبعت] بعقب k تثبت corr. Sch | أصولها وفروعها] فروعها أصولها ELBP || ٢ إيمانه] ايما منه G(!) إيماننا B إمانته Ka || ٣ اطّردت فروعه على] لزمة فروعه ELBP || ٦ في الأشياء الطبيعية. وإنّ هذا ليس رأي موسى] om. ELBP || ٧ ذا] لذي ELBP || ٨ رأيه] رأيته G | أنّ] om. G || ١٠ فرع] om. Ka | لازم] لاحق Ka || ١١ يخبط] يخلط corr. Sch || ١٤ يختار] إلا add. B | المادّة] om. B || ١٦ ومما] Ka G? ومثله Sch ومنذ BELP || ١٧ وتقسيط] وبقسط Ka

From all this one knows, of necessity, that the grapelike tunic of the eye has been perforated for the purpose of vision,[209] that the bones are hard and dry in order to provide solid support, and likewise all that exists in the bodies of living beings, or rather everything that exists, as the prophets who came after Moses—peace be upon him—have said that God has made all that He created with wisdom.[210] Galen understood only this one of Moses' opinions, that is, that something can suddenly exist in a manner contrary to the course of nature, like the transformation of a rod into a serpent[211] and of dust into lice.[212] Therefore, it is possible according to him that ashes are instantaneously transformed into a horse or an ox, and this is true and it is the opinion of Moses—peace be upon him. All these are necessary consequences of the principles in which Moses—peace be upon him—believes, and that is that the world was created. For the meaning of the world being created is that God—may He be exalted—alone, without anything beside Him, is the primordial and eternal one, that He has created the world after complete nonexistence and has brought into existence this heaven and all that is in it, and the first matter that is below the heaven, that He has formed from it water, air, earth, and fire, that He has shaped the celestial globe with its different spheres according to His will, and that He has shaped these elements and all that is composed of them with these [different] natures that we perceive, for He is the giver of forms by which they get their nature. This is the principle of the doctrine of Moses—peace be upon him. Since the first matter, according to Him, was brought into existence after nonexistence and was then shaped [into its forms], it is possible that God, who brought it into existence, will destroy it once He has made it. Likewise, it is possible that He will change its nature and the nature of everything that is composed of it and will give it instantly a nature different from the regular one, just as He brought it into existence instantly.

فيعلم من هذه الجملة بالضرورة أنّ العين إنّما ثقبت منها الطبقة العنبية للإبصار وأنّ العظام إنّما صلبت وجفّفت ليصحّ الاعتماد عليها وكذلك كلّ ما في أجسام الحيوان بل كلّ ما في الوجود كما قال الأنبياء أتباع موسى عليه السلام إنّ كلّ ما خلق اللّه بحكمة صنعه. وكان جالينوس فهم هذه الواحدة من رأي موسى وهي كون الشيء دفعة على غير المجرى الطبيعي كانقلاب العصا ثعبانا والتراب قملا. ولذلك يمكن عنده أن يصير الرماد فرسا أو ثورا دفعة وهذا صحيح وهو رأي موسى عليه السلام. وهذه كلّها فروع لازمة لأصل يعتقده موسى عليه السلام وهو أنّ العالم محدث لأنّ معنى حدوث العالم هو أنّ اللّه تعالى هو القديم الأزلي وحده لا غيره معه وأنّه أحدث العالم بعد عدم محض وأوجد هذه السماء وكلّ ما فيها وأوجد المادّة الأولى دون السماء وكوّن منها ماء وهواء وأرضا ونارا وطبع هذا الفلك على هذه الأدوار المختلفة كما شاء وطبع هذه الأسطقسّات وكلّ ما تركّب منها على هذه الطبائع التي نشاهدها إذ هو معطيها الصور التي بها صارت لها طبيعة. هذا هو أصل مذهب موسى عليه السلم. وإذا كانت المادّة الأولى عنده أوجدت بعد العدم وطبعت على ما طبعت فيجوز أن يعدمها اللّه موجدها بعد أن أوجدها وكذلك يجوز أن يغيّر طبيعتها وطبيعة كلّ شيء تركّب منها ويجعل لها طبيعة غير هذه المستقرّة دفعة كما أوجدها دفعة.

---

٤ وكان] وكأن Sch || ٥ ولذلك] وكذلك Sch || ٦ وهذا صحيح] om. ELBP || ٨ الأزلي] الأوّل EL || كلّ ما فيها وأوجد المادّة الأولى دون السماء] om. B || ١١ صارت] اتصورت B || ١٢ بعد] عند P

Thus, according to Moses—peace be upon him—the change of anything that belongs to the natural world of coming into being and passing away from its present condition falls under the category of being possible, and God possesses the power and will to effect this. If God—may He be exalted—wishes to maintain this world in its present state for all eternity and forever and ever, He can do so. And if He wishes to annihilate it all so that nothing remains besides Himself—may He be exalted—He can do so and has the power for it. If He wishes to retain it in its [present] nature in all its particulars [he can do so], and [if He wishes] to change an existing particular of an existing thing from its natural course, He can do so. All the miracles are of this kind.[213] Therefore the perception of one miracle on the part of him who perceives it is a stringent proof for the creation of the world. I mean by miracle here [those cases] in which there appears the existence of a thing not in accordance with the normal and permanent nature of its existence. It is of two types, either that of a thing that has the property of being always formed by certain degrees and under certain conditions is formed contrary to these normal conditions and is transformed instantly, like the transformation of the rod into a serpent, of dust into lice, of water into blood,[214] of air into fire,[215] and the noble holy hand [of Moses] turning white,[216] all of which occurred instantly; or that of a thing the production of which cannot occur at all according to the nature of this established [world], like the manna that was so hard that it could be ground and made into bread,[217] but melted and became liquid when the sun warmed it, together with the other miracles of the manna related by the Torah. All these and similar miracles fall under the category of the possible, because the existence of the world in the way in which it was produced is [a] possible [thing] itself. But according to the opinion of someone who professes that the world is eternal, all these things that are possible with us are impossible for him. For someone who believes in the eternity [of the world] says that this world, in its entirety, was made by God, that is, that He is the cause of its existence, and that this world in its present state is a necessary consequence of the existence of the Creator, just as the thing caused is a necessary consequence of the cause that is only to be found together with it, like the day being the necessary consequence of the sunrise and the shadow being the necessary consequence of an erect object, and similar cases.[218]

ولذلك كلّ ما في طبيعة الكون والفساد فتغيّره عمّا هو عليه عند موسى عليه السلام من باب الممكن الذي يوصف الله بالقدرة عليه وتتعلّق به المشيئة. إن شاء الله تعالى إبقاء هذا العالم على ما هو عليه لدهر الداهرين وأبد الأبدين أبقاه وإن شاء أن يعدم الكلّ ولا يبقى سواه تعالى فعل وهو القادر على ذلك. وإن شاء أن يبقيه على طبيعته في جميع جزئياته ويغيّر كون ما من جزئيات الكون عن مجرى طبيعته فعل. والمعجزات كلّها من هذا القبيل هي. ولذلك تكون مشاهدة المعجزة الواحدة عند من شاهدها برهانا قطعيا على حدث العالم. أعني بالمعجزة هاهنا ما بان فيه كونه على غير طبيعة الكون المعتادة دائما وهو نوعان: إمّا أن يتكوّن الشيء الذي شأنه أن يتكوّن على تدريجات مخصوصة وبأحوال مخصوصة دائما على غير تلك الأحوال المعتادة بل ينقلب دفعة كانقلاب العصا ثعبانا والتراب قملا والماء دما والهواء نارا واليد الكريمة المقدّسة بيضاء وكان جميع ذلك دفعة. وإمّا أن يحدث ما ليس في طبيعة هذا الوجود المستقرّ أن يتكوّن فيه مثل ذلك الحادث أصلا كالمنّ الذي كان من الصلابة في حيز أن يطحن ويخبز منه خبزا وإذا حميت عليه الشمس ذاب وسال وسائر ما نصّت التوراة في المنّ من المعجزات. كلّ هذه وأشباهها من باب الممكن إذ والعالم كان وجوده على ما أوجد بإمكان. وأمّا على رأي من يقول بقدم العالم فكلّ هذه الممكنات عندنا هي عنده ممتنعة وذلك أنّ معتقد القدم يقول إنّ هذا العالم بجملته الله هو فاعله أيّ علّة وجوده وهذا العالم على ما هو عليه لزم عن وجود البارئ كلزوم المعلول للعلّة التي لم تفارقها قطّ يعني كلزوم النهار عن طلوع الشمس أو لزوم الظلّ عن القائم وما أشبه ذلك.

---

١ ولذلك] وكذلك Sch | فتغيّره] تغيّره k فغيّره Sch تغيّره corr. Sch || ٣ أبقاه . . . وأبد الأبدين (٦٥)] om. B כאן חסר $B^1$ || ٦ شاهدها] يشاهدها Ka || ١٢ حيز] حين om. ELSch | أن] om. LP | حميت] حمت LP || ١٣ التوراة . . . الأشياء الممكنة ومن الممكنة (٦٧)] om. E || ١٤ والعالم] العالم corr. Ka Sch | أوجد] وجد L || ١٥ القدم] ($G^1$=) الدمم(G?) اللزوم Ka | الله] om. Ka Sch G

(65) Someone who holds this opinion says that movement can neither be generated nor perish; therefore the heaven is, according to him, eternal and the first matter [is] neither generated nor perishable, [but] has been and will be forever in the same condition as it is. And all that differs from this natural world of generation and decay is impossible according to him. Therefore it is impossible, according to him, that something is generated instantly whose nature is not such that it can be generated instantly, and that a thing can be generated whose generation does not belong to the nature of this matter, and that any condition of the conditions of what exists in the upper or lower [world] can be changed from its condition.

It is apparent to anyone who understands the necessary consequences of the opinions that for someone who believes in the eternity of the world in this manner God has no novel will nor choice, and nothing can possibly exist on which He can exert His power and will,[219] so that, for instance, He cannot bring us rain on one day and withhold it on another day, according to His will, because the rainfall in this established nature is consequential upon the formation of the vapors and the air that bring it about or withhold it. All this is consequential upon the formation of matter over which God can exert no influence. This means that he cannot simply bring about that which is impossible in matter, and he cannot create anything that is impossible in its forms of existence, since the matter has not been created but exists necessarily in this manner for all eternity and forever and ever. It should [thus] be clear to you what the consequences are of the opinions of those who believe in the eternity of the world as well as the consequences of [the opinions] of those who believe in its creation.

(66) But this Galen, [a] feebleminded and inexact [man], who is ignorant in most of the things he speaks about except for the medical art, repeatedly says and explains that he is skeptical on this [point], namely, the fundamental principle of the creation of the world, and does not know whether it is eternal or created. I wish I knew how he can be skeptical on this principle when he has built his whole discussion of the hair of the eyelashes and eyebrows on the principle of the eternity of the world. Therefore he says that anything that is impossible in matter is impossible [for God to bring about] and one cannot attribute to Him the power over it, even if He wished so a million times. He further states that [His] will is not sufficient, unless the matter is appropriate.

(٦٥) فصاحب هذا الرأي يقول إنّ الحركة غير كائنة ولا فاسدة فلذلك السماء عنده قديمة والمادّة الأولى غير كائنة ولا فاسدة ولم تزل ولا تزال أبدا هكذا على هذه الطبيعة. وكلّ ما يخالف هذه الطبيعة الكون والفساد فهو ممتنع عنده فلذلك فليس ممكن عنده أن يتكوّن دفعة ما ليس في طبيعته أن يتكوّن دفعة ولا أن يتكوّن ما ليس في طبيعة هذه المادّة أن يتكوّن ولا تتغيّر حالة من حالات الوجود العلوي والسفلي عمّا هو عليه.

وبيّن هو عند من يفهم ما يلزم عن الآراء أنّ القائل بقدم العالم على هذا النحو ليس للّه مشيئة حادثة ولا اختيار ولا في الوجود ممكن تتعلّق به قدرته وإرادته حتّى أنّه مثلا لا يقدر أن يأتينا بمطر يوما ما أو يمنعه يوما ما بحسب إرادته إذ نزول المطر في هذه الطبيعة المستقرّة تابع لتهيّء الأبخرة والهواء الموجبين له أو المانعين منه. وكلّ ذلك تابع لتهيّء المادّة التي لا فعل للّه فيها أعني أنّ كلّ ما يعتاص في المادّة فلا يقدر أن يسهله وما يمتنع في أكوانها لا يقدر أن يوجده إذ ليست المادّة كوّنت بل هكذا وجودها اللازم لها دهر الداهرين وأبد الأبدين. فقد بان لك ما يلزم من الآراء لمن يعتقد قدم العالم وما يلزم لمن يعتقد حدوث العالم.

(٦٦) وهذا جالينوس المخرّف الغير محصّل الجاهل لأكثر ما يتكلّم فيه خارجا عن صناعة الطبّ يقول ويصرّح مرّات أنّه شكّاك في هذه، قاعدة حدث العالم ولا يعلم هل هو قديم أو محدث. فيا ليت شعري كيف هو شكّاك في هذا الأصل وطرد قوله كلّه هنا في كلامه في شعر الأشفار والحاجبين على أصل قدم العالم ولذلك يقول إنّ كلّ ما هو معتاص في المادّة فغير ممكن ولا يوصف اللّه بالقدرة عليه ولو شاء ذلك ألف ألف مرّة. وقال إنّ ليس المشيئة كافية إلا أن توافق المادّة.

---

٢ ولا تزال] om. L | تزال] يزول Ka || ٣ فليس ممكن] ليس من الممكن LP || ٦ العالم] العامل G || ٨ يأتينا بمطر] يوتي المطر Ka | إرادته] إراده G || ١٠ يمتنع ... ولا تعرّضت في (٨٦)] om. P || ١١ لها] om. L || ١٢ بان] اللّه add. G del G[1] | لك] om. B || ١٣ المخرّف] المخزف (!)B المنحرف Sch | الغير محصّل] الغر Ka || ١٤ قاعدة] المقعدة B

(67) He says that God is the principle of the creation of all created things, as Moses has said, in addition to the principle that resides in the matter from which they have been created. These are Galen's very words, and therefore he believes in the eternity of the world and, likewise, in the eternity of God, and that both of them are principles for the creation of everything that is created. This is the belief in the eternity of the world of which Galen says is subject to skepticism. Therefore he should also have been skeptical whether the sudden creation of a horse from dust is possible, as Moses—peace be upon him—says, or impossible, as say those who pass judgment in favor of the eternity of the world. That he is skeptical[220] about the principle but passes judgment in favor of [the possibility] of a necessary consequence is proof of his ignorance about the fact that that consequence is intrinsically connected to that principle.

Similarly, his statement that there are things that are impossible for God in themselves is an acknowledgment of the eternity of matter. The most amazing thing is his saying that God knew that it was best for the eyebrows not to grow long, and his saying that God only wishes possible things to occur, and from the possible [things] he only chooses the best. [As to] that knowledge, will, and choice that are attributed to God, according to him, and as to the existence of things that are possible for God [to bring about]: I wish I knew on which of the two fundamental principles he has based his saying and decided his judgment, on the belief in the eternity or on that in the creation of the world.

(68) I have explained to you that, according to the belief in the eternity of the world, there does not remain with God either will or choice, and there is no possible thing in existence that He could choose or produce. But what he [Galen] has said in these sayings is correct according to the opinion that both world and matter are created. Therefore you should consider how he confuses in what he says things that are consequences of the doctrine of the creation of the world with [other] things that are consequences of the doctrine of the eternity of the world and thinks that all this is one belief and one opinion, whereas he is skeptical about the question whether the world is eternal or created. All that he said in his confused statement is clear and evident to him, but they are his particular belief and something he is convinced of. This is clear proof that he is ignorant about the[221] principles and their necessary consequences he is speaking about and that he pays only little attention to his own words.

(٦٧) وقال إنّ اللّه مبدأ خلق كلّ مخلوق كما قال موسى وزيادة المبدأ الذي من قبل المادّة التي منها خلق. هذا نصّ جالينوس فهو إذاً يعتقد قدم المادّة كقدم اللّه وأنّهما مبدآن لخلق كلّ ما خلق. وهذا هو القول بقدم العالم الذي يعتقد جالينوس أنّ الأمر في ذلك مشكوك فيه فلذلك كان يلزمه أن يشكّ أيضا هل كون الفرس من الرماد دفعة ممكن كما يقول موسى عليه السلام أو ممتنع كما يقول من يبتّ القضية بقدم العالم. فكونه شكّ في الأصل وبتّ القضية في الفرع دليل على جهله بلزوم هذا الفرع لذلك الأصل.

وكذلك قوله إنّ من الأشياء أشياء في أنفسها غير ممكنة عند اللّه هو القول بقدم المادّة. وأعجب الأمور قوله لمّا علم اللّه أنّ شعر الحاجبين الأصلح له أن لا يطول وقوله إنّما يشاء اللّه أن تكون الأشياء الممكنة ومن الممكنة لا يختار إلا أجودها. يا ليت شعري هذا العلم والمشيئة والاختيار الذي يوصف بها اللّه عنده وكون في الوجود أمور ممكنة عند اللّه، على أيّ القاعدتين بنى قوله هذا وبتّ الحكم فيه، على رأي القدم أو على رأي حدث العالم.

(٦٨) وقد بيّنت لك أنّ على رأي اعتقاد قدم العالم ليس يبقى للّه لا مشيئة ولا اختيار ولا ثمّ في الموجودات ممكن يمكنه أن يختاره أو يحدثه. وإنّما يصحّ ما قاله في هذه الأقاويل على رأي حدث العالم وكون المادّة محدثة. فتأمّل كيف يخلط في كلامه أشياء تلزم عن القول بحدث العالم مع أشياء تلزم عن القول بقدم العالم ويظنّ الكلّ اعتقادا واحدا ورأيا واحدا وهل العالم قديم أو محدث مشكوك فيه عنده. وكلّ ما قال في هذا الكلام المختلط هو بيّن واضح عنده وهو الإيمان الخاصّ وبتّ القضية فيه فهذا دليل واضح على جهله بأصول ما تكلّم فيه وفروعه وقلّة تأمّله لما يقول.

٥ شكّ] شاكّ L || ٦ دليل] واضح add. L || ٨ وقوله] إلى قوله L || ١٢ ليس] لم B || ١٧ الإيمان] om. Ka

This was my aim in this chapter and nothing else. I did not endeavor in this chapter to refute those who believe in the eternity [of the world], to make them doubt and to expose them, as I have composed a number of expositions of these subjects in my compositions on the Divine Law.

(69) Says Moses: In a previous aphorism I spoke about human diseases.[222] My[223] aim in this aphorism is to give you some very useful advice concerning your opinions and beliefs. That is that if any man informs you about things that he has witnessed and observed with his own eyes,[224] even if that person is according to you most trustworthy and honest and has excellent intellectual and moral qualities, you should consider [carefully] what he tells you. If he wants with his account of his observation to strengthen an opinion that he has or a doctrine he believes in, distrust him in what he says that he observed and let not your mind become confused by those stories. Rather, consider those opinions and doctrines according to the requirements of sound judgment without paying attention to what he says that he saw with his own eyes, regardless whether this assertion is advanced by a single person or by a group of persons holding that opinion. For the ambition [to have his opinions accepted] induces a person to ugly things, especially in the case of controversy and disputation.

(70) I have only made this statement as an introduction to what I will remind you of concerning the matter of Galen, this[225] learned and eminent man. You know that according to his opinion there are three major organs—the heart, the brain, and the liver—and that none of these three fundamental organs derive their particular power from another organ in whatever way. But, as you know, the opinion of Aristotle and his followers is that the only major organ is the heart, and that the heart sends a power to every singular organ [and] with this power those organs perform their particular function. Therefore, according to Aristotle, the heart sends a power to the brain [and] with this power the brain performs its function, namely, providing sensation and motion to the other parts of the body. Similarly, [concerning] the

وهذا كان غرضنا في هذا الفصل لا غير ولا تعرّضت في هذا الفصل ولا لردّ على من قال بقدم ولا لتشكيك عليه ولا لتشنيع إذ قد تقدّم لي في هذه الأغراض عدّة أقاويل في التآليف الشرعية.

(٦٩) قال موسى: قد تقدّم لي الكلام في الفصل الذي قبل هذا في الأمراض الإنسانية وغرضي في هذا الفصل نصيحتك بنصيحة نافعة لك جدّا في آرائك واعتقاداتك. وهو أنّ كلّ شخص يخبرك بأمور شاهدها وأدركها حسّا وإن كان ذلك الشخص عندك في غاية الصدق والعدالة وفضيلة النطق والخلق فتأمّل ما يخبرك به. فإن كان يريد بما ذكر أنّه رآه تقوية رأي يراه أو مذهب يعتقده فاتّهمه في ما ذكر أنّه شاهده ولا تشوش أفكارك بتلك الأخبارات بل اعتبر تلك الآراء والمذاهب بحسب ما يقتضيه النظر من غير التفات لما ذكر أنّه شوهد عيانا سوى كان ذلك المخبّر واحدا أو جماعة من أهل ذلك الرأي لأنّ الهوى يحمل الإنسان على أشياء قبيحة وبخاصّة عند المخاصمة والمنازعة.

(٧٠) وإنّما قدّمت لك هذه المقدّمة لما أنبّهك عليه من أمر جالينوس هذا العالم الفاضل. قد علمت رأيه في الأعضاء الرئيسة أنّها ثلاثة: القلب والدماغ والكبد وأنّ هذه الثلاثة مبادئ ليس يستفيد منها أحدها قوته الخصيصة به من عضو آخر بوجه. ومذهب أرسطو وتباعه كما علمت هو أنّ العضو الرئيس وحده هو القلب وأنّ القلب يبعث قوة إلى كلّ عضو من الأعضاء، بتلك القوة يفعل ذلك العضو فعله الخاصّ به ولذلك القلب عند أرسطو يبعث قوة إلى الدماغ، بتلك القوة يفعل الدماغ فعله وهو إعطاء الحسّ والحركة لسائر الأعضاء. وكذلك

---

١ غير] الأخير E | ولا لرد] لا للرد EL لا لرد B || ٢ لتشكيك] تشكيك G للتشكيك ELB التشكيك Ka | لتشنيع] للتشنيع ELB تشنيع Sch التشنيع Ka || ٤ الإنسانية] النفسانية Ka || ٥ آرائك] رأيك Ka || ٧ أنّه رآه] om. EL || ٨ تقوية] يقوّي Ka | يراه] بداه Ka || ١١ والمنازعة] om. ELBP || ١٥ وأنّ] ومن EL || ١٧ إعطاء] يعطي EL ?P

faculties of imagination, rational thought, and memory that exist in the brain, these faculties exist in the brain and perform their functions thanks to that principle that the brain derives from the heart. And this is correct when one looks into it, because the brain—and similarly every organ—only carries out its functions while it lives its particular perfect life, and the heart is [the organ] that provides [the brain] with the power for its particular life.[226]

(71) Others than us have sufficiently discussed this matter. Galen thinks this faculty of sensation [and] motion, as well as rational thought, memory, and imagination, has its first principle in the brain and that the heart does not participate in this at all, meaning that no power of sensation or motion reaches the brain [from the heart]. You[227] know his constant argumentation concerning this opinion in all his books. His endeavor to prove the correctness of his opinion led him to relate the following in the second treatise of his book *On the Doctrines of Hippocrates and Plato*. Listen to what he says there.

He says: It is possible to expose the heart, press it, crush[228] it, or remove it completely without piercing the two chest cavities. It was a custom for most sacrifices to be offered in this way. And animals could be observed—once their heart was removed and placed on the altar[229]—to breathe and bellow vehemently and to flee until they suffered from a hemorrhage and died. These are his words.[230]

(72) Be amazed, you who belong to the community of those who engage in speculation. How can we believe him in [what he says in] this statement and at the same time believe him in what he says in the fifth [treatise] of *De locis affectis*, and [this last] statement be correct? For there he remarks that it is in any case unavoidable that the heart suffers harm when death occurs. And death is consequential upon an excessive dyscrasia of the heart. But a severe dyscrasia of the heart that is specific for the homogeneous parts is not followed by quick death. But when it is specific for the composite organs, it is followed by sudden death. These are his words there.[231]

قوة التخيّل والفكر والذكر الموجودة في الدماغ بذلك المبدأ الذي يستفيده الدماغ من القلب توجد فيه هذه القوى وتفعل أفعالها وهذا هو الصحيح عند النظر لأنّه إنّما يفعل الدماغ أفعاله وكذلك كلّ عضو إنّما يفعل أفعاله وهو حيّ الحياة الكاملة الخصيصة به والقلب هو الذي يبعث له قوة الحياة الخصيصة به.

(٧١) وقد تكلّم في هذا غيرنا بما فيه كفاية وجالينوس يرى أنّ هذه القوة الحسّ والحركة وكذلك الفكر والذكر والتخيّل مبدأها الأوّل في الدماغ ولا للقلب في ذلك مشاركة أصلا أعني أنّه لا تصل قوة إلى الدماغ بها يحسّ أو يتحرّك. وقد علمت خصومته الدائمة على هذا الرأي في جميع كتبه فوصل به الاجتهاد في تصحيح رأيه هذا أن حكى في المقالة الثانية من كتابه في آراء أبقراط وأفلاطون ما حكى واسمع ما قال هناك.

قال: يمكن أن يكشف عن القلب ويعصر أو يشقّ أو يقتلع بجملته من غير أن يثقب تجويفي الصدر. وقد جرت العادة في أكثر الضحايا أن يفعل ذلك فيها وينظر الحيوان وقلبه قد اقتلع ووضع في موضع القرابين والحيوان يتنفّس ويصيح صياحا شديدا ويهرب حتّى يجحف به انبثاق الدم فيموت. هذا نصّه.

(٧٢) فاعجبوا يا معشر أهل النظر كيف نستطيع أن نصدّقه في هذا الخبر مع تصديقنا له بما ذكر في خامسة التعرّف وهو الحقّ وهو قوله هناك إنّ لا بدّ على كلّ حال أن ينال القلب آفة عند حلول الموت والموت هو تابع لإفراط سوء مزاج القلب فما كان من سوء مزاج القلب عظيم القدر وخاصّ بالأعضاء المتشابهة الأجزاء فليس يتبعه موت عاجلا. وما هو منه خاصّ بالأعضاء المركّبة فالموت يتبعه فجأة. هذا نصّه هناك.

---

١ يستفيده] يقتنيه Ka || ٦ الأوّل] الأولى G || ٧ يتحرّك] يحرّك ELBP || ١٠ يقتلع] يقلع G || ١١ أكثر] هذا Ka || ١٣ يجحف] يحجو Ka || ١٥ وهو الحقّ] om. B | إنّ] انه Ka | ينال] تصال إلى Ka || ١٧ القدر] المقدار LBP

Galen wants us to believe in both statements at the same time. One [statement] is that if the heart suffers from a severe dyscrasia, because it is a composite organ, that is when [superfluous] matter streams into it that changes its temperament or causes a swelling [and] the living being dies suddenly. And the second statement is that the heart can be pressed or crushed or removed and thrown into a different place, yet the animal lives, bellows, runs, and breathes until he is killed by an excessive loss of blood, as he states in this other statement. Perhaps we could also say to him that, since his death only results from the harm caused by the loss of blood, if we would grasp the edges of the [pulsatile] vessels from which the blood is flowing with our hands for a long time, the animal would remain alive while he has no heart. This is astonishing!

Consider to what consequences a person is necessarily led when he wants to support his opinion. One of the things that should be pointed out is that if[232] what he says is correct, it would not be a decisive argument for refuting Aristotle's opinion that the principle of sensation and motion comes from the heart. For [the truth is that] the root (i.e., the heart) that provides a certain power may be eliminated and [yet] that power remains for a certain time but then ceases because that which replenishes it has ceased [to be active]. This is comparable to a well that is suddenly filled up and the water that flowed from it remains in channels that water and moisten the surrounding area until that water comes to an end.

One can also see how [in the case of] some dead persons their body remains warm for an hour like the heat of [the body] of living persons even though their heart has stopped [beating]. This is because that heat is that which emanated from the heart before it stopped, but then [this heat] dwindles away and dissolves because it finds none to replenish it. Likewise,[233] some animals after being decapitated [still] move their limbs through that strength that remains in their nerves until it is exhausted. So, too, we say to him that the principle that the heart sends to the brain remains there for a short time after the heart is gone until that strength ceases to be. The only thing that befalls us from these stories [by Galen] is that they are repulsive and difficult to accept, nothing else.

و يريد منّا جالينوس أن نصدّقه في القولين جميعا أحدهما هو أنّ القلب إذا ساء مزاجه جدّا من حيث هو عضو مركّب وذلك بأن تنصبّ له مادّة تغيّر مزاجه أو تورمه فيموت الحيوان فجأة. والقول الآخر وهو أنّ القلب يعصر أو يشقّ أو يقتلع و يرمى في موضع آخر والحيوان حيّ يصيح ويجري و يتنفّس حتّى يقتله كثرة خروج الدم كما ذكر في هذا القول الآخر. ولعل نقول له أيضا إذ وموته إنّما يتبع إجحاف خروج الدم لعلّنا لو مسكنا أطراف تلك العروق التي يخرج منها الدم بأيدينا مدّة طويلة لدام الحيوان حيّا وهو لا قلب له. وهذا عجيب.

فاعتبر ما يوجبه للإنسان نصرة رأيه وممّا يجب أن ينبّه عليه أنّه لو صحّ ما ذكره لما كان له في ذلك حجّة قطعية يبطل بها رأي أرسطو في أنّ مبدأ الحسّ والحركة من القلب لأنّه قد يبطل الأصل المعطي لقوة ما وتبقى تلك القوة مدّة ما وتنفد بعد ذلك لانقطاع الممدّ لها كعين ماء تطمّ دفعة و يبقى الماء الذي قد جرى منها في مجرى تروي وترطّب ما حولها حتّى ينفد ذلك الماء.

أنت ترى بعض الأموات يبقى جسمه حارّا ساعة كحرارة الأحياء و إن كان قد سكن قلبه لأنّ تلك الحرارة هي التي استفادها من القلب قبل سكونه وهي تنفد وتنحلّ إذ لا تجد ما يمدّها. وكذلك يحرّك بعض الحيوان أعضاءه بعد قطع رأسه بتلك القوة الحاصلة في العصب حتّى تنفد. كذلك نقول له إنّ المبدأ الذي بعثه القلب إلى الدماغ بقي فيه مديدة يسيرة بعد ذهاب القلب حتّى نفدت تلك القوة. فما حصلنا من هذه الحكايات إلا على الشناعة البعيدة من القبول لا غير.

وأمّا كيف يخرج القلب ولا ينثقب أحد تجويفي الصدر فهو أن يشقّ من المنحر في آخر

---

٥ إجحاف] احجاف Ka || ٦ حيّا] فيها EL || ٨ يوجبه للإنسان] يوجب الإنسان E | نصرة رأيه] نصره ورأيه G || ٩ قد] يمكن أن L يكون أن add. E || ١٠ الممدّ ($=G^1$) ] المواد ELP المدد G الممدّ لها] المد لها الممد Ka | تطمّ] تضم EL || ١١ مجرى] مجراه EL || ١٣ لأنّ] لكن Ka | إذ لا] ولا G || ١٥ له] om. Ka || ١٦ الحكايات] الحكاية ELBP

But how can one take out the heart without perforating one of the chest cavities? This can only be done by splitting the site of the throat at the back of the neck and by gently pulling out the heart from its membrane therethrough. And then the membrane of the heart is left as it is, connected to the back and chest. [Such an operation] is very difficult if one tries to do it after the death of an animal. But when the animal is [still alive] as he (i.e., Galen) mentions, it is something that is most unlikely. He only made this assumption to support his opinion, nothing else. God is all-knowing.

العنق ويتلطّف من هناك في إخراج القلب من غلافه ويترك غلاف القلب كما هو متّصل بالظهر والصدر. وهذا في غاية العسر إذا فعلته بعد موت الحيوان وأمّا في حال حياته كما ذكر فهو أمر في غاية البعد. وإنّما هذا فرض فرض لنصر الرأي لا غير. واللّه أعلم.

---

١ هو] MS P ends here || ٢ العسر] جدّا add. ELB | إذا فعلته] فعله EL || ٣ هذا فرض فرض] كان هذا فرض k هذا فكان فرض G? | واللّه أعلم] تمّ الكتاب والحمد لربّ العالمين وقع الفراغ منه في العشر الأوّل من شهر الأوّل سنة תקי״ב من الخليقة وكتب لنفسه بخطّ يده أصغر الأطبّاء مخلوف ولد **אלחזן שמואל דמנשי זלה״ה** نفعه اللّه بما فيه وكشفه على أسراره ومعانيه وسرره في سائر أفعاله لما يرضيه ونجحه في كلّ مقاصده الدنيائيّة والأخروية ورقّاه إلى المدار الشريفة العلويّة ليحصل إلى السعادة الأبديّة الدائما والغير منقضية إنّه على ذلك قدير وبلاغه به جدير والحمد لواهب العقل كما هو مستحقّه لا إلاه سواه تبارك وتعالى B | أعلم] تمّت المقالة والحمد للّه وكمل كتاب الفصول للرأيس الأكمل والعالم الأوحد موسى بن ميمون بن عبيد اللّه الإسرائيلي القرطبي رحم اللّه عنه وكان الفراغ من نسخه في شهر مايه سنة ألف وثلاثة مائة واثنين وستين لتأريخ الصغر وذلك بمدينة طليطلة حرسها اللّه وكتبها يوسف بن اسحق بن شبتاي الإسرائل add. L تمّت المقالة الخامسة والعشرون والحمد للّه ربّ العالمين وبتمامها كمل جميع كتاب الفصول للرئيس الأجل ربينو موسى ابن ميمون القرطبي رضي اللّه عنه وقدس روحه وكان الفراغ من نسخة هذا الكتاب في العشر الأوسط من شهر فبرير ألذي من سنة ألف وثلثة مائة وثمانين لتأريخ الروم وافقه كب **אדר ראשון** الذي من سنة خمسة آلاف ومائة وتسعة وأربعين لتأريخ الخليقة كتبه لنفسه ولمن شاء إليه سعده موسى ابن يهودة بن شوشان وكان كتبه بمدينة القلعة <. . .> add. E تمّت المقالة الخامسة والعشرين وبتمامها تمّ كتاب الفصول التي جمعها موسى بن عبيد اللّه الاسرائيلي القرطبي في الطبّ. نقلت هذه النسخة من نسخة نقلت من [G$^{1}$?] نسخة بخطّ أبي المعاني يوسف بن عبد اللّه وهو ابن أخت المصنّف المذكور ووجدت فيها مكتوب: كتبت هذه المقالة الخامسة والعشرون بعد وفاة المولى الرئيس خالي ولم يرتّبها كما فعل بالمقالات الأوّل جميعها لأنّه تحرّر (*يحرّر) التعاليق التي بخطّه وبعد ذلك أبيّضها وأحرّرها بين يديه وكان نسخ هذه المقالة في أوّل سنة اثنين وستّمائة وللّه الحمد والمنّة (G (fol. 273, end aphorism 25.55

# Notes to the English Translation

## The Twenty-Second Treatise

1. "We find medicines that are effective through their powers": Cf. Galen, *De theriaca ad Pisonem* 4: τὰ δὲ καὶ μικτὸν ἐν τῇ οὐσίᾳ τὴν δύναμιν ἔχοντα (ed. Kühn, 14:225). Also cf. ed. and trans. Richter-Bernburg, 109a (Arabic edition), 64 (German translation): وبعضها يفعل بقوة أو قوى فيه (and other [medicines] are effective through one or more powers they contain). The Arabic title *ilā Qayṣar* is a corruption of *ilā Fīṣun*; see Steinschneider, "Griechische Ärzte," 292 n. 55; and Ullmann, *Medizin im Islam*, 49 n. 51.

2. Galen, *De theriaca ad Pisonem* 4 (ed. Kühn, 14:225).

3. Galen, *De theriaca ad Pisonem* 9 (ed. Kühn, 14:240; ed. and trans. Richter-Bernburg, 113a–114a [Arabic edition], 75–76 [German translation]).

4. Galen, *De theriaca ad Pisonem* 9 (ed. Kühn, 14:240; ed. and trans. Richter-Bernburg, 113a–114a [Arabic edition], 75–76 [German translation]).

5. Galen, *De theriaca ad Pisonem* 9 (ed. Kühn, 14:240; ed. and trans. Richter-Bernburg, 113b [Arabic edition], 75 [German translation]).

6. Galen, *De theriaca ad Pisonem* 9 (ed. Kühn, 14:241; ed. and trans. Richter-Bernburg, 114a [Arabic edition], 76 [German translation]).

7. Galen, *De theriaca ad Pisonem* 9 (ed. Kühn, 14:242–43; ed. and trans. Richter-Bernburg, 114a [Arabic edition], 76 [German translation]).

8. Galen, *De theriaca ad Pisonem* 9 (ed. Kühn, 14:240; ed. and trans. Richter-Bernburg, 113b [Arabic edition], 75 [German translation]). This remedy is quoted by the fourteenth-century Jewish physician R. Moshe Narboni in his medical encyclopedia entitled *Sefer Oraḥ Ḥayyim*, fol. 23a, according to the translation by Nathan ha-Meʾati. For more on this encyclopedia, see Bos, "R. Moshe Narboni."

9. Galen, *De theriaca ad Pisonem* 9 (ed. Kühn, 14:240–41; ed. and trans. Richter-Bernburg, 113b [Arabic edition], 75 [German translation]); cf. Narboni, *Sefer Oraḥ Ḥayyim*, fol. 23a.

10. Galen, *De theriaca ad Pisonem* 9 (ed. Kühn, 14:240; ed. and trans. Richter-Bernburg, 113b [Arabic edition], 75 [German translation]); cf. Narboni, *Sefer Oraḥ Ḥayyim* fol. 22a.

11. "Shrimp" (*irbiyān*): Cf. Galen, *De theriaca ad Pisonem* 9: κάρις (ed. Kühn, 14:242; ed. and trans. Richter-Bernburg, 114a [Arabic edition], 76, 151 n. 75 [German translation]).

12. Galen, *De theriaca ad Pisonem* 9 (ed. Kühn, 14:242; ed. and trans. Richter-Bernburg, 114a [Arabic edition], 76 [German translation]).

13. Galen, *De theriaca ad Pisonem* 9 (ed. Kühn, 14:241; ed. and trans. Richter-Bernburg, 113b [Arabic edition], 75 [German translation]).

14. Galen, *De theriaca ad Pisonem* 9 (ed. Kühn, 14:241; ed. and trans. Richter-Bernburg, 113b [Arabic edition], 76 [German translation]).

15. Galen, *De theriaca ad Pisonem* 9 (ed. Kühn, 14:242; ed. and trans. Richter-Bernburg, 114a [Arabic edition], 76 [German translation]).

16. Galen, *De theriaca ad Pisonem* 9 (ed. Kühn, 14:242; ed. and trans. Richter-Bernburg, 114a [Arabic edition], 76 [German translation]).

17. Galen, *De theriaca ad Pisonem* 9 (ed. Kühn, 14:242; ed. and trans. Richter-Bernburg, 114a [Arabic edition], 76 [German translation]); cf. Narboni, *Sefer Oraḥ Ḥayyim*, fol. 47b.

18. Galen, *De theriaca ad Pisonem* 9 (ed. Kühn, 14:242; ed. and trans. Richter-Bernburg, 114a [Arabic edition], 76 [German translation]).

19. "it reduces the swelling of the spleen": Cf. Galen, *De theriaca ad Pisonem* 9: σπλῆνα τήκει (ed. Kühn, 14:241); and ed. and trans. Richter-Bernburg, 113b: يزيل الطحال العظيم. It is possible that يزيل is a corrupt reading of يذبل.

20. Galen, *De theriaca ad Pisonem* 9 (ed. Kühn, 14:242; ed. and trans. Richter-Bernburg, 113b [Arabic edition], 75 [German translation]); cf. Narboni, *Sefer Oraḥ Ḥayyim*, fol. 51b.

21. Galen, *De theriaca ad Pisonem* 9 (ed. Kühn, 14:242; ed. and trans. Richter-Bernburg, 113b [Arabic edition], 75 [German translation]); cf. Narboni, *Sefer Oraḥ Ḥayyim*, fol. 82a.

22. Galen, *De theriaca ad Pisonem* 9 (ed. Kühn, 14:242; ed. and trans. Richter-Bernburg, 114a [Arabic edition], 76 [German translation]); cf. Narboni, *Sefer Oraḥ Ḥayyim*, fol. 82a.

23. Galen, *De theriaca ad Pisonem* 9 (ed. Kühn, 14:242; ed. and trans. Richter-Bernburg, 114a [Arabic edition], 76 [German translation]); cf. Narboni, *Sefer Oraḥ Ḥayyim*, fol. 82a.

24. "for intestinal ulcers": Cf. Galen, *De theriaca ad Pisonem* 9: δυσεντερικοῖς (for those suffering from dysentery; ed. Kühn, 14:241); and ed. and trans. Richter-Bernburg, 113b: من الخلفة الكائنة من قروح الأمعاء (for diarrhea resulting from intestinal ulcers).

25. "Castoreum": A desiccated excretion of the glands of the genital apparatus of the *Castor fiber*; see Maimonides, *Glossary of Drug Names* 79 (trans. Rosner, 65).

26. "shivers" (*kuzāz*): Cf. Galen, *De theriaca ad Pisonem* 9 (ed. Kühn, 14:241): σπασμούς (convulsions).

27. Galen, *De theriaca ad Pisonem* 9 (ed. Kühn, 14:241; ed. and trans. Richter-Bernburg, 113b [Arabic edition], 75 [German translation]).

28. "[this remedy] somewhat alleviates the pain": Cf. Galen, *De theriaca ad*

*Pisonem* 10 (ed. Kühn, 14:246): ἀπαλλάττονται τοῦ κινδύνου ([those bitten by the viper] are delivered from danger); also cf. ed. and trans. Richter-Bernburg, 115b: سكّنت الألم (it alleviates the pain).

29. Galen, *De theriaca ad Pisonem* 10 (ed. Kühn, 14:246; ed. and trans. Richter-Bernburg, 115b).

30. "marcasite stone": Galen, *Ad Glauconem de medendi methodo* 2.6 (ed. Kühn, 11:107), speaks about a pyrite stone (τοῦ πυρίτου λίθου).

31. "as if it is an act of magic": Cf. Galen, *Ad Glauconem de medendi methodo* 2.6 (ed. Kühn, 11:107): ὡς τὸ πρᾶγμα παραπλήσιον εἶναι μαγείᾳ.

32. Galen, *Ad Glauconem de medendi methodo* 2.6 (ed. Kühn, 11:107); cf. Narboni, *Sefer Oraḥ Ḥayyim*, fols. 82a–b. See also Bos, introduction to Maimonides, *Medical Aphorisms* (ed. and trans. Bos), 1:xxvi; and Bos, "Medical Aphorisms: Towards a Critical Edition," 45–47.

33. Galen, *De simplicium medicamentorum temperamentis ac facultatibus* 6.10 (ed. Kühn, 11:859–60). It should be noted that Galen explains the effectivity of this means in a rational way (εὔλογον), namely, that it worked through the fact that the child either inhaled certain particles that fell out from the root or inhaled the air tempered and changed by the root. See Temkin, *Falling Sickness*, 25. See also Maimonides, *Guide of the Perplexed* 3.37 (ed. and trans. Pines, 2:544); and Schwartz, "Magiyah, madda$^{c}$ nisyoni u-metodah madda$^{c}$it," 35–36. Also cf. Ibn Janāḥ, *Kitāb al-Talkhīṣ* (forthcoming), no. 761: فاونيا، يقال إنّه ورد الحمير، وقد امتحنّا أصله فلم نجد فيه خاصّية الفاونيا <في النفع للمصروعين> *Fāwaniyā* (peony) is said to be *ward al-ḥamīr* (lit. "rose of the donkeys"). We have experimented with its root, but we were not able to verify that it has the sympathetic property of *fāwaniyā*, <which is to say a positive effect on epileptics>.

34. "Asafetida [gum resin of *Ferula assa-fetida*]": Cf. Galen, *De simplicium medicamentorum temperamentis ac facultatibus* 6.10 (ed. Kühn, 11:860): ὁ Κυρηναῖος ὀπός (resin of a plant growing in the Cyrenaica). This plant called σίλφιον (silphion) disappeared from the market in the beginning of the time of the Roman emperors and was then replaced by the asafetida. For this remedy with asafetida, see Narboni, *Sefer Oraḥ Ḥayyim*, fol. 24a.

35. "[will dry up]": Cf. Galen, *De simplicium medicamentorum temperamentis ac facultatibus* 6.10 (ed. Kühn, 11:860): ξηραίνει.

36. "if one takes some of the threads that were dyed with purple hailing from the purple-fish, and that were used for choking a viper, and wraps them around the neck of someone who suffers from an inflammation of the tonsils or from any other inflammation in the neck, you see that it is beneficial for it in an amazing way": Cf. Narboni, *Sefer Oraḥ Ḥayyim*, fol. 25a.

37. "hailing from the purple-fish": Lit. "hailing from the sea." Cf. Galen, *De simplicium medicamentorum temperamentis ac facultatibus* 6.10 (ed. Kühn, 11:860): ἀπὸ θαλασσίας πορφύρας.

38. Galen, *De simplicium medicamentorum temperamentis ac facultatibus* 6.10 (ed. Kühn, 11:860).

39. For this remedy, see Durling, "Excreta as a Remedy," 30; and Maimonides, *Guide of the Perplexed* 3.37 (ed. and trans. Pines, 2:544).

40. "angina and inflammation of the throat": Cf. Galen, *De simplicium medicamentorum temperamentis ac facultatibus* 10.2 (ed. Kühn, 12:291): συνάγχας; and Ullmann, *Wörterbuch zu den griechisch-arabischen Übersetzungen*, 654.

41. "[red-hot]": Cf. Galen, *De simplicium medicamentorum temperamentis ac facultatibus* 10.2 (ed. Kühn, 12:292): διαπύρος.

42. Galen, *De simplicium medicamentorum temperamentis ac facultatibus* 10.2 (ed. Kühn, 12:291–92).

43. Galen, *De simplicium medicamentorum temperamentis ac facultatibus* 10.2 (ed. Kühn, 12:293–94).

44. Cf. Narboni, *Sefer Oraḥ Ḥayyim*, fol. 44a. "Or [the attack] is milder than usual": Missing in Narboni's quotation of these remedies.

45. Galen, *De simplicium medicamentorum temperamentis ac facultatibus* 10.2 (ed. Kühn, 12:295).

46. "knee": Narboni, *Sefer Oraḥ Ḥayyim*, fol. 51b, reads, following Nathan ha-Me᾿ati: "neck" (*ẓawwar* = *raqaba*; Arabic text: *rukba*).

47. "Do not use this therapy for those with a soft [body], like women, children and eunuchs": Galen, *De simplicium medicamentorum temperamentis ac facultatibus* 10.2 (ed. Kühn, 12:298), remarks that this medicine is too sharp for women who live in the city, for children, or in general for those with soft flesh.

48. "The excrements of a goat [mixed] with barley meal and kneaded with vinegar dissolve hard tumors, tumors of the knee and spleen. Do not use this therapy for those with a soft [body], like women, children . . .": Cf. Narboni, *Sefer Oraḥ Ḥayyim*, fol. 51b.

49. Galen, *De simplicium medicamentorum temperamentis ac facultatibus* 10.2 (ed. Kühn, 12:301); cf. Galen, *De theriaca ad Pisonem* 9 (ed. Kühn, 14:241); and Durling, "Excreta as a Remedy," 30; see also Narboni, *Sefer Oraḥ Ḥayyim*, fol. 49b.

50. Galen, *De simplicium medicamentorum temperamentis ac facultatibus* 10.2 (ed. Kühn, 12:301–2); cf. Narboni, *Sefer Oraḥ Ḥayyim*, fol. 94b.

51. Galen, *De simplicium medicamentorum temperamentis ac facultatibus* 10.2 (ed. Kühn, 12:302–3); Durling, "Excreta as a Remedy," 29; see also Narboni, *Sefer Oraḥ Ḥayyim*, fol. 76a.

52. This quotation does not appear in Galen, *De simplicium medicamentorum temperamentis ac facultatibus* 10, but in 11 (ed. Kühn, 12:342), as stated in the translations by Nathan ha-Me᾿ati and Zeraḥyah ben Isaac ben She᾿altiel Ḥen. See also Narboni, *Sefer Oraḥ Ḥayyim*, fol. 14a.

53. Cf. Narboni, *Sefer Oraḥ Ḥayyim*, fol. 96a. "Vinegar": Following the Hebrew translation by Nathan ha-Me᾿ati, Narboni reads: strong vinegar.

54. Galen, *De simplicium medicamentorum temperamentis ac facultatibus* 10.2 (ed. Kühn, 12:303).

55. Galen, *De simplicium medicamentorum temperamentis ac facultatibus* 11.1 (ed. Kühn, 12:356). See also Maimonides, *On Poisons* 56 (ed. and trans. Bos, 36–37).

56. Galen, *De simplicium medicamentorum temperamentis ac facultatibus* 11.1 (ed. Kühn, 12:335); cf. Narboni, *Sefer Oraḥ Ḥayyim*, fol. 25b.

57. Galen, *De simplicium medicamentorum temperamentis ac facultatibus* 11.1 (ed. Kühn, 12:360); cf. Narboni, *Sefer Oraḥ Ḥayyim*, fol. 44a.

58. Cf. Narboni, *Sefer Oraḥ Ḥayyim*, fol. 92b.

59. Cf. Narboni, *Sefer Oraḥ Ḥayyim*, fol. 57a.

60. Galen, *De simplicium medicamentorum temperamentis ac facultatibus* 11.1 (ed. Kühn, 12:363).

61. "next to its cutting effect it dissolves [and at the same time] checks the dissolution process": Cf. Galen, *De compositione medicamentorum secundum locos* 1.8 (ed. Kühn, 12:465): πρὸς τῷ διαφορεῖν ἀναστέλλειν τε καὶ ἀποκρούεσθαι τὸ ἐπιρρέον (next to the dissolving effect, it checks and repels what is flowing). It is possible that the Arabic text should read *annahu jama$^{c}$a ma$^{c}$a taqṭī$^{c}$ihi wa-taḥlīlihi annahu mānī$^{c}$ li-tajallub mā tajallaba*.

62. "checks the dissolution process": Lit. "checks the flow of what is flowing," i.e., falling apart, dissolving. Thus it does not fall apart completely.

63. Galen, *De compositione medicamentorum secundum locos* 1.8 (ed. Kühn, 12:465).

64. The standard *dirham* is 3.125 grams. See Hinz, *Islamische Masse und Gewichte*, 3.

65. One ounce is 37.5 grams in Egypt and 33.85 grams in Iraq; see Hinz, *Islamische Masse und Gewichte*, 35.

66. Galen, *De compositione medicamentorum secundum locos* 9.2 (ed. Kühn, 13:242); cf. Narboni, *Sefer Oraḥ Ḥayyim*, fol. 51b.

67. Abū Marwān $^{c}$Abd al-Malik ibn Zuhr (d. 1161), known in the West as Avenzoar, was one of the foremost physicians of the Western Caliphate. He was born in Seville, where he spent most of his life, and was in the service of the Almoravid dynasty (see Colin, *Avenzoar*, 23–41; Ullmann, *Medizin im Islam*, 162–63; *Encyclopaedia of Islam*, new ed., 3:977–78; and Kuhne Brabant, "Abū Marwān b. Zuhr: Un professionel"). Ibn Zuhr is frequently quoted by Maimonides, who regarded him highly. In *On the Elucidation of Some Symptoms and the Response to Them* 2 (ed. and trans. Bos, forthcoming), Maimonides praises him as unique in his generation and as one of the greatest observers (but see as well "Medicinische Schwanengesang" [ed. Kroner, 88–89]), and in *On Poisons* 78 (ed. and trans. Bos, 54) he remarks, "All this was mentioned and verified by the venerable Abū Marwān b. Zuhr, may God have mercy on him, with his lengthy experience, because he was the greatest among men in testing drugs and one who devoted himself to this more than any other. He was able to do so more than any other because of his great wealth and his skill in the medical art." (See Maimonides, *On Asthma* 9.1 [ed. and trans. Bos, 1:40, 131 n. 2]; and *Medical Aphorisms* 20.67 [ed. and trans. Bos, 4:87–88]). See also Bos, "Maimonides' Medical Works and Their Contributions," 251–52, 259–60.

68. "His son": I.e., Abū Bakr Muḥammad ibn $^{c}$Abd al-Malik ibn Zuhr al-Ḥafīd, a physician just like his father, but foremost known as a poet, who died in Marrakūsh in 1198/99; see *Encyclopaedia of Islam*, new ed., 3:978–79; and Ullmann, *Medizin im Islam*, 163.

69. "*Book on the Facilitation [of Treatment and Diet]*": I.e., Ibn Zuhr, *Kitāb al-taysīr* (ed. Al-Khouri).

70. "*Book on Foodstuffs*": I.e., Ibn Zuhr, *Kitāb al-aghdhiya* (ed. and trans. García Sánchez).

71. "one of the Andalusian kings": I.e., the Caliph Abū Muḥammad ᶜAbd al-Muʾmin ibn ᶜAlī, who ruled from 524 to 558 (1130–63 CE); cf. Ullmann, *Medizin im Islam*, 201; and Maimonides, *Medical Aphorisms* 20.67 (ed. and trans. Bos, 4:87–88).

72. Abū al-ᶜAlāʾ ibn Zuhr (d. 1131); cf. Colin, *Avenzoar,* 16–22; Ullmann, *Medizin im Islam*, 162; *Encyclopaedia of Islam*, new ed., 3:976–77. The *Kitāb al-Tadhkira* was edited and translated by Colin as *La Teḏkira d'Abū al-ᶜAlāʾ* in 1911, but on the basis of her research into the existing manuscripts of this text, Álvarez Millán, "Corpus médico-literario de los Banū Zuhr," 174–75, suggests that the author of this text was not the elder Abū al-ᶜAlāʾ ibn Zuhr, but rather his son, Abū Marwān. See also Maimonides, *Medical Aphorisms* 13.44 (ed. and trans. Bos, 3:49), where Maimonides quotes some *waṣāyā* (rules in hortatory form) by Abū l-ᶜAlāʾ ibn Zuhr, and *Medical Aphorisms* 20.68–81 (ed. and trans. Bos, 4:87–91), where he quotes a variety of foodstuffs from the *Kitāb al-Tadhkira*.

73. "The ingestion of nine granules of emerald, pulverized and filtered, in a mouthful of water on an empty stomach stops the diarrhea caused by poisons": Cf. Ibn Zuhr, *Kitāb al-taysīr* (ed. Al-Khouri, 8–9); *Kitāb al-aghdhiya* (ed. and trans. García Sánchez, 105); and Narboni, *Sefer Oraḥ Ḥayyim*, fol. 100b. See also Maimonides, *On Poisons* 19 (ed. and trans. Bos, 18).

74. "granules" *(ḥabbāt)*: One granule is approximately 0.0446 grams; cf. Hinz, *Islamische Masse und Gewichte*, 12–13.

75. "stops the diarrhea caused by poisons": Ibn Zuhr, *Kitāb al-taysīr* (ed. Al-Khouri, 8), remarks that it cures the diarrhea caused by a purging drug or a poisonous humor, and in the *Kitāb al-aghdhiya* (ed. and trans. García Sánchez, 105), he remarks that it resists all poisons.

76. "diarrhea": Following Nathan ha-Meʾati, Narboni, *Sefer Oraḥ Ḥayyim*, fol. 100b, reads "affliction" (*pegaᶜ* = آفة **L**).

77. "If it is hung [around the neck] of someone suffering from diarrhea or lientery, it cures him": Cf. Ibn Zuhr, *Kitāb al-taysīr* (ed. and trans. García Sánchez, 9).

78. "If the emerald is hung [around the neck], it strengthens the stomach and is beneficial for epilepsy. If it is kept in the mouth, it strengthens the teeth and the stomach": Cf. Ibn Zuhr, *Kitāb al-taysīr* (ed. Al-Khouri, 12).

79. "The criteria for [the application of] the emerald are the same as those for the theriac. It should not be taken together with food, but there should be an interval of nine hours between them": Cf. Ibn Zuhr, *Kitāb al-taysīr* (ed. Al-Khouri, 9); and Narboni, *Sefer Oraḥ Ḥayyim*, fol. 100b.

80. "nine": Ibn Zuhr, *Kitāb al-taysīr* (ed. Al-Khouri, 9): seven.

81. Ibn Zuhr, *Kitāb al-taysīr* (ed. Al-Khouri, 12), 64–65: "to look into the eyes of wild asses perpetuates the health of one's eyesight, and prevents the formation of a cataract; it is a wonderful property given by God for the perpetuation of the health of the eyes; this is undoubtedly true. [...] One should often look into the eyes of wild asses that are alive, for it has a specific wonderful property which I have tested myself. The physicians said that the vapor of its flesh, if it is cooked with saffron, is good for that. By applying this treatment continuously it is possible that vapor is dissolved and that healing occurs[?]." Cf. Maimonides, *On the Regimen of Health* 4.28 (ed. and trans. Bos, forthcoming): "The wild ass has a great

specific property in strengthening vision; this has been verified by experience. The consumption of its flesh and holding one's eyes over the vapor of its cooking meat strengthens vision and opens obstructions of the hollow nerves, and if one looks into the eyes of the wild ass for a long time, it strengthens vision and removes its defects. This has been verified by experience."

82. "The consumption of the heads of hares, as much as one is able to eat them, is beneficial for trembling. I found by experience that it is also beneficial for numbness and hemiplegia": Cf. Ibn Zuhr, *Kitāb al-taysīr* (ed. Al-Khouri, 12); cf. also Maimonides, *On the Regimen of Health* 4.27 (ed. and trans. Bos, forthcoming): "The best of game meat is the gazelle; similarly the hare. It has virtues that have been verified by experience, that is, eating its brain is beneficial for tremor, and in the same way its flesh in general is good for tremor and diseases of the nerves."

83. "I found by experience that the drinking of water in which mastic has been cooked protects against diseases of the liver and stomach, and that the drinking of water in which watermelon seed has been cooked protects against [kidney] stones": Cf. Ibn Zuhr, *Kitāb al-taysīr* (ed. Al-Khouri, 12): "I found by experience that the drinking of water in which mastic has been cooked protects against diseases of the liver and stomach." Cf. Narboni, *Sefer Oraḥ Ḥayyim*, fol. 46b.

84. "gold": Ibn Zuhr, *Kitāb al-taysīr* (ed. Al-Khouri, 12): pure gold (*dhahab ibrīz*).

85. "and that if one cooks therewith or throws [some of it] into a cooked dish, it strengthens the body in general": Cf. Ibn Zuhr, *Kitāb al-taysīr* (ed. Al-Khouri, 12): "If a dish is cooked and washed dinars are put into it, the dish acquires strength beneficial for the body in general"; another version reads: "If a dish is cooked in a golden pot, the dish acquires strength beneficial for the body in general." Cf. Narboni, *Sefer Oraḥ Ḥayyim*, fol. 31a: "If [a dish is] cooked with gold or if gold is put into a dish, it strengthens the heart and the body in general."

86. "[I also found by experience] that the application of a poultice of fresh rose blossoms to the eyes protects against ophthalmia": Ibn Zuhr, *Kitāb al-taysīr* (ed. Al-Khouri, 12–13).

87. "The anointment of the eyelids with rose syrup made with sugar strengthens vision": Cf. Narboni, *Sefer Oraḥ Ḥayyim*, fol. 20a. The fourteenth-century French surgeon Guy de Chauliac possibly refers to the Latin translation of this remedy for strengthening vision in his *Chirurgia Magna* (1:230, lines 1–2; 2:188).

88. "mace": I.e., the false aril of the nut of the nutmeg tree (*Myristica fragrans* Houtt.).

89. "mint [*Mentha*]": For the different species of mint, see *Encyclopaedia of Islam*, new ed., 12:309–10.

90. Cf. Ibn Zuhr, *Kitāb al-taysīr* (ed. Al-Khouri, 13).

91. "Constant anointing of the spine of the back with sweet almond oil, lukewarm, protects against the bending [of the body] that occurs to the elderly": Cf. Ibn Zuhr, *Kitāb al-taysīr* (ed. Al-Khouri, 13); and Narboni, *Sefer Oraḥ Ḥayyim*, fol. 74b.

92. "It has been verified by experience that the consumption of turnip [*Brassica rapa*], boiled, sharpens vision": Cf. Ibn Zuhr, *Kitāb al-taysīr* (ed. Al-Khouri, 14).

93. "turnip [*Brassica rapa*]": The Arabic *lift* can also refer to rape (*Brassica napus*); cf. *Wörterbuch der klassischen arabischen Sprache* 2:970a, line 30. Cf. also

Maimonides, *Medical Aphorisms* 20.47, 72, and 85 (ed. and trans. Bos, 4:77–78, 87–88, 93–94).

94. "The consumption of the heads of sparrows and especially the male ones, and similarly the consumption of turnips cooked either in meat or alone, and similarly [the consumption of] carrots, and similarly the consumption of young pigeons that are able to fly, and similarly the ingestion of juice of chick-peas (*Cicer arietinum* and var.)—each of these substances on its own is good for strengthening [the lust for] sexual intercourse": Cf. Ibn Zuhr, *Kitāb al-taysīr* (ed. Al-Khouri, 14); and Narboni, *Sefer Oraḥ Ḥayyim*, fols 60b–61a.

95. "sparrows": The Arabic term *ᶜaṣāfīr* can also have the more general meaning of small birds.

96. "and washing the bottom after defecation with lukewarm sweet water protects against hemorrhoids": Cf. Narboni, *Sefer Oraḥ Ḥayyim*, fol. 41a: "And washing the bottom with lukewarm sweet water protects against hemorrhoids."

97. Cf. Ibn Zuhr, *Kitāb al-taysīr* (ed. Al-Khouri, 14).

98. Cf. Ibn Zuhr, *Kitāb al-taysīr* (ed. Al-Khouri, 14); and Narboni, *Sefer Oraḥ Ḥayyim*, fol. 74b.

99. "The consumption of radish [*Raphanus sativus* and var.] and cabbage [*Brassica oleracea*] eliminates hoarseness": Cf. Narboni, *Sefer Oraḥ Ḥayyim*, fol. 25a.

100. "the consumption of roasted quince [*Cydonia oblonga*] after meals gives energy and joy. The consumption of citron peel strengthens the heart, and its seeds are beneficial against poisons. Lemon peel is [also] beneficial against poisons, as are the leaves of its tree": Cf. Narboni, *Sefer Oraḥ Ḥayyim*, fol. 31a.

101. "The consumption of citron peel strengthens the heart, and its seeds are beneficial against poisons. Lemon peel is [also] beneficial against poisons, as are the leaves of its tree": Cf. Maimonides, *On Poisons* 67 (ed. and trans. Bos, 44): "Lemon peel, if eaten, has the specific property of being beneficial against poisons. The leaves of the lemon tree, if imbibed as a decoction, have a similar effect."

102. Cf. Ibn Zuhr, *Kitāb al-taysīr* (ed. Al-Khouri, 15).

103. "The consumption of *al-murrī al-naqīᶜ* and vinegar removes the causes for the development of worms in the abdomen. The consumption of peaches [*Amygdalus persica*], in spite of its harmful effects, is beneficial against vapor [arising] from the stomach. Similarly, field eryngo [*Eryngium campestre*] has about the same effect": Cf. Ibn Zuhr, *Kitāb al-taysīr* (ed. Al-Khouri, 15–16).

104. "*al-murrī al-naqīᶜ* ": Cf. Waines, "*Murrī*: The Tale of a Condiment," 382: "a kind of fermented infusion of cereal grains."

105. "The consumption of peaches [*Amygdalus persica*], in spite of their harmful effects, is beneficial against vapor [arising] from the stomach. Similarly, field eryngo [*Eryngium campestre*] has about the same effect. The smelling of peaches brings [someone] around, and the drinking of the juice of their leaves kills worms": Cf. Narboni, *Sefer Oraḥ Ḥayyim*, fol. 42b.

106. "The smelling of peaches brings [someone] around, and the drinking of the juice of their leaves kills worms": Cf. Ibn Zuhr, *Kitāb al-aghdhiya* (ed. and trans. García Sánchez, 48).

107. "If mustard [*Brassica nigra*] oil is dripped into a deaf ear, hearing returns": Cf. Ibn Zuhr, *Kitāb al-taysīr* (ed. Al-Khouri, 16): "If a small drop of mustard oil is dripped into the deaf ear every three days, it restores the hearing." See also Narboni, *Sefer Oraḥ Ḥayyim*, fol. 20b.

108. "and the immersion in lukewarm olive oil is beneficial for all pains of the body": Ibn Zuhr, *Kitāb al-taysīr* (ed. Al-Khouri, 16); and Narboni, *Sefer Oraḥ Ḥayyim*, fol. 74b.

109. "If the inner coat of the stomach of the male bustard is dried and mixed with collyria, it has the specific property of being beneficial against a cataract in the eye": Cf. Ibn Zuhr, *Kitāb al-aghdhiya* (ed. and trans. García Sánchez, 16).

110. "The coat of the stomach of the ostrich has the specific property, if one takes thereof, of being beneficial for those suffering from a stomach disease and for crumbling [kidney] stones": Cf. Ibn Zuhr, *Kitāb al-aghdhiya* (ed. and trans. García Sánchez, 17).

111. Cf. Ibn Zuhr, *Kitāb al-aghdhiya* (ed. and trans. García Sánchez, 18). See also Narboni, *Sefer Oraḥ Ḥayyim*, fol. 13a. "Strengthen the soul": Ibn Zuhr, *Kitāb al-aghdhiya* (ed. and trans. García Sánchez, 18): hearten and strengthen the soul (*yushajji*ᶜ*u al-qulūb wa-yashuddu al-nufūs wa-yuqawwīhā*).

112. "If the penis is rubbed with hedgehog fat, it gives a strong erection and provides increased pleasure during sexual intercourse": Cf. Ibn Zuhr, *Kitāb al-aghdhiya* (ed. and trans. García Sánchez, 25); and Narboni, *Sefer Oraḥ Ḥayyim*, fol. 61a.

113. "If the penis of a hedgehog is dried, pulverized, and ingested, it gives a strong erection. The penis of a male deer has a similar effect [if dried, pulverized, and ingested] by its specific property": Ibn Zuhr, *Kitāb al-aghdhiya* (ed. and trans. García Sánchez, 26); and Narboni, *Sefer Oraḥ Ḥayyim,* fol. 61a.

114. Cf. Ibn Zuhr, *Kitāb al-aghdhiya* (ed. and trans. García Sánchez, 49); and Narboni, *Sefer Oraḥ Ḥayyim*, fol. 27b.

115. "The acidic inner part of the citron eliminates thirst, vigorously subdues yellow bile": Cf. Ibn Zuhr, *Kitāb al-aghdhiya* (ed. and trans. García Sánchez, 50); "The acidic inner part of the citron eliminates thirst, vigorously subdues yellow bile, and strengthens the soul. Myrobalan has the specific property of being beneficial for the stomach": Cf. Narboni, *Sefer Oraḥ Ḥayyim*, fol. 33b.

116. "and strengthens the soul": Ibn Zuhr, *Kitāb al-aghdhiya* (ed. and trans. García Sánchez, 49), ascribes this property to lemon peel.

117. "Myrobalan": I.e., laxative fruits of the Combretaceae family, namely, *Terminalia chebula* Retz. or *Terminalia citrina* Roxb.; cf. Maimonides, *Glossary of Drug Names* 112 (trans. Rosner, 86–87). The properties of myrobalan and those of aloe in aphorism 22.54 below have been swapped in Ibn Zuhr, *La Tedkira d'Abū al-*ᶜ*Alā*ᵓ, 22: Myrobalan has the specific property of being harmful for the anus, and aloe has the specific property of being beneficial for the stomach. Maimonides' version is evidently correct; cf. Ibn al-Bayṭār, *Al-Jāmi*ᶜ *li-mufradāt*, 2:108: If administered alone, it [i.e., aloe] is harmful for the anus.

118. "The drinking of half a *dirham* of balsam of Mecca [*Commiphora opobalsamum*] counteracts all poisons": Cf. Ibn Zuhr, *Kitāb al-aghdhiya* (ed. and trans. García Sánchez, 105). See also Maimonides, *On Poisons* 26 (ed. and trans. Bos, 20–21).

119. "drinking": Ibn Zuhr, *Kitāb al-taysīr* (ed. Al-Khouri, 45), speaks about balsam oil (*duhn al-balsān*).

120. According to Ibn Zuhr, *Kitāb al-taysīr* (ed. Al-Khouri, 45), the carnelian is good against cavities in the teeth.

121. "Broad beans [*Vicia faba*] have the specific property of corrupting the mind. Milk has the specific property of being harmful for the brain": Cf. Ibn Zuhr, *La Teḏkira d'Abū al-ʿAlāʾ* (ed. and trans. Colin, 22).

122. "Aloe [*Aloe vera*] [has the specific property] of being harmful for the anus": Cf. Ibn Zuhr, *La Teḏkira d'Abū al-ʿAlāʾ* (ed. and trans. Colin, 22); see n. 117 to aphorism 22.52 above.

123. "Colocynth [*Citrullus colocynthis*] [has the specific property] of being harmful for the liver": Cf. Ibn Zuhr, *La Teḏkira d'Abū al-ʿAlāʾ* (ed. and trans. Colin, 22); and Narboni, *Sefer Oraḥ Ḥayyim*, fol. 45a.

124. "Figs [*Ficus carica*] have the specific property of producing lice. Service tree [*Sorbus domestica*] [has the specific property of being beneficial] for weakness of the liver": Once again it seems that Ibn Zuhr, *La Teḏkira d'Abū al-ʿAlāʾ* (ed. and trans. Colin, 21), has swapped the properties of figs and service tree: Service tree has the specific property of producing lice and figs [have the specific property of being beneficial] for weakness of the liver; and that Maimonides' version as extant in **GS** is the correct one, contrary to the version preserved in **BELOU**, which accords with *La Teḏkira d'Abū al-ʿAlāʾ*; cf. Ibn al-Bayṭār, *Al-Jāmiʿ li-mufradāt*, 1:202 (citing al-Rāzī, *Fī dafʿ maḏārr al-aghdhiya*): Dried figs [...] soften the stools and expel the putrefying superfluities to the pores so that many lice originate in those who eat them constantly. See also, following the Hebrew translation by Nathan ha-Meʾati, Narboni, *Sefer Oraḥ Ḥayyim*, fol. 45a: Figs have the specific property of weakening the liver.

125. "Almonds [*Prunus dulcis*] have the specific property of preserving the substance of the brain, while their moisture preserves the organs in an amazing way, without producing abnormal moisture": Cf. Narboni, *Sefer Oraḥ Ḥayyim*, fol. 118a.

126. "Rose jam has the specific property of strengthening the lungs": Cf. Narboni, *Sefer Oraḥ Ḥayyim*, fol. 28b.

127. Cf. Ibn Zuhr, *La Teḏkira d'Abū al-ʿAlāʾ* (ed. and trans. Colin, 20–21).

128. "Agarwood [*Aquilaria malaccensis*] has the specific property of being beneficial for the stomach and of strengthening it, and it eliminates a bad smell from the mouth. Artichoke [*Cynara cardunculus* and var.] perfumes winds [and] breath from the body. Smelling narcissus eliminates children's epilepsy. Its smell has the same effect as that which Galen attributes to peony [*Paeonia officinalis*]": Cf. Ibn Zuhr, *La Teḏkira d'Abū al-ʿAlāʾ* (ed. and trans. Colin, 20); "Indian aloeswood [*Aquilaria agallocha* and var.] has the specific property of being beneficial for the stomach and of strengthening it": Cf. Narboni, *Sefer Oraḥ Ḥayyim*, fols 33b–34a.

129. "breath" (*arwāḥ*): Cf. Ibn Zuhr, *La Teḏkira d'Abū al-ʿAlāʾ* (ed. and trans. Colin, 20 [Arabic text: *arfāʿ*], 63 [French translation: *parties supérieures*]). It seems that Maimonides has preserved a better version and that Colin's version should be emendated accordingly.

130. "narcissus": For the relevant different varieties, see Schmucker, *Pflanzliche und mineralische Materia Medica*, no. 766; and Dioscurides, *Dioscurides triumphans* 4.147 (ed. and trans. Dietrich, 2:663).

131. Cf. Galen, *De simplicium medicamentorum temperamentis ac facultatibus* 6.2 (ed. Kühn, 11:859); and aphorism 22.18 above.

132. These remedies are quoted by Narboni, *Sefer Oraḥ Ḥayyim*, fol. 23b.

133. The physician al-Tamīmī (d. 980), hailing from Jerusalem, moved to Egypt in 970 to serve the vizier Ya<sup>c</sup>qūb ibn Killis. His pharmaceutical manual, entitled *Kitāb al-murshid fī jawāhir al-aghdhiya wa-quwā l-mufradāt min al-adwiya* (Guide to the substances of the foods and the powers of the simple drugs), has been preserved only partly and is, except for the section on stones (see Schönfeld, *Über die Steine*), still in manuscript. In his *Medical Aphorisms* 20.82–89 (ed. and trans. Bos, 4:91–94), Maimonides quotes other beneficial foods and medicines from al-Tamīmī with the argument that he "allegedly had much experience. Although most of his statements are taken from others and although sometimes he wrongly understands the words of others, he still, in general, mentions many properties of various foods and of medications." (Maimonides, *Medical Aphorisms* 20.82 (ed. and trans. Bos, 4:91).

134. "craving for clay": For this phenomenon occurring to women during pregnancy, see Maimonides, *Medical Aphorisms* 16.23 (ed. and trans. Bos, 4:11–12); and Ibn al-Jazzār, *On Sexual Diseases* 15 (ed. Bos, 57–58 [introduction], 184–85 [Arabic text], 287 [English translation]).

135. "If beef is boiled with vinegar, it has the specific property of being beneficial for jaundice, of expelling yellow bile, and of stopping diarrhea of bilious matter": Narboni, *Sefer Oraḥ Ḥayyim*: If beef is boiled with vinegar, it has the specific property of stopping diarrhea (fol. 37a); If beef is boiled with vinegar, it has the specific property of being beneficial for jaundice, of expelling yellow bile (fol. 47b).

136. "tellin [*Tellinae*]": Cf. Dioscurides, *Dioscurides triumphans* 2.5 (ed. and trans. Dietrich, 2:199–200).

137. Cf. Maimonides, *On Coitus* 6, 8 (ed. and trans. Bos, forthcoming).

138. "arum" (*lūf*): The Arabic term indicates various species of arum and other plants. Cf. *Wörterbuch der klassischen arabischen Sprache*, 2:1786–88; and Dioscurides, *Dioscurides triumphans* 2.149 (ed. and trans. Dietrich, 2:313–16).

139. Quoting this recipe from Nathan ha-Me<sup>ᵓ</sup>ati's Hebrew translation, Narboni remarks that it seems to him that Maimonides has omitted one condition necessary for its successful application, since he tested it and it did not work that way. See Bos, "R. Moshe Narboni," 235.

140. "St. John's wort [*Hypericum perforatum*]" (*al-dādhī*, i.e., *al-dādhī al-rūmī*): Cf. Dioscurides, *Dioscurides triumphans* 3.7 (ed. and trans. Dietrich, 2:352 n. 6); and Maimonides, *Glossary of Drug Names* (trans. Rosner), no. 115.

141. "lichen [*Alectoria usneoides*] is beneficial for palpitation of the heart caused by black bile. Women should sit in a decoction [prepared] therefrom": Cf. Narboni, *Sefer Oraḥ Ḥayyim*, fol. 30a.

142. "[for uterine diseases]": Cf. Dioscurides, *Pedanii Dioscuridis Anazarbei* (ed. Wellmann) 1.21; and Ibn al-Bayṭār, *Al-jāmi<sup>c</sup> li-mufradāt* 1:49–50; French translation in Leclerc, no. 85.

143. "Galingale [*Cyperus longus*] has the specific property of liquefying, dissolving, and crumbling [kidney] stones, and it stimulates micturition": Cf. Narboni, *Sefer Oraḥ Ḥayyim*, fol. 57b.

144. "If rock crystal is burned, pulverized, washed, and imbibed [in a dose of] one ounce with two *mithqāls* of the milk of a donkey, it is beneficial for trembling, tremor, and phthisis. If a salve therefrom [prepared] with water is put on the breast, it makes the milk flow": Cf. Narboni, *Sefer Oraḥ Ḥayyim*, fol. 31b, following the Hebrew translation by Nathan ha-Me'ati: If rock crystal is burned, pulverized, and crushed with marble and dripped in water on the breast, it makes the milk flow.

145. One *mithqāl* is 4.46 grams.

## The Twenty-Third Treatise

1. "unknown": neglected **BELO**.

2. Maimonides' text seems to be a summary of Galen's discussion in *De curandi ratione per venae sectionem* 4, 6, 7, and 8 (ed. Kühn, 11:259, 266–69, 273–74); for this treatise, see Steinschneider, "Griechische Ärzte," 289, no. 45; and Ḥunayn, *Über syrische und arabische Galen-Übersetzungen* (ed. Bergsträsser, no. 71).

3. Galen, *De plenitudine* 8, 10, and 11 (ed. Kühn, 7:548, 564, 572).

4. "Therefore, understand that [this is what I mean] when I speak of a surplus of chymes and of a surplus of blood": Cf. Galen, *De plenitudine* 10 (ed. Kühn, 7:566): ὅθεν ἐγὼ κἀν τοῖς ἔμπροσθεν ἠξίουν ὡσαύτως ἀκούειν, εἴτε τοὺς χυμοὺς πλεονάζειν, εἴθ' αἷμα φήσαιμι.

5. "The chyme that Galen calls 'raw' in his *De multitidune*, and of which he says that dropsy of the flesh develops from this chyme, and that it is this chyme that settles in the urine similar to cooked broad bean [*Vicia faba*] groats": Cf. Galen, *De plenitudine* 11 (ed. Kühn, 7:575).

6. "dropsy of the flesh": I.e., anasarca.

7. Galen, *In Hippocratis Epidemiarum librum* 6 *commentarius* 2 (ed. Wenkebach and trans. Pfaff, 108–10); Latin translation in Deller, "Epidemienkommentare," 535, no. 72.

8. In his *Hippokrates' "De humoribus,"* Deichgräber showed that this commentary is a forgery dating from the Renaissance, probably from the hand of Rasarius. Deichgräber pointed out that Maimonides' quotations—in the form of the old Latin translation—were used by Rasarius for reconstructing parts of the text. By comparing these quotations with parallels from Oribasius, Deichgräber also showed how problematic it is to distinguish between the Maimonidean and the genuine Galenic elements. This quotation does not appear in Galen, *In Hippocratis De humoribus commentarius* (ed. Kühn, 16:1–206).

9. Galen, *In Platonis Timaeum* 2 (ed. Schröder, 4–5; ed. and trans. Larrain, 212–13).

10. Galen, *Ad Glauconem de medendi methodo* 2.9 (ed. Kühn, 11:120).

11. This quotation does not appear in the spurious text edited by Kühn; see aphorism 23.5 above.

12. Galen, *De consuetudinibus* (ed. Schmutte, 16, 18). German translation from the Arabic (cf. ed. and trans. Klein-Franke, 145) by Pfaff in Schmutte, 45–46; English translation in Klein-Franke, 132–33.

13. Galen, *De alimentorum facultatibus* 3.38 (ed. Helmreich, 382, lines 1–3).

14. Galen, *De simplicium medicamentorum temperamentis ac facultatibus* 5.15 (ed. Kühn, 11:755).

15. Galen, *De symptomatum differentiis liber* 5 (ed. Kühn, 7:75): ὀνομάζω δὲ τὴν μὲν διὰ λάφυγγος ὁλκήν τε καὶ αὖθις ἔκπεμψιν τοῦ πέριξ ἀέρος, ἀναπνοήν · τὴν δὲ καθ' ὅλον τὸ σῶμα, διαπνοήν. Galen's *De morborum causis et symptomatibus* consists of six books: *De morborum differentiis, De causis morborum liber, De symptomatum differentiis liber, De symptomatum causis* 1, *De symptomatum causis* 2, and *De symptomatum causis* 3 (cf. Ullmann, *Medizin im Islam*, 42, no. 22).

16. Galen, *De morborum differentiis* 5 (ed. Kühn, 6:853–54).

17. Galen, *De compositione medicamentorum secundum locos* 10.2 (ed. Kühn, 13:332). For the Arabic *mayāmir*, coined after the Syriac *mēmra*, see Ullmann, *Medizin im Islam*, 48, no. 50.

18. Aphorisms 23.15–16: Cf. **C**: "He says that of these [diseases] comprehensive in their occurrence there are such that occur often and constantly in one city—they are called 'endemic'—and such that occur to the general [population] during the change of the air in a certain season [of the year], and these are called 'general.'" Galen's commentary on this treatise by Hippocrates (*In Hippocratis De aere aquis locis commentarius*) survives only in an Arabic translation (ed. Strohmaier, forthcoming) and in a Hebrew translation by Solomon ha-Me'ati (ed. and trans. Wasserstein; for our quotation see 19, 203). I thank Professor Strohmaier for providing me with photocopies of the passages from the forthcoming edition.

19. Galen, *In Hippocratis Epidemiarum librum 1 commentarius* 2 (ed. Wenkebach and trans. Pfaff, 56, lines 11–22); Latin translation in Deller, "Epidemienkommentare," 521, no. 4.

20. "not because of the fact that": "it does not mean" **G**.

21. Galen, *In Hippocratis Epidemiarum librum 6 commentarius* 1 (ed. Wenkebach and trans. Pfaff, 9, lines 9–28); Latin translation in Deller, "Epidemienkommentare," 531, no. 55.

22. "in the case of fevers that are related to the substance of the organs": Cf. Galen, *De marcore* 1 (ed. Kühn, 7:668): ἔν τισι τῶν ἑκτικῶν πυρετῶν.

23. "Such a temperament": I.e., predominantly dry and heat.

24. Galen, *De marcore* 1 (ed. Kühn, 7:667–68).

25. "and the marasmus called 'syncopal' occurs to someone who suffered from syncope": Cf. Galen, *De marcore* 5 (ed. Kühn, 7:686): τῷ συγκοπώδει δὲ ἐπειδὰν ἐν συγκοπῇ γενηθέντες ἐκφευγούσιν ἐν τῷ παραυτίκα τὸ τοῦ κινδύνου σφοδρὸν ὑπολείπεται δ' αὐτοῖς τι τῆς συγκοπώδους διαθέσεως.

26. "[The cold marasmus, on the other hand, which is a condition similar to old age, results in cases where]": Cf. Galen, *De marcore* 5 (ed. Kühn, 7:687): ὁ δὲ ψυχρὸς μαρασμὸς ὁ τὴν τοῦ γήρως ἔχων διάθεσιν ἐκ μεταπτώσεως γίνεται.

27. Galen, *De marcore* 5 (ed. Kühn, 7:686–87).

28. "*De tremore, palpitatione, rigore et convulsione*": Cf. Galen, *De tremore, palpitatione, rigore et convulsione* (ed. Kühn, 7:584–642).

29. In his quotation of the Arabic title for this treatise, Sezgin, *Geschichte des arabischen Schrifttums*, 3:135 n. 139, actually gives *riʿsha* instead of *riʿda*.

30. "physicians": Lit. "people."

31. Galen, *De symptomatum causis* 2.2 (ed. Kühn, 7:149–53).

32. This text could not be identified in Galen, *De pulsibus libellus ad tirones* (ed. Kühn, 8:453–92); see, however, aphorism 23.23 below. For the Arabic name of *De pulsibus libellus ad tirones*, see Ullmann, *Medizin im Islam*, 44, no. 32.

33. Galen, *De symptomatum causis* 1.5 (ed. Kühn, 7:108–9, 111).

34. "windpipe": Cf. Galen, *De compositione medicamentorum secundum locos* 7.1 (ed. Kühn, 13:5): ἀρτηρίαν.

35. "larynx": Cf. Galen, *De compositione medicamentorum secundum locos* 7.1 (ed. Kühn, 13:5): λάρυγγα.

36. "pharynx": Cf. Galen, *De compositione medicamentorum secundum locos* 7.1 (ed. Kühn, 13:5): φάρυγγα.

37. Galen, *De compositione medicamentorum secundum locos* 7.1 (ed. Kühn, 13:5).

38. The Hebrew translator Zeraḥyah ben Isaac ben Sheʾaltiel Ḥen has added an interesting note to his translation of this particular text that gives us insight into the problem facing him and his colleagues in finding Hebrew equivalents to the Arabic technical terminology employed: "Says the translator: I know that one should not translate this text from the Rabbi, of blessed memory, at all, since in our Hebrew language I cannot find [equivalents for] the terms mentioned here. For these three [kinds of] membranes as they are found in the Arabic language, namely the three mentioned in this place: *aghshiyya*, *ṣifāqāt*, and *ṭabaqāt*—although in Hebrew one [uses the terms] *qelippot* and *qerumot* for them—anyhow only the term *qerum* is applicable to them in the Hebrew language. For the term *qelippah* is not at all applicable to any of these three [membranes], because it is mostly used for the peels of edible fruits. For this reason I truly know that my translation does not at all elucidate nor clarify what the Rabbi, of blessed memory, wants to say. May the reader accept this apology of mine for the embarrassment caused to him just by this text on the explanation of the membranes." See aphorism 24.107 below for a comment on the problem of finding Hebrew equivalents to the Arabic terms for milk products.

39. Galen, *De febrium differentiis* 1.9 (ed. Kühn, 7:306).

40. Galen's *De pulsu* [*magno*] *(Megapulsus)* encompasses four books, each consisting of four treatises: *De differentia pulsuum, De dignoscendis pulsibus, De causis pulsuum,* and *De praesagitione ex pulsibus*. Maimonides' quote appears in Galen, *De causis pulsuum* 2.3 (ed. Kühn, 9:66); cf. Ullmann, *Medizin im Islam*, 43.

41. Galen, *De differentia pulsuum* 1.10 (ed. Kühn, 8:523–24); cf. Maimonides, *Medical Aphorisms* 4.11 (ed. and trans. Bos, 1:63).

42. Galen, *De differentia pulsuum* 1 (ed. Kühn, 8:493–565).

43. "'Continuous' fevers and 'perpetual' [fevers] are synonyms. Similarly, the [fever] called 'synochous' is continuous, as is the continuous burning [fever]": Cf. Galen, *De crisibus* 2.6 (ed. Kühn, 9:664; ed. Alexanderson, 141, lines 12–14): οὐδε γὰρ, εἰ συνόχον ὀνομάζει τις αὐτὸν ὥσπερ ἔνιοι τῶν ἰατρῶν, ὅλῳ τῷ γένει διοίσει τῶν

καυσωδῶν πυρετῶν ἕνεκά τε τῆς προσηγορίας (And if someone calls it [i.e., continuous fever] "synochous," as some physicians [do], it would not be different from the total class of ardent fevers, because of this appellation).

44. Galen, *De crisibus* 2.6 (ed. Kühn, 9:664; ed. Alexanderson, 141, lines 12–14).

45. Galen, *De febrium differentiis* 2.7 (ed. Kühn, 7:350–51).

46. "Inflammations may occur in the muscles of the ribs after which fever arises": Cf. Galen, *De locis affectis* 5.3 (ed. Kühn. 7:326; English translation in Siegel, 147): ἕτεραι δ' εἰσὶν ὀδύναι πλευρῶν ἅμα πυρετοῖς (There are other [types of] pain of the ribs combined with fever).

47. Galen, *De locis affectis* 5.3 (ed. Kühn, 7:326–27).

48. "There are five kinds of it: moist, dry, biting, intermediate, and moderate": Cf. Galen, *In Hippocratis de victu acutorum commentaria quattuor* 2.1 (ed. Helmreich, p. 164, line 32–p. 165, line 2: ἔστι δ' αὐτῶν ἔνια μὲν ὑγρὰ τελέως, ἔνια δὲ ξηρά, τινὰ δ' ἐξ ἀμφοῖν μικτά, δακνώδη δ' ἄλλα ἢ ἄδηκτα καί τινα τρίτα κἀνταῦθα σύμμικτα (Some of them are completely moist, some dry, some mixed from both, others are biting or not biting, and a third [type] mixed from both of them).

49. "The dry one is the one that is prepared with rags heated over a fire or with wormwood [*Artemisia* spp.] or with roasted millet [*Panicum miliaceum*]. The biting one is that which is prepared with salt heated in bags or with bitter vetch [*Vicia ervilia*] and the like": Cf. Galen, *In Hippocratis de victu acutorum commentaria quattuor* 2.6 (ed. Helmreich, 168, lines 1–7).

50. "The strength of bitter vetch is sufficient for cutting, concocting, and dissolving the thickness of the humors": Cf. Galen, *In Hippocratis de victu acutorum commentaria quattuor* 2.5 (ed. Helmreich, 167, lines 12–13).

51. "The moderate [hot compress] is such that one can touch with it the body of a living being, such as a child or a puppy and the like": Missing in Galen, *In Hippocratis de victu acutorum commentaria quattuor* 2.

52. "The intermediate one is that prepared with barley and bitter vetch; they should be pulverized and boiled with acid vinegar mixed with it to a degree that is stronger than could be drunk. Put this in a bag and apply it as a hot compress to the parts of the body [you want to treat]. The same [should be done] with bran": Cf. Galen, *In Hippocratis de victu acutorum commentaria quattuor* 2.5 (ed. Helmreich, 167, lines 1–4).

53. Galen, *De methodo medendi* 7.6 (ed. Kühn, 10:491; ed. and trans. Johnston and Horsley, 2:288 [Greek text], 289 [English translation]): ἡ δὲ σύμμετρος ἐπὶ τούτων τρίψις ἐστίν, ὡς θερμῆναι τὸ σῶμα (The rubbing is moderate in these cases so as to warm the body).

54. Cf. **C**: "Hippocrates says: Every city which is situated towards the rising of the sun is healthier than that city which is situated towards the *Farqadain* [i.e., β and γ of Ursa minor], and then that city that is situated towards the hot winds." Cf. Solomon ha-Me'ati's Hebrew translation of Galen, *Commentary on Airs, Waters, Places* (ed. and trans. Wasserstein, 40, 225).

55. "*namla* [shingles]": Cf. Galen, *In Hippocratis Aphorismos commentarius* 6 (ed. Kühn, 18A:72).

56. "*ākila* [canker]": Cf. *In Hippocratis Aphorismos commentarius* 6 (ed. Kühn, 18A:72): φαγεδαίνας. See aphorisms 23.48–49 below.

57. Galen, *In Hippocratis Aphorismos commentarius* 6 (ed. Kühn, 18A:72).

58. "*ʿAbīṭ*" (*ghabīṭ* **GL**): Cf. Galen, *De tumoribus praeter naturam* 2 (ed. Kühn, 7:710): θρόμβος (clot of blood); and Ullmann, *Wörterbuch zu griechisch-arabischen Übersetzungen*, 472: θρόμβος: عبيط دم.

59. Galen, *De tumoribus praeter naturam* 2 (ed. Kühn, 7:710).

60. Cf. Galen, *De tumoribus praeter naturam* 4 (ed. Kühn, 7:718): ἔστι δὲ καὶ ἡ σύριγξ ὀνομαζομένη στενὸς καὶ προμήκης κόλπος, ὁμοίως τοῖς ἄλλοις κόλποις προστελλομένη τε καὶ αὖθις ἀφίσταμένη δι' ἐπιρροὴν περιττωμάτων.

61. Galen, *Ad Glauconem de methodo medendi* 2.10 (ed. Kühn, 11:125); cf. Maimonides, *Medical Aphorisms* 15.45 (ed. and trans. Bos, 3:65).

62. Galen, *De tumoribus praeter naturam* 6 (ed. Kühn, 7:719).

63. Galen, *De febrium differentiis* 1.5 (ed. Kühn, 7:288–89).

64. "If humors stream from the openings of the vessels into the spaces that have no flesh or muscles and the bodily part is soaked with those humors just as a sponge is soaked with liquids, this is called 'inflammation'": Cf. Galen, *De tumoribus praeter naturam* 2 (ed. Kühn, 7:713–14).

65. "If the pus corrodes parts of the flesh and the like and a cavity is formed in that place into which pus accumulates, it is called 'abscess'": Cf. Galen, *De tumoribus praeter naturam* 3 (ed. Kühn, 7:715).

66. "If those corrupt matters inside the abscess are surrounded by a cover similar to a membrane, it is called *dubayla* [cystic abscess]": Cf. Galen, *De tumoribus praeter naturam* 5 (ed. Kühn, 7:718–19).

67. "If the humor is only in the skin, it is called 'furuncle,' and it is very hot. If it is deep in the body, it is very malignant, and then it is similar to an abscess. The only difference between it and an abscess lies in its hardness": Cf. Galen, *De tumoribus praeter naturam* 15 (ed. Kühn, 7:729).

68. "The term swelling" (*khurāj*): Cf. Galen, *In Hippocratis Epidemiarum librum 6 commentarius* 1 (ed. Wenkebach and trans. Pfaff, 7, line 23): τὸ τοῦ οἰδήματος ὄνομα (the term *swelling*).

69. "every type of swelling": Cf. Galen, *In Hippocratis Epidemiarum librum 6 commentarius* 1 (ed. Wenkebach and trans. Pfaff, p. 7, line 24–p. 8, line 1): ἅπαντας τοὺς παρὰ φύσιν ὄγκους (all unnatural swellings). This quotation does not appear in Deller's Latin translation.

70. "Pustules": Cf. Galen, *In Hippocratis Epidemiarum librum 6 commentarius* 2 (ed. Wenkebach and trans. Pfaff, 95, line 8): ἐξανθήματα.

71. "tumors": Cf. Galen, *In Hippocratis Epidemiarum librum 6 commentarius* 2 (ed. Wenkebach and trans. Pfaff, 95, line 8): φυμάτα.

72. Galen, *In Hippocratis Epidemiarum librum 6 commentarius* 2 (ed. Wenkebach and trans. Pfaff, 95, lines 8–10, 17–21; 96, lines 12–14); Latin translation in Deller, "Epidemienkommentare," 534, no. 70.

73. "If the matter streaming to a part of the body is a superfluity composed of blood and yellow bile, both of which are warmer than they should be, or if that which streams to it is only blood but blood that is boiling hot, of a fine

consistency, the illness developing therefrom is called 'erysipelas'": Cf. Galen, *Ad Glauconem de medendi methodo* 2.1 (ed. Kühn, 11:74–75).

74. "'Scirrhus' is the name of a hard tumor that develops from a thick, viscous humor that settles in those parts in which the [tumor] occurs. It is of two types: that which is absolutely insensible and incurable and that which is a little bit sensible and is hard to cure": Cf. Galen, *Ad Glauconem de medendi methodo* 2.6 (ed. Kühn, 11:103–4).

75. Cf. Ibn Janāḥ, *Kitāb al-Talkhīṣ* (forthcoming), no. 683: سقيروس هو الورم الصلب من كتاب الأعضاء الآلمة (*Sqīrūs* [σκῖρος/scirrhus] is a hard swelling [*waram ṣulb*], according to [sc. Galen's] *Book on Affected Parts* [*al-Aʿḍāʾ al-ālima*]).

76. "And the sites where the tumor becomes very large and the blood is congested in it and the respiration becomes so small that one reaches a point that the patient dies are called "gangrenes" as long as they are in a stage of mortification but have not [actually] died. Their therapy consists of evacuating the blood that became congested in that part of the body by a deep scarification and by making incisions in it in [several] places until as much blood as possible is extracted": Cf. Galen, *Ad Glauconem de medendi methodo* 2.11 (ed. Kühn, 11:135–36).

77. "'hard erysipelas'": Cf. Galen, *De methodo medendi* 14.3 (ed. Kühn, 10:953; ed. and trans. Johnston and Horsley, 3:434–35): σκιρρῶδες ἐρυσίπελας (scyrrhous erysipelas).

78. "'soft erysipelas'": Cf. Galen, *De methodo medendi* 14.3 (ed. Kühn, 10:952; ed. and trans. Johnston and Horsley, 3:434–35): ἐρυσίπελας οἰδηματῶδες (edematous erysipelas).

79. Galen, *De methodo medendi* 14.3 (ed. Kühn, 10:952–53; ed. and trans. Johnston and Horsley, 3:434–35).

80. Galen, *De methodo medendi* 14.6 (ed. Kühn, 10:962; ed. and trans. Johnston and Horsley, 3:450–51).

81. Galen, *De compositione medicamentorum per genera* 1.18 and 4.1.14 (ed. Kühn, 13:449, 652–53, 750–51); for the title *Qaṭājānas*, cf. Ullmann, *Medizin im Islam*, 48–49, no. 50.

82. Galen, *De tumoribus praeter naturam* 9 (ed. Kühn, 7:724); cf. Anastassiou and Irmer, eds., *Hippokrateszitate in übrigen Werken Galens*, 2:366.

83. Galen, *De tumoribus praeter naturam* 12 (ed. Kühn, 7:726).

84. Galen, *Ad Glauconem de medendi methodo* 2.12 (ed. Kühn, 11:140); cf. Maimonides, *On Hemorroids* 2.1 (ed. and trans. Bos, 8–9).

85. Galen, *De tumoribus praeter naturam* 12–13 (ed. Kühn, 7:726–27). See aphorism 23.35 above.

86. "Canker is an ulcer[ous sore] that corrodes [the flesh] deep inside, while herpes is an ulcer[ous disease] that corrodes on the outside": Cf. Galen, *In Hippocratis De humoribus commentarius* 3.26 (ed. Kühn, 16:460–61). See aphorism 23.35 above.

87. "herpes" (*mā̆sharā*): Cf. Galen, *In Hippocratis De humoribus commentarius* 3.26 (ed. Kühn, 16:460–61): ἕρπητας. According to Richter, "Über allgemeine Dermatologie des ʿAlī ibn al-ʿAbbās," 485 n. 4, *māsharā* is "erysipelas" (following Brockelmann, *Lexicon Syriacum*, 408).

88. "Lanolin": οἴσυπος; cf. Dioscurides, *Dioscurides triumphans* 2.61 (ed. and trans. Dietrich, 2:236).

89. "the filthy wool": ἔρια οἰσυπηρά; cf. Dioscurides, *Dioscurides triumphans* 2.60–61 (ed. and trans. Dietrich, 2:235–36) and aphorism 23.89 below. See as well Bos, Hussein, Mensching, Savelsberg, *Medical Synonym Lists from Medieval Provence*, 174-75 (Dalet 10); and Ibn Janāḥ, *Kitāb al-Talkhīṣ* (forthcoming), no. 315: زوفا رطب هو دسم الصوف من كتاب قطاجانس. *Zūfā raṭb* is the wool grease (*dasam al-ṣūf*), according to (sc. Galen's) "Composition of drugs according to kind" (*Qāṭājānis*). This section does not appear in Galen, *In Hippocratis De humoribus commentarius* 3.

90. For this spurious commentary, see aphorism 23.5 above.

91. "Anasarca": I.e., dropsy in the flesh: cf. Galen, *De locis affectis* 5.7 (ed. Kühn, 8:353): ἀνὰ σάρκα.

92. "'leucophlegmasia'": Cf. Galen, *De locis affectis* 5.7 (ed. Kühn, 8:353): λευκοφλεγματίας.

93. "*al-ḥaban*": Cf. Lane, *Arabic-English Lexicon*, 506: "The dropsy [...] The yellow water [of the blood; i.e. the serum: a superabundant effusion of which, in the body, constitutes dropsy]"; Galen, *De locis affectis* 5.7 (ed. Kühn, 8:353): ὑδέρους. Cf. Ibn Janāḥ, *Kitāb al-Talkhīṣ* (forthcoming), no. 402: الحبن الأبيض هو اللحمي (the white dropsy [*ḥaban abyaḍ*] is the flesh-dropsy (*laḥmī*)].

94. "*jam*ᶜ *al-mā*ʾ": I.e., accumulation of fluid. Cf. Ibn Janāḥ, *Kitāb al-Talkhīṣ* (forthcoming), no. 403: الحبن الرطب هو الزقي. (The moist dropsy [*ḥaban raṭb*] is the wineskin-like dropsy (*ziqqī*).

95. "tympanites": Cf. Galen, *In Hippocratis Aphorismos commentarius* 4.11 (ed. Kühn, 17B:669): τυμπανίας; i.e., dropsy, in which the abdomen is stretched like a drum by gas, fluid, or both.

96. "'dry dropsy'": Cf. Maimonides, *Commentary on Hippocrates' Aphorisms* 4.11 (ed. and trans. Bos, forthcoming): "Says Hippocrates: Those who suffer from constant colic, pains around the navel, and pain in the loins that are not alleviated with purgatives or with something else will eventually develop dry dropsy. Says the commentator: If [those pains] are not alleviated through [medical] treatment, it indicates that a bad temperament prevails in those organs and has settled in them. This results in tympanites, and this is the [hydrops] that he calls 'dry,' contrary to ascites in which there is water. Ascites originates from excessive cold." Cf. Ibn Janāḥ, *Kitāb al-Talkhīṣ* (forthcoming), no. 404: الحبن اليابس هو الطبلي عن إسحاق بن عمران (The dry dropsy [*ḥaban yābis*] is the drumlike dropsy [*ṭablī*], according to Isḥāq ibn ᶜImrān).

97. Galen, *In Hippocratis Aphorismos commentarius* 4.11 (ed. Kühn, 17B:669).

98. "A swelling occurs when thin phlegm accumulates": Cf. Galen, *De tumoribus praeter naturam* 9 (ed. Kühn, 7:723–24). Note that Ibn Janāḥ in *Kitāb al-Talkhīṣ* actually calls the swelling originating from thin phlegm انتفاخ (inflation [emphysema]); cf. aphorism 23.52 below: الانتفاخ هو الورم المتولّد عن البلغم الرقيق عن جالينوس (*Intifāḫ* [inflation] is, according to Galen, a swelling [*waram*] arising from thin phlegm).

99. "The illness called 'gangrene' is the beginning of the mortification of the solid parts of the body, except for the bones. If the bones perish as well, the illness is called 'sphacelus'": Cf. Galen, *De tumoribus praeter naturam* 11 (ed. Kühn, 7:726).

100. "'sphacelus'": Cf. Galen, *De tumoribus praeter naturam* 11 (ed. Kühn, 7:726): σφάκελος.

101. "inflation [emphysema]": Cf. Galen, *De methodo medendi* 14.7 (ed. Kühn, 10:963; ed. and trans. Johnston and Horsley, 3:450–53): ἐμφυσήματα.

102. "swelling [edema]": Cf. Galen, *De methodo medendi* 14.7 (ed. Kühn, 10:963; ed. and trans. Johnston and Horsley, 3:450–53): οἰδήματα.

103. Galen, *De methodo medendi* 14.7 (ed. Kühn, 10:963; ed. and trans. Johnston and Horsley, 3:450–53).

104. "Alopecia": Cf. Galen, *De compositione medicamentorum secundum locos* 1.2 (ed. Kühn, 12:382): ἀλωπεκία; i.e., a disease like mange in foxes, in which hair falls out (cf. Liddell and Scott, *Greek-English Lexicon*, 75).

105. "ophiasis": Cf. Galen, *De compositione medicamentorum secundum locos* 1.2 (ed. Kühn, 12:382): ὀφίασις; i.e.. a bald place on the head, of serpentine or winding form (cf. Liddell and Scott, *Greek-English Lexicon*, 1278).

106. Galen, *De compositione medicamentorum secundum locos* 1.2 (ed. Kühn, 12:382).

107. "*saʿfa* [cradle cap]": Cf. Galen, *De compositione medicamentorum secundum locos* 1.8 (ed. Kühn, 12:463): ἀχώρ.

108. "'honeycomb'": Cf. Galen, *De compositione medicamentorum secundum locos* 1.8 (ed. Kühn, 12:464): κηρίον. This ulceration is called "honeycomb" because the perforations have the size of the combs of bees, while the fluid contained in them has the consistency of honey.

109. Galen, *De tumoribus praeter naturam* 15 (ed. Kühn, 7:728).

110. Galen, *De tumoribus praeter naturam* 15 (ed. Kühn, 7:729).

111. "'sarcocele'": I.e., a fleshy excrescence on the testicles; cf. Galen, *De tumoribus praeter naturam* 15 (ed. Kühn, 7:729): σαρκοκήλη.

112. "'hydrocele'": I.e., water in the scrotum; cf. Galen, *De tumoribus praeter naturam* 15 (ed. Kühn, 7:729): ὑδροκήλη.

113. "Epiplocele": I.e., hernia of the omentum; cf. Galen, *De tumoribus praeter naturam* 15 (ed. Kühn, 7:729): ἐπιπλοκήλη.

114. "enterocele": I.e., intestinal hernia; cf. *De tumoribus praeter naturam* 15 (ed. Kühn, 7:729): ἐντεροκήλη.

115. Galen, *De tumoribus praeter naturam* 15 (ed. Kühn, 7:729).

116. Galen, *In Hippocratis Epidemiarum librum 2 commentarius* 2 (ed. Wenkebach and trans. Pfaff, 251, lines 20–25).

117. "that raving is a mild form of delirium": Cf. Galen, *In Hippocratis Epidemiarum librum 3 commentarius* 1 (ed. Wenkebach and trans. Pfaff, p. 1, line 22–p. 2, line 1): εἴπερ οὖν ἐλήρησεν ὁ Πυθίων, εὔδηλον ὅτι μετρίως παρεφρόνησεν. See as well Maimonides, *Commentary on Hippocrates' Aphorisms* 7.9: "Says Hippocrates: If delirium or spasms occur as a result of a flow of blood, it is a bad sign. Says the commentator: After an evacuation [of blood] a delirium develops because the brain is disturbed in its movements and is then constantly weak. Hippocrates calls a mild delirium 'raving.'"

118. Galen, *In Hippocratis Aphorismos commentarius* 2.3 (ed. Kühn, 17B:457).

119. "lethargy" (*al-birsām* [*sirsām*] *al-bārid wa-huwa līthārghūs*): For the terminology, see Dols, *Majnūn: The Madman*, 57–58. Cf. Ibn Janāḥ, *Kitāb al-Talkhīṣ*

(forthcoming), no. 1023: †التيرغس† هو الشرسام البارد من التقسيم للرازي . (†Al-tīrġus† [*recte al-līṭarġus* leg., λήθαργος, lethargy] is a "cold phrenitis" [*shirsām bārid*], according to al-Rāzī's *Taqsīm*.)

120. "If the brain only becomes warm qualitatively or in combination with [superfluous] matter, sleeplessness develops": Cf. Galen, *In Hippocratis Aphorismos commentarius* 2.3 (ed. Kühn, 17B:457): οὕτω δὲ καὶ ἀγρυπνίαι γίνονται μὲν διὰ θερμασίαν τοῦ πρώτου μορίου τῶν αἰσθητικῶν, ἀλλ' ἤτοι κατὰ δυσκρασίαν μόνην ἢ καὶ χυμοῦ χολώδους πλεονάσαντος (Thus sleeplessness develops through heat affecting the principal part of the brain where the senses are located, [or when there is a general affection of the whole body,] which can take the form of a general dyscrasia or simply an excess of bile).

121. Galen, *In Hippocratis Aphorismos commentarius* 2.3 (ed. Kühn, 17B:457).

122. This quotation does not appear in Galen, *De pulsu parva*, i.e., *De pulsibus libellus ad tirones* 9 (ed. Kühn, 8:453–91).

123. "the psychical pneuma": Galen, *In Hippocratis Aphorismos commentarius* 2.43 (ed. Kühn, 17B:542), speaks about the psychical faculty.

124. "severity": Lit. "size."

125. Galen, *In Hippocratis Aphorismos commentarius* 2.43 (ed. Kühn, 17B:541–42).

126. Galen, *In Platonis Timaeum* 4 (ed. Schröder, 29–30; ed. and trans. Larrain, 213).

127. Galen, *In Hippocratis Epidemiarum librum* 3 *commentarius* 3 (ed. Wenkebach and trans. Pfaff, 138, lines 24–25); Latin translation in Deller, "Epidemienkommentare," 530, no. 49; cf. Dols, *Majnūn: The Madman*, 29–31.

128. "melancholic delusion" (*al-waswās al-sawdāwī*): Cf. Lane, *Arabic-English Lexicon*, 2940: "A certain disease [i.e., melancholia, in which is a doting in the imagination and judgment, a sort of delirium . . .] arising from a predominance of the black bile, attended with confusion of the intellect"; Dols, *Majnūn: The Madman*, 50; and Maimonides, *Medical Aphorisms* 2.16 (ed. and trans. Bos, 1:31).

129. This statement could not be retrieved in Galen, *In Hippocratis Epidemiarum librum* 6 *commentarius* 3; a possible source is Galen, *In Hippocratis Aphorismos commentarius* 3.24 and 4.2 (ed. Kühn, 17B:627, 659); see also Dols, *Majnūn: The Madman*, 50.

130. "'torpor'" (*istighrāq*): Cf. Galen, *De symptomatum differentiis liber* 3 (ed. Kühn, 7:60): κάρος (heavy sleep, torpor).

131. "bad" (*munkar*): Cf. Galen, *De symptomatum differentiis liber* 3 (ed. Kühn, 7:60): μοχθηρός.

132. "Loss of reasoning [power] is called 'amentia'": Cf. Galen, *De symptomatum differentiis liber* 3 (ed. Kühn, 7:60): τῆς διανοητικῆς ἐνεργείας ἡ μὲν οἷον παράλυσις, ἄνοια.

133. Cf. Galen, *De symptomatum differentiis liber* 3 (ed. Kühn, 7:60). Galen's *De morborum causis et symptomatibus* consists of six books: *De morborum differentiis*, *De causis morborum liber*, *De symptomatum differentiis liber*, *De symptomatum causis* 1, *De symptomatum causis* 2, and *De symptomatum causis* 3 (cf. Ullmann, *Medizin im Islam*, 42, no. 22).

134. "the 'hypochondriac illness' and the 'flatulent illness'": Cf. Galen, *De locis affectis* 3.10 (ed. Kühn, 8:185): ὑποχονδριακόν τε καὶ φυσῶδες νόσημα.

135. Galen, *De locis affectis* 3.10 (ed. Kühn, 8:192): ὑποχονδριακόν [...] καὶ φυσῶδες.

136. Galen, *De locis affectis* 3.10 (ed. Kühn, 8:185, 192).

137. "*bayḍa* and *khūdha* [helmet]": I.e., a chronic headache affecting the total head; cf. Galen, *De locis affectis* 3.13 (ed. Kühn, 8:204): Οὐ μὴν οὐδὲ περὶ τῆς ὀνομαζομένης ὑπὸ τῶν ἰατρῶν κεφαλαίας ἀμφισβητήσειεν ἄν τις, ὡς οὐκ ἂν εἴη τῆς κεφαλῆς τὸ νόσημα. Trans. Siegel, *Galen on the Affected Parts*, 99: "No one, of course, will dispute that *kephalaia*, as the physicians call it, is a disease of the head." Arabic translation by Ḥunayn ibn Isḥāq (MS London, Wellcome Library, MS WMS. Or. 14a, fol. 82a: وكذلك أيضا العلّة التي يسمّيها الأطبّاء البيضه والخوذة ما من أحد يشكّ فيها ولا يرتاب بها فيقول إنّها ليست مرضا من أمراض الرأس. Cf. Thies, *Erkrankungen des Gehirns*, 40–41; and Maimonides, *Medical Aphorisms* 15.14 (ed. and trans. Bos, 3:59). See also Ibn Janāḥ, *Kitāb al-Talkhīṣ* (forthcoming), no. 269: داء البيضة هو الصداع المشتمل على <جملة> الرأس (*Dāʾ al-bayḍa* is a headache [*ṣudāʿ*] which afflicts the head as a whole).

138. This text does not appear in Galen, *De usu partium* 3, but in *De locis affectis* 3.13 (ed. Kühn, 8: 204, as in n. 137).

139. Galen, *De locis affectis* 5.4 (ed. Kühn, 8:329). See also Dols, *Majnūn: The Madman*, 30.

140. "severe stuporific attacks" (*subāt mustaghriq*): Cf. Galen, *De methodo medendi* 13.21 (ed. Kühn, 10:931; ed. and trans. Johnston and Horsley, 3:404–5): καταφορὰς βαθείας (deep somnolence).

141. "'stupor'": Cf. Galen, *De methodo medendi* 13.21 (ed. Kühn, 10:931; ed. and trans. Johnston and Horsley, 3:404–5): ἀποπληξίας (apoplexies).

142. "'torpor'" (*istighrāq*): Cf. Galen, *De methodo medendi* 13.21 (ed. Kühn, 10:931; ed. and trans. Johnston and Horsley, 3:404–5): κάρους (torpors).

143. "'catalepsy'": Cf. Galen, *De methodo medendi* 13.21 (ed. Kühn, 10:931; ed. and trans. Johnston and Horsley, 3:404–5): κατοχάς (catalepsies).

144. Galen, *De methodo medendi* 13.21 (ed. Kühn, 10:931; ed. and trans. Johnston and Horsley, 3:404–5).

145. "and that the physicians call 'extension'": I.e., extension of the pupil; this explanatory note is from Maimonides and does not appear in Galen's text.

146. Galen, *De usu partium* 10.1 (ed. Helmreich, 2:55); cf. Ibn Janāḥ, *Kitāb al-Talkhīṣ* (forthcoming), no. 628: الانتشار في العين هو اتّساع الحدقة من الأدوية في ذكر النبات الذي يقال له سطوبي(*Al-intishār* [synchysis, lit. "widening"] of the eye is a dilation [*ittisāʿ*] of the pupil [*ḥadaqa*]—from the entry on the plant called στοιβή in [sc. Galen's] *Drugs* [*al-Adwiya*]).

147. "chemosis": I.e., a swelling of the cornea resembling a cockleshell; cf. Galen, *De symptomatum causis* 1.2 (ed. Kühn, 7:101): χήμωσις.

148. "pterygium": I.e., a winglike membrane growing over the eye from the inner corner; cf. Galen, *De symptomatum causis* 1.2 (ed. Kühn, 7:101); and Maimonides, *Medical Aphorisms* 15.21, 24 (ed. and trans. Bos, 3:60–61).

149. Galen, *De symptomatum causis* 1.2 (ed. Kühn, 7:101); cf. Ibn Janāḥ, *Kitāb al-Talkhīṣ* (forthcoming), no. 306: الوردينج، رأيتُ في بعض التراجم أنّه انتفاخ في العين والجفن حتّى يصير كأنّه وردة، وقرأتُ في كتاب العلل والأعراض لجالينوس أنّه يحدث في الملتحم علّة يقال لها خيموسيس وهو نوع من الرمد يقال له الوردينج، وفي الحاوي إنّه ورم (٩٢ آ) يحدث في الملتحم عظيم، يتحوّل منه الجفن إلى داخل حتّى لا يقدر العليل أن يفتح عينه (*Al-wardīnaj* [chemosis]. I have seen in some dissertations that it is an edema [*intifāḫ*] of the eye and the lids, which looks like a rose [*warda*]. I have read in Galen's *Book on Causes and Symptoms* [*Kitāb al-ʿilal wa-l-aʿrāḍ*]: In the conjunctiva [*multaḥim*] there occurs a disease called *ḫīmūsīs* [χήμωσις], which is a

variety of conjunctivitis [*ramad*]. It is also called *wardīnaj*. In [al-Rāzī's] *Ḥāwī*: It is a severe swelling [*waram*], which occurs in the conjunctiva. The lids curve inwards, wherefore the patient cannot open his eye).

150. "*mūsaraj* [prolapse]": I.e., of the iris; cf. Galen, *De compositione medicamentorum secundum locos* 4.1, 2, and 4 (ed. Kühn, 12:705, 709, 716): πρόπτωσις.

151. "The pus that originates behind the hornlike tunic is called *kumna*": Cf. Galen, *De compositione medicamentorum secundum locos* 4.4 (ed. Kühn, 12:716).

152. *kumna*: I.e., hidden [matter]; cf. Maimonides, *Medical Aphorisms* 15.25 (ed. and trans. Bos, 3:61).

153. "The eyelids that become thick and hard and whose color turns red and whose hairs fall off is an illness that is called *sulāq* [ptilosis]: Cf. Galen, *De compositione medicamentorum secundum locos* 4.8 (ed. Kühn, 12:799).

154. "*sulāq* [ptilosis]": Cf. Ibn Janāḥ, *Kitāb al-Talkhīṣ* (forthcoming), no. 693: السلاق في العين هي العلّة التي تغلظ وتصلب وتحمرّ منها الأجفان وتتناثر أشفارها من كتاب الميامر (*Al-sulāq* of the eye [blepharitis/ptilosis] is the disease in which the eyelids become swollen, hard, and red, and the eyelashes fall off—from [Galen's] *Book on the Composition of Drugs according to Places* [*Kitāb al-Mayāmir*]).

155. "If the flesh in the inner angle of the eye disappears, it is an illness that is called *damᶜa* [rhyas]": Cf. Galen, *De compositione medicamentorum secundum locos* 4.8 (ed. Kühn, 12:774). Maimonides clarifies the Galenic term ῥυάς (a wasting of flesh at the great canthus, causing a continuous weeping discharge). Ibn Janāḥ, *Kitāb al-Talkhīṣ* (forthcoming), no. 273: الدمعة هي ذوبان لحمة المأق الأكبر من مآقي العين من كتاب الميامر (*Al-damᶜa* [lit. "the tear"] is a melting away [*dawabān*] of the flesh of the greater canthus of the canthi of the eye, according to the *Book on the Composition of Drugs according to Places* [*Mayāmir*]).

156. "A fistula occurring in the inner angle of the eye is called *gharab* [*Fistula lachrimalis*]": Cf. Galen, *De compositione medicamentorum secundum locos* 5.2 (ed. Kühn, 12:820): αἰγίλωψ.

157. "*gharab* [*Fistula lachrimalis*]": Cf. Ibn Janāḥ, *Kitāb al-Talkhīṣ* (forthcoming), no. 625: ناسور هو الخراج الذي يخرج في مآقي العين الأكبر من كتاب الميامير لجالينوس، ويقال له ريشة (*Nāsūr* [fistula] is an abscess [*ḫurāj*] occurring in the greater canthi of the eye [*maʾāqī al-ᶜayn al-akbar*], according to Galen's *Book on the Composition of Drugs according to Places* [*Mayāmīr*]; and it is also called *rīsha* [feather]).

158. "Callous hardenings on the face are called *naḥīlāt*": The callous hardenings Maimonides refers to are possibly small hard swellings or warts that Galen, *De compositione medicamentorum secundum locos* 5.3 (ed. Kühn, 12:823), calls ἴονθοι.

159. Galen, *De compositione medicamentorum secundum locos* 3.1 (ed. Kühn, 12:655).

160. "*nāṣūr*": Normally means fistula; cf. aphorism 23.72 above.

161. Galen, *De compositione medicamentorum secundum locos* 3.3 (ed. Kühn, 12:678, 681).

162. Nowadays aphthae are specks, flakes, or blisters on the mucous membranes (or in the mouth or gastrointestinal tract or on the lips), characteristic of some diseases (as thrush). But in ancient and medieval times they were superficial ulcers in the mouth and on the tongue, but also on a woman's genitals and the trachea. Cf. Grmek, *Diseases in the Ancient Greek World*, 149.

163. "corrosion" (*ākila*): Cf. Galen, *De compositione medicamentorum secundum locos* 6.9 (ed. Kühn, 12:988): νομή (spreading ulcer).

164. Galen, *De compositione medicamentorum secundum locos* 6.9 (ed. Kühn, 12:988).

165. "*naghānigh*": I.e., m. stylopharyngeus, hyopharyngeus?; cf. Ibn al-ʿAbbas al-Majūsi, "Livre royal (*al-malakī*)" 3.4 (ed. and trans. de Koning, 248–49, esp. 249 n. 3).

166. This quotation from Galen's lost treatise *De voce* [*et hanelitu*] escaped the attention of ed. Baumgarten, "Galen über die Stimme," 98: "Eine Durchsicht der Aphorismen des Moses Maimonides trug ebenfalls nichts ein."

167. Galen, *De locis affectis* 4.6 (ed. Kühn, 8:249).

168. Galen, *De causis pulsuum* 4.21 (ed. Kühn, 9:196).

169. "uninterruptedly": Cf. Galen, *De compositione medicamentorum secundum locos* 7.6 (ed. Kühn, 13:106): πυκνόν (thick).

170. Galen, *De compositione medicamentorum secundum locos* 7.6 (ed. Kühn, 13:105–6).

171. "dyspnea": (*ḍīq al-nafas wa-ʿasr al-nafas*): The synonymous Arabic terms represent Greek στενοχωρία; cf. Galen, *De compositione medicamentorum secundum locos* 7.6 (ed. Kühn, 13:105).

172. Galen, *De compositione medicamentorum secundum locos* 7.6 (ed. Kühn, 13:105–6).

173. Cf. Galen, *De symptomatum differentiis liber* 4 (ed. Kühn, 7:65–67).

174. "excessive dissolution": Cf. Galen, *De symptomatum causis* 1.7 (ed. Kühn, 7:132): κένωσις πλείων δι' ὅλου τοῦ σώματος (a major evacuation of the entire body).

175. Galen, *De symptomatum causis* 1.7 (ed. Kühn, 7:132); cf. Maimonides, *Commentary on Hippocrates' Aphorisms* 2.21 (ed. and trans. Bos, forthcoming): "Says Hippocrates: Drinking *sharāb* alleviates [cures] hunger. Says the commentator: With *sharāb* he means 'wine' and with 'hunger' he means 'canine appetite,' for the drinking of wine that has a strong warming effect and relieves this hunger. Canine appetite originates either from a cold temperament of the stomach alone or from an acid humor that has been absorbed by its substance. Wine, as mentioned, cures both [conditions] together."

176. "nausea": Arabic *tahawwuʿ*; Ibn Janāḥ, *Kitāb al-Talkhīṣ* (forthcoming), no. 1024: التهوّع هو الحركة إلى القيء من كتاب الأعضاء الآلمة، وهو عند أهل اللغة القيء بلا كلفة، كذا ذكره صاحب كتاب العين. (*Al-tahawwuʿ* is the impulse to vomit (*al-ḥaraka ilā l-qayʾ*), according to (Galen's) "Book on affected parts" (*Al-aʿḍā al-ālima*). According to the lexicographers, it is vomiting without exertion (i.e., spontaneous); the author of the *Kitāb al-ʿayn* mentioned this.

177. "distress": Cf. Galen, *De symptomatum causis* 2.3 (ed. Kühn, 7:173): τὸ κέρχνειν (roughness, hoarseness).

178. "soul is upset": I.e., stomach is upset; cf. Maimonides, *Medical Aphorisms* 9.51, 55 (ed. and trans. Bos, 2:70–71).

179. "distress": Cf. Galen, *De symptomatum causis* 2.3 (ed. Kühn, 7:173): κέρχνος (roughness, hoarseness).

180. Galen, *De symptomatum causis* 2.3 (ed. Kühn, 7:173).

181. "disturbance": Lit. "cause."

182. Galen, *De symptomatum causis* 3.2 (ed. Kühn, 7:217–18).

183. "in terms of what is taken first and what is taken later": Explanatory note by Maimonides, not found in Galen, *De locis affectis* 5.6 (ed. Kühn, 8:344).

184. Galen, *De locis affectis* 5.6 (ed. Kühn, 8:344); cf. Maimonides, *On Asthma* 5.4 (ed. and trans. Bos. 1:26).

185. Maimonides' text possibly goes back to Galen's statement in *De pulsibus libellus ad tirones* 12 (ed. Kühn, 8:489–90) that the pulse of those who suffer from cold of the cardia of the stomach and from pressure on it by a large amount of food or by nonbiting humors becomes very rare, slow, small, and weak and that patients suffering from bulimia have a similar pulse. Cf. Maimonides, *Medical Aphorisms* 4.20 (ed. and trans. Bos, 1:65). Cf. Ibn Janaḥ, *Kitāb al-Talkhīṣ* (forthcoming), no. 692: بوليموس هو الغَشْي وتفسيره الجوع من رسالة جالينوس إلى إغلوقن. *Būlīmūs* (βούλιμος) is the swoon (*ghashy*); its meaning is "hunger," according to Galen's letter to Glaucon.

186. "an upset stomach": Lit. "an upset soul"; cf. Galen, *De compositione medicamentorum secundum locos* 8.2 (ed. Kühn, 13:127): οἷς ἐπιγίνεται ναυτία (who are affected by nausea); see also aphorism 23.82 above.

187. Galen, *De compositione medicamentorum secundum locos* 8.2 (ed. Kühn, 13:127–28).

188. Galen, *De compositione medicamentorum secundum locos* 8.1 (ed. Kühn, 13:122).

189. Galen, *De compositione medicamentorum secundum locos* 8.6 (ed. Kühn, 13:192–93).

190. "When speaking of 'spleen patients,' physicians mean those patients whose spleen is affected by induration and calcification without an inflammation": Galen, *De compositione medicamentorum secundum locos* 9.2 (ed. Kühn, 13:239).

191. "The illness that is really called 'dysentery'": I.e., dysentery in a strict sense. — "The illness that is really called 'dysentery' is an ulceration of the intestines": Cf. Ibn Janāḥ, *Kitāb al-Talkhīṣ* (forthcoming), no. 271 : دوسنطاريا هو قروح الأمعاء من كتاب المارستان للرازي (*Dūsanṭāriyā* [δυσεντερία, dysentery] are intestinal ulcers [*qurūḥ al-amʿāʾ*], according to al-Rāzī's *Book on the Hospital* [*Kitāb al-Māristān*]).— "The illness that is really called 'dysentery' is an ulceration of the intestines, and this ulceration is either simple without putrfaction or with putrefaction": Galen, *De compositione medicamentorum secundum locos* 9.5 (ed. Kühn, 13:288).

192. [The illness] that the physicians usually call 'spreading ulcer' is a cankerous sore": Galen, *De compositione medicamentorum secundum locos* 9.5 (ed. Kühn, 13:288).

193. "'spreading ulcer'": Cf. Galen, *De compositione medicamentorum secundum locos* 9.5 (ed. Kühn, 13:288): νομή.

194. "Lanolin is the fatty wool": Cf. aphorism 23.49 above.

195. The term "lanolin" appears in several places in Galen, *De compositione medicamentorum secundum locos* 9.6 (ed. Kühn, 13:308–9, 311–12).

196. "unchanged": I.e., undigested.

197. Galen, *In Hippocratis Epidemiarum librum 1 commentarius* 2 (ed. Wenkebach and trans. Pfaff, 68, lines 10–13); Latin translation in Deller, "Epidemienkommentare," 522, no. 7.

198. "a severe pricking pain" (*waḥzan shadīdan*): Cf. Galen, *De locis affectis* 6.2 (ed. Kühn, 8:383): σφοδρὰς ἐντάσεις (severe tension).

199. "an urge to relieve oneself": Cf. Galen, *De locis affectis* 6.2 (ed. Kühn, 8:383): προθυμίας ἰσχυρᾶς. For *qiyām*, cf. Freytag, *Lexicon arabico-latinum*, 3:518: "Alvi deiectio vel fluctus."

200. Galen, *De locis affectis* 6.2 (ed. Kühn, 8:383).

201. Galen, *De symptomatum causis* 2.5 (ed. Kühn, 7:187).

202. "abdominal affections": Cf. Galen, *De locis affectis* 6.2 (ed. Kühn, 8:388): αἱ κοιλιακαὶ [...] διαθέσεις (bowel conditions).

203. Galen, *De locis affectis* 6.2 (ed. Kühn, 8:388).

204. "What is really called 'dysentery'": I.e., dysentery in a strict sense.

205. Galen, *De locis affectis* 6.2 (ed. Kühn, 8:381); see aphorism 23.89 above.

206. Galen, *De locis affectis* 6.3 (ed. Kühn, 8:394).

207. Galen, *De propriorum animi cuiuslibet affectuum dignotione et curatione* 9 (ed. Kühn, 5:45–46).

208. Galen, *In Hippocratis Aphorismos commentarius* 5.46 (ed. Kühn, 17B:839).

209. "*raḥā*": Lit. "millstone," a hard formation in a woman's womb, after Greek: μύλη; cf. Galen, *De methodo medendi* 14.13 (ed. Kühn, 10:987; ed. and trans. Johnston and Horsley, 3:486–87); cf. also Liddell and Scott, *Greek-English Lexicon*, 1152.

210. Galen, *De methodo medendi* 14.13 (ed. Kühn, 10:987; ed. and trans. Johnston and Horsley, 3:486–87). Cf. Nathan ha-Meʿati's glossary to his Hebrew translation of Ibn Sīnā's *Kitāb al-Qānūn*, Resh 2 (Bos, *Novel Medical and General Hebrew Terminology*, 2:119, 159: רחיים הוא חולי ברחם נקרא כן (RḤYYM [millstone, (hand) mill]). This is an illness of the womb. It is called thus RḤYYM).

211. This text does not appear in Galen, *De compositione medicamentorum secundum locos* 1, but in *De antidotis* 1.1 (ed. Kühn, 14:1).

212. Galen, *De compositione medicamentorum per genera* 5 (ed. Kühn, 13:763).

213. "cyclamen [*Cyclamen purpurascens* and var.]": Cf. Galen, *De simplicium medicamentorum temperamentis ac facultatibus* 5.14 (ed. Kühn, 11:750): κυκλάμινος. The Arabic *shajarat Maryam* normally refers to *Chrysanthemum balsamita*, but Maimonides identifies this plant as "cyclamen" (cf. Dioscurides, *Dioscurides triumphans* 2.148 and 3.130 [ed. and trans. Dietrich, 2:310–13, 492–93], and Maimonides, *Glossary of Drug Names* 364 [trans. Rosner, 287–88]).

214. Galen, *De simplicium medicamentorum temperamentis ac facultatibus* 5.14 (ed. Kühn, 11:749–50).

215. Galen, *De simplicium medicamentorum temperamentis ac facultatibus* 5.12 (ed. Kühn, 11:743–45).

216. "stinging or urticating caterpillar of the pinewoods": Cf. Galen, *De simplicium medicamentorum temperamentis ac facultatibus* 5.15 (ed. Kühn, 11:756): πιτυοκάμπη (cf. Liddell and Scott, *Greek-English Lexicon*, 1409: "prob. the processional caterpillar").

217. "aconite [*Aconitum napellus*]": For the Arabic *qātil al-dhiʾb* (wolf killer), cf. Dioscurides, *Dioscurides triumphans* 4.68 (ed. and trans. Dietrich, 2:581–83, esp. n. 2).

218. Galen, *De simplicium medicamentorum temperamentis ac facultatibus* 5.15 (ed. Kühn, 11:754–56).

219. "The king's nut is the edible nut [i.e., walnut, *Juglans regia*]. The small nut is the hazelnut [*jillawz*], that is, *bunduq* [*Corylus avellana*]": Cf. Galen, *De bonis malisque sucis* 5 (ed. Helmreich, 409, lines 13–14).

220. "edible nut [i.e., walnut, *Juglans regia*]" (*al-jawz al-maʾkūl*): Cf. Maimonides, *Glossary of Drug Names* 82 (trans. Rosner, 67–69); and Schmucker, *Pflanzliche und mineralische Materia medica*, no. 208.

221. "The small nut is the hazelnut [*jillawz*], that is, *bunduq* [*Corylus avellana*]": Cf. Maimonides, *Glossary of Drug Names* 43 (trans. Rosner, 35).

222. "sorghum [*Sorghum bicolor*] is called *shaylam* by the ancients": Cf. Galen, *De bonis malisque sucis* 7 (ed. Helmreich, 414, lines 13–14); for sorghum, cf. Galen, *De bonis malisque sucis* 7 (ed. Helmreich, 414, line 13): ἔλυμος; and Dioscurides, *Dioscurides triumphans* 2.82 (ed. and trans. Dietrich, 2:248–49).

223. "*shaylam*": It is possible that the Arabic *shaylam*, which stands for darnel, *Lolium temulentum,* is a corruption of the Greek μελίνη (Galen, *De bonis malisque sucis* 7 [ed. Helmreich, 414, line 13]); cf. Liddell and Scott, *Greek-English Lexicon*, 1097: "ἔλυμος; Italian millet, *Setaria italica*."

224. "millet [*Panicum miliaceum*] is type of sorghum": Cf. Galen, *De bonis malisque sucis* 7 (ed. Helmreich, 414, line 15); Maimonides, *Glossary of Drug Names* 70 (trans. Rosner, 59); and Dioscurides, *Dioscurides triumphans* 2.81 (ed. and trans. Dietrich, 2:247–48).

225. "Concentrated grape juice is the must that has been extremely well cooked": Cf. Maimonides, *Glossary of Drug Names* 84 (trans. Rosner, 70).

226. Galen, *De victu attenuante* 12 (ed. Kalbfleisch, 446, lines 27–28).

227. "[soft] fat and suet [i.e., hard fat]": Cf. Galen, *De alimentorum facultatibus* 3.10 (ed. Helmreich, 343, line 14): πιμελή καὶ στέαρ.

228. "because of its age": Cf. Galen, *De alimentorum facultatibus* 3.10 (ed. Helmreich, 343, lines 16–17): διὰ μακρὰν παλαιότητα.

229. Galen, *De alimentorum facultatibus* 3.10 (ed. Helmreich, 343, lines 4–11).

230. "Sour milk is [the milk] from which only the buttery part has been removed and that was then left until it turned sour": An exact source to this statement could not be identified. Galen deals with sour milk extensively in *De alimentorum facultatibus* 3.15 (ed. Helmreich, p. 349, line 23–p. 353, line 20).

231. "'moderately boiled'" (*mutarajjaj*): Lit. "trembling"; cf. Galen, *De alimentorum facultatibus* 3.21 (ed. Helmreich, 359, line 25): τρομητά (trembling, moderately boiled, of eggs).

232. "soft-boiled egg" (*nīmbirisht*): Cf. Vullers, *Lexicon persico-latinum*, 1393: "ovum sorbile, semicoctum"; and Ibn Lūqā, *Risāla fī tadbīr* (ed. and trans. Bos, 90 n. 39).

233. "'the one that can be supped'": Cf. Galen, *De alimentorum facultatibus* 3.21 (ed. Helmreich, 359, line 25): ῥοφητά.

234. Galen, *De alimentorum facultatibus* 3.21 (ed. Helmreich, 359, lines 23–25).

235. "Such a kind of wine is [similar to the water that is] suitable and fit for preparing honey water from it, which is called 'hydromel'": Cf. Galen, *De alimentorum facultatibus* 3.21 (ed. Helmreich, 359, lines 23–25): παραπλήσιοί πως ὄντες

ὕδασι τοῖς εἰς τὸ καλούμενον ὑδρόμηλον ἐπιτηδείοις ([white wines are] similar to the kinds of water that are suitable for the preparation of the so-called “hydromel”).

236. Galen, *De alimentorum facultatibus* 3.39 (ed. Helmreich, 383, lines 7–9).

237. “*dūgh*”: Cf. Ibn Janāḥ, *Kitāb al-Talkhīṣ* (forthcoming), no. 245: الدوغ هو مخيض البقر كان حامضًا أو غير حامضٍ عن مسيح، وهو عند الإسرائيلي الرائب، وقد أشار الرازي فيه إلى مثل هذا في المنصوري، وقال يحيى بن ماسويه: هو اللبن الحامض المنزوع الزبد المتّخذ من لبن الغنم (*Al-dūġ* is—according to Masīḥ—cow’s buttermilk [*maḫīḍ*], be it sour or not. According to al-Isrāʾīlī it is curdled milk [*rāʾib*]. Al-Rāzī held a similar view about it in his *Manṣūrī*. Yaḥyā ibn Māsawayh: It is the sour milk from which the butter has been extracted. It is made from ewe’s and goat’s milk [*laban al-ġanam*]). The Persian term *dūgh* (Freytag, *Lexicon arabico-latinum*, 2:71) or *dawgh* (Maimonides, *Sharḥ asmāʾ al-ʿuqqār* 104 [ed. and trans. Meyerhof, 53; English translation in Rosner, no. 83]) stands for “churned sour milk, whey, butter-milk” (Steingass, *Comprehensive Persian-English Dictionary*, 545). The Arabic equivalent of the Persian loanword is *makhīḍ* (Freytag, *Lexicon arabico-latinum*, 3:158a; Ibn Sayyār al-Warrāq, *Annals of the Caliphs’ Kitchens* [trans. Nasrallah, 588]: “sour buttermilk left after churning sour yoghurt and extracting its butter”). Ibn Janāḥ’s sources allude to the fact that fresh buttermilk ferments and becomes sour (*ḥāmiḍ*). Al-Isrāʾīlī dedicated a chapter of his *Kitāb al-aghḏiya* (ed. al-Ṣabbāḥ, 558) to the sour milk called *dūgh*. The definition as curdled milk is not found there. The beginning of Ibn Janāḥ’s entry was copied by Maimonides, *Sharḥ asmāʾ al-ʿuqqār* 104 (ed. and trans. Meyerhof, 53; English translation in Rosner, no. 83): *Dawghun huwa makhīḍu labani l-baqari iḏā ḥamuḍa* (It is the cream of cow’s milk turned sour). Cf. Ibn al-Bayṭār, *al-Jāmiʿ li-mufradāt*, 1:409: *al-dūgh huwa makhīḍ al-baqar*. See also Nathan’s glossary to his Hebrew translation of Ibn Sīnā’s *Kitāb al-qānūn*, Dalet 9 (Bos, *Novel Medical and General Hebrew Terminology*, 2:112, 133): דוג הוא מטעם נעשה מחלב מסוכסך (“DWG. I.e., a dish prepared from churned milk”).

238. “*kashk*”: Cf. Vullers, *Lexicon Persico-Latinum*, 2:842: “lac acidum siccatum s. oxygala siccata”; Dozy, Supplément aux dictionnaires arabes, 1:472: “sorte de fromage qu’on tire du lait aigre.” According to Aubaile-Sallenave, “*Al-Kishk*,” the term had the basic meaning of “curdled milk” and was then used at different times and in different cultures for a wide variety of products, both hard and soft, prepared from this milk. Thus it could refer to dried yogurt or sour milk, a dried product obtained from buttermilk, a black dried product used as a condiment, or a soft product: cheese, curd, sour milk, and whey. In addition it was used as a by-product from cereal (barley gruel or broth, barley bread), and for a complex preserved food from cereals and a dried sour product, and was then usually called *kishk*.

239. “*rāʾib*”: Cf. Ibn Janāḥ, *Kitāb al-Talkhīṣ* (forthcoming), no. 557: ماء الرائب هو الذي يعلو على الرائب إذا شُمّس من كتاب الجدري للرازي (*Māʾ al-rāʾib* [water of curdled milk] is [the liquid] appearing on the surface of curdled milk [*rāʾib*] if it is exposed to the sun—from al-Rāzī’s *Book on Smallpox* [*Kitāb al-judarī*]).

240. “*al-māst*”: Cf. Ibn al-Bayṭār, *Al-Jāmiʿ li-mufradāt*, 2:421; Dozy, *Supplément aux dictionnaires arabes*, 2:564–65; and Ibn Sayyār al-Warrāq, *Annals of the Caliphs’ Kitchens* (trans. Nasrallah, 589): “sour and thick yogurt made with rennet.” See also Ibn Janāḥ, *Kitāb al-Talkhīṣ* (forthcoming), no. 558: الماست هو أقوى حموضةً من الرائب

عن الإسرائيلي، وفي الأدوية المركّبة: إنّ الماست بالفارسية هو الرائب بنفسه، والماست منه حلو ومنه حامض ومنه مرّ
(*Al-māst* [soured milk] is sourer than curdled milk [*rā*ᵓ*ib*], according to al-Isrāᵓīlī. From the *Compound Drugs* [*al-Adwiya al-murakkaba* (sc. by Galen?)]: Persian *māst* is a synonym of *rā*ᵓ*ib*. There are sweet, sour, and bitter varieties of *māst*).

241. "*al-ḥāzir*": Cf. Lane, *Arabic-English Lexicon*, 560: "Sour or acid, or applied to milk, it means more than *ḥāmiḍ*."

242. "*aqiṭ*": Cf. Lane, *Arabic-English Lexicon*, 70: "A preparation of dried curd, a preparation of, or thing made from milk of sheep or goats, which has been churned, and of which the butter has been taken, cooked, and then left until it becomes concrete [...], or milk which is dried, and has become hard like stone; with which one cooks; or a thing made from milk, being a kind of cheese"; see also Ibn Sayyār al-Warrāq, *Annals of the Caliphs' Kitchens* (trans. Nasrallah, 585): "somewhat sour yogurt cheese made by heating sour yogurt and leaving it aside until whey separates from the solids. To drain the liquid, a round woven mat of date palm fronds, called sufra khūṣ, is used to spread the cheese pieces on it [...] The resulting piece of cheese is called 'aqiṭa.'" See also Aubaile-Sallenave, "Al-Kishk," 130: "In certain Arabic-speaking countries, *aqit* 'is made from curdled milk, dried in irregular pieces and then pounded for use' (Kazimirski 1860)." The Hebrew translator Zeraḥyah ben Isaac ben Sheᵓaltiel Ḥen comments on his translation of this aphorism: "Says the translator: Of all these nine names [of substances] which are the result and product of milk which he mentioned in this section, I can only find two [equivalents] in the Hebrew language, namely: *he-ḥalav* and *miẓ he-ḥalav* because the term *ḥem*ᵓ*ah* is not part of these nine [terms], and the terms *he-ḥalav ha-niqpa* and *he-ḥalav he-ḥamuẓ* are derivative terms: *ha-niqpa* from *ha-haqpa*ᵓ*ah* and *he-ḥamuẓ* from *ha-ḥimmuẓ*. For this reason I have mentioned all these nine terms in the Arabic language, and they are milk, which is the highest class with seven species derived from the milk beneath it, and each of the seven is different from the others; one can also call them 'individuals' when using the term 'species' for milk. The nine terms, including the seven species of milk for which I do not know a Hebrew name except for *miẓ ḥalav,* are respectively: *makhīḍ*, i.e., [milk] from which the butter has been removed, and the rest is [called] *maḥīḍ*; it is also called *dūgh*. The third term mentioned by him is *kashk*, the fourth *maṣl*, the fifth *rā*ᵓ*ib* and is also called *māsit*, the sixth *ḥāriz* (= *ḥāzir*), and the seventh *al-aqiṭ*." For another comment on the problem of finding Hebrew equivalents for Arabic technical terms, see aphorism 23.25 above.

243. Ibn al-Tilmīḏ's *Ikhtiyārāt al-Ḥāwī* (*Selections from "*[*the Kitāb*] *al-Ḥāwī"*) has been lost and appears in bibliographical literature as *Ikhtiyārāt Kitāb al-Ḥāwī lil-Rāzī* (*Selections from al-Rāzī's "Kitāb al-Ḥāwī"*); cf. Ibn Abī Uṣaybiᶜah, *ᶜUyūn al-anbā*ᵓ (ed. Riḍā, 371). Maimonides' quotation of the section on milk could not be retrieved from al-Rāzī, *Kitāb al-Ḥāwī*, 21.2:414–59. On Amīn al-Daula Abū ᵓal-Ḥasan Hibāt Allah ibn al-Tilmīḏ, a Christian Arab physician of Baghdad (d. 1154/65), see *Encyclopaedia of Islam*, new ed., 3:956–57; and Ullmann, *Medizin im Islam*, 163–64, and especially Kahl, *Dispensatory of Ibn at-Tilmīḏ*, 7–19. See also Maimonides, *Elucidation of Some Symptoms* 1.8 (ed. and trans. Bos, forthcoming), where he quotes "the exhilarating drink" composed by Ibn al-Tilmīḏ.

244. "If the watery part of milk is boiled and the fatty parts that separate from it through the boiling are taken from it, it is called *al-lawr*": Ibn al-Bayṭār, *Al-jāmi*ʿ *li-mufradāt*, 2:415, quotes a variety of recipes with *mā*ʾ *al-jubn* in the name of Ibn al-Tilmīḏ.

245. "*al-lawr*": From Persian *lōr*; cf. Vullers, *Lexicon persico-latinum*, 2:1103a; and *Wörterbuch der klassischen arabischen Sprache*, 2:1747a: "term for a kind of cheese." Cf. Ibn Janāḥ, *Kitāb al-Talkhīṣ* (forthcoming), no. 518: اللور بالراء هو شيء يعمل من ماء الجبن، وذلك أنّه يؤخذ منه مقدار ما، فيُصبّ عليه لبن حليب ويطبخ حتّى يخثر ويصير في قوام الشيراز، كذا رأيتُ في بعض الكتب. وقال أبو الفتوح: إنّما يطبخ ماء الجبن مع اللبن الحليب حتّى تبتدئ الرغوة فلا تزال كذلك، تؤخذ تلك الرغوة وتلقى في القدور يجتمع منها شيء كثيف وهو دسم جدًّا، يؤكل بالعسل إذا كان رطبًا وبالتمر الدنس، وإذا يبس كان كالجبن في يبسه إلّا أنّ طعمه غير طعم الجبن (*Al-lawr*—written with *rā*ʾ—is something made from whey [*mā*ʾ *al-ğubn*]. A certain quantity of it is taken; then fresh milk [*laban ḥalīb*] is poured on it. It is boiled until it thickens and becomes similar in consistency to curd (*shīrāz*)—this is what I read in some books. Abū l-Futūḥ said: In fact, whey and fresh milk are boiled until froth begins to emerge. This froth, which continues [to emerge], is skimmed off and put in vessels. It solidifies into a thick and very greasy substance. When it is still moist it can be eaten together with honey and low-quality dates [*tamr danis*]. When it becomes dry it resembles cheese, as regards its dryness, but its taste is different from that of cheese).

246. Galen, *In Platonis Timaeum* 2 (ed. Schröder, 7; ed. and trans. Larrain, 213–14).

## The Twenty-Fourth Treatise

1. "commented upon by Galen": The authenticity of this lost commentary by Galen is uncertain. It is not mentioned by Ḥunayn ibn Isḥāq in his list of Galen translations; perhaps he learned about it only afterwards. It is mentioned only by Ibn Abī Uṣaybiʿah, *ʿUyūn al-anbā*ʾ (ed. Riḍā, 149); see Meyerhof, "Echte und unechte Schriften Galens," 542, no. 56; Dietrich, *Medicinalia Arabica*, 241; and Ullmann, "Zwei spätantike Kommentare." See also Bos, introduction to Maimonides, *Medical Aphorisms* (ed. and trans. Bos), 1:xxi.

2. On the Greek philosopher Porphyry of Tyre (ad 234–305), especially in the Arabic tradition, see *Encyclopaedia of Islam*, new ed., 2:948–49.

3. This text quoted by Maimonides is probably part of the manuscript Manissa, Kitapsaray 1815 described by Dietrich, *Medicinalia Arabica*, 237–42, which bears the title *Kitāb Abuqrāṭ fī ʿilāj aujā*ʾ *an-nisā wa-ʿilalihinna mimmā fassar-ahu Hirmis al-hakīm wa-Jālīnūs*. This text is, as Dietrich, *Medicinalia Arabica*, 241, states, a mixture of Galenic medicine and Hermetic superstition. For this and the next aphorism, see Ullmann, "Zwei spätantike Kommentare," 250–51.

4. Maimonides' quotation from the end of this treatise is unique, as it does not survive in any other source. Only the first part of this work—originally consisting of five parts—survives in an Arabic translation by Ḥunayn ibn Isḥāq: Galen, *Über die medizinischen Namen* (ed. and trans. Meyerhof and Schacht); cf. Strohmaier, "Syrischer und arabischer Galen," 2013.

5. Galen, *On Examinations* 6.5–6 (ed. Iskandar, 82, lines 11–15; 84, lines 1–5). Maimonides' text seems to be a summary of part of the case history related by Galen.

6. Galen, *De anatomicis administrationibus* 7.13 (ed. Kühn, 2:632–33).

7. Galen, *De usu partium* 8.9 (ed. Helmreich 1:481, line 22–p. 482, line 1).

8. "*raṭl*": For its varying weight, see Hinz, *Islamische Masse und Gewichte*, 27–33; cf. Galen, *De curandi ratione per venae sectionem* 7 (ed. Kühn, 11:315): λίτρα (pound).

9. Galen, *De curandi ratione per venae sectionem* 23 (ed. Kühn, 11:314–15). For the role played by dreams of patients as a diagnostic tool in Galen's medical system, see Oberhelman, "Dreams in Graeco-Roman Medicine," 139–44.

10. "Guinea worms": Cf. Galen, *De locis affectis* 6.3 (ed. Kühn, 8:392–93): δρακόντια (little snakes); Ullmann, *Islamic Medicine*, 81: "Enlightening is the case of the guinea-worm, also called the Medina-worm (*Dracunculus medinensis*), a parasite which attacks human beings [...] Galen had only heard from many people that in a place in Arabia there were 'little snakes' (*drakontia*) that had a 'nerve-like' nature similar to intestinal worms in colour and thickness. He says that he himself has never seen them and can therefore say nothing exactly either about their origin or their nature"; and Ibn Lūqā, *Risāla fī tadbīr* 13 (ed. and trans. Bos).

11. "Tihāma": Cf. Galen, *De locis affectis* 6.3 (ed. Kühn, 8:392): Ἀραβία.

12. Galen, *De locis affectis* 6.3 (ed. Kühn, 8:392–93).

13. Galen, *De locis affectis* 6.4 (ed. Kühn, 8:412).

14. Galen, *De purgantium medicamentorum* [*facultate*] 4 (ed. Kühn, 11:336–37); cf. Narboni, *Sefer Oraḥ Ḥayyim*, fol. 95b.

15. "[clots of] blood" (*ghabīṭ*): Cf. Galen, *De tumoribus praeter naturam* 4 (ed. Kühn, 7:718): θρόμβος. See also aphorism 23.36 above.

16. "a honeylike mucous nasal discharge": Cf. Galen, *De tumoribus praeter naturam* 4 (ed. Kühn, 7:718): χυλός μελιτώδης, καὶ μυξώδης.

17. "living creatures that originate from putrefaction": For the underlying concept of spontaneous generation, see Ibn Lūqā, *Risāla fī tadbīr* (ed. and trans. Bos, 146–47 n. 350).

18. Galen, *De tumoribus praeter naturam* 4 (ed. Kühn, 7:718).

19. Galen, *In Hippocratis Epidemiarum librum* 1 *commentarius* 1 (ed. Wenkebach and trans. Pfaff, 33, lines 4–6); Latin translation in Deller, "Epidemienkommentare," 521, no. 2.

20. Cf. Galen, *In Hippocratis Epidemiarum librum* 2 *commentarius* 4 (ed. Wenkebach and trans. Pfaff, p. 341, line 43–p. 342, line 1). Instead of "eggplant," Wenkebach and Pfaff read "melon."

21. On Ibn Riḍwān (eleventh century), renowned physician, medical author, and polemist in Cairo, see *Encyclopaedia of Islam*, new ed., 3:906a–907a. The source of this statement by Ibn Riḍwān could not be identified.

22. Maimonides' opinion that the eggplant was unknown to the Greeks was shared by most Arab botanists, Ibn Riḍwān being a notable exception. However, in modern research the question is open to debate—some, like Clement-Mullet or Meyerhof and Sobhy, defending the opinion that the Greeks did know this plant, and others, like Leclerc, attacking this opinion; for a summary account of

this question, see al-Ghāfiqī, *"Book of Simple Drugs"* (ed. and trans. Meyerhof and Sobhy, 283–87).

23. Galen, *In Hippocratis Epidemiarum librum 2 commentarius* 4 (ed. Wenkebach and trans. Pfaff, 344, lines 24–34); Latin translation in Deller, "Epidemienkommentare," 525–26, no. 27.

24. "ounces": One ounce is 1/12 *raṭl* and corresponds to Greek οὐγκία.

25. Galen, *In Hippocratis Epidemiarum librum 6 commentarius* 3 (ed. Wenkebach and trans. Pfaff, p. 167, lines 9–11, 25–p. 168, lines 2, 6–8); Latin translation in Deller, "Epidemienkommentare," 536, no. 78.

26. Galen, *In Hippocratis Epidemiarum librum 6 commentarius* 4 (ed. Wenkebach and trans. Pfaff, 246, lines 3–6); Latin translation in Deller, "Epidemienkommentare," 537, no. 84.

27. Galen, *In Hippocratis De humoribus commentarius* 1.18 (ed. Kühn, 16:173). For this commentary, see aphorism 23.5 above.

28. This statement is quoted by von Krzowitz, *Historia ophtalmiae omnis aevi observata medica continens*, following Friedenwald, *Jews and Medicine,* 1:208 n. 36.

29. Cf. Galen, *On Problematic Movements* 8.16 (ed. Nutton and Bos). **G** has an additional marginal text: "Says Moses: The Ḥamdanite sultans were in Egypt [read: Mosul?], and the ruler was Nāṣir al-Dawla. He complained about a colic, but [his disease] thwarted all efforts of the physicians and no cure was found for him. Then the Sultan schemed to murder him and designated a man who had a dagger [to do so]. When he [i.e., Nāṣir] entered an antechamber of the palace, the man jumped upon him and hit him [with the dagger] at the lower end of the hip. The point of the dagger hit the intestine in which the colic was, and as result of this the [putrid] humor it contained was excreted. Then God cured him; he recovered and became very healthy."

30. "[throughout the whole night. I learned the truth by experience and had to believe it. I walked]": Cf. Galen, *De motu musculorum* 2.4 (ed. Kühn, 4:435–36): δεῆσάν ποτε δι' ὅλης νυκτὸς ὁδοιπορῆσαι, τῇ πείρᾳ τἀληθὲς ἔμαθον, ἠναγκάσθην πιστεύειν.

31. Galen, *De motu musculorum* 2.4 (ed. Kühn, 4:435–36).

32. Galen, *De motu musculorum* 2.6 (ed. Kühn, 4:446–47).

33. "he convulsed": Cf. Galen, *De motu musculorum* 2.6 (ed. Kühn, 4:449): βραχὺ κυλινδηθείς ("he rolled over slowly").

34. Galen, *De motu musculorum* 2.6 (ed. Kühn, 4:449).

35. "pregnant for some months": Galen, *On Examinations* 13 (trans. Iskandar, 131, lines 17–18): "in her fourth month of pregnancy."

36. Galen, *On Examinations* 13 (ed. Iskandar, 130, lines 13–14; 132, lines 1–5).

37. Galen, *De theriaca ad Pisonem* 2 (ed. Kühn, 14:218–19; ed. and trans. Richter-Bernburg, 16–17 [Arabic text], 59 [German translation]).

38. "but he was very fearful of an incision": Cf. Galen, *De theriaca ad Pisonem* 2 (ed. Kühn, 14:219): ὀκνηρότερον εἶχες πρὸς τὴν τομήν ("you [i.e., his father] were very reluctant to have it incised").

39. Galen, *De theriaca ad Pisonem* 2 (ed. Kühn, 14:219; ed. and trans. Richter-Bernburg, 17 [Arabic text], 59 [German translation]).

40. "breast": Arm[s] **BGU**.

41. Galen, *De theriaca ad Pisonem* 8 (ed. Kühn, 14:236–37; ed. and trans. Richter-Bernburg, 36–38 [Arabic text], 72–73 [German translation]).

42. Galen, *De theriaca ad Pisonem* 11 (ed. Kühn, 14:253–54; ed. and trans. Richter-Bernburg, 58–59 [Arabic text], 85 [German translation]).

43. Galen, *De theriaca ad Pisonem* 12 (ed. Kühn, 14:256; ed. and trans. Richter-Bernburg, 62 [Arabic text]), 87–88 [German translation]).

44. Galen, *De theriaca ad Pisonem* 16 (ed. Kühn, 14:281; ed. and trans. Richter-Bernburg, 91–92 [Arabic text), 104–5 [German translation]); cf. Narboni, *Sefer Oraḥ Ḥayyim*, fol. 125a.

45. Galen, *De theriaca ad Pisonem* 11 (ed. Kühn, 14:254–55; ed. and trans. Richter-Bernburg, 59–60 [Arabic text], 86 [German translation]).

46. "testicles": I.e., the ovaries.

47. "Thus female swine are castrated by our countrymen in Athens but also by other nations": Cf. Galen, *On Semen* 1.16 (ed. and trans. De Lacy, 122, lines 2–4; 123, lines 1–2): τὰς γοῦν θηλείας ὗς εκτέμνουσιν οἱ παρ' ἡμῖν, οὐ μόνον ἐπὶ τῆς 'Ασίας, ἀλλὰ κἀν τοῖς ὑπερκειμένοις ἔθνεσιν ἄχρι Καππαδοκίας (Thus our countrymen castrate female swine, not only in Asia, but also in the nations that lie above us as far as Cappadocia).

48. "to cut [around] both the flanks": Cf. Galen, *On Semen* 1.16 (ed. De Lacy, 122, line 11): περισχίζειν τὰς λαγόνας ἑκατέρας.

49. Galen, *On Semen* 1.16 (ed. De Lacy, 120, line 29; 122, lines 1–12).

50. Galen, *On Semen* 2.1 (ed. De Lacy, 152, lines 10–13).

51. Galen, *De locis affectis* 6.5 (ed. Kühn, 8:420; trans. Siegel, 185): "While I was occupied with these thoughts I encountered the following story of a woman who had been a widow for a long time. Besides some other disturbances she was afflicted with nervous tension. When a midwife told her that her womb was pulled up, she thought that she should employ remedies customarily used for this ailment. On application the heat of this medicine and the contact with her sexual organs provoked [uterine] contractions associated with the pain and pleasure similar to that experienced during intercourse. As a result the woman secreted a large quantity of heavy semen and thus lost the bothersome complaints."

52. Galen, *De alimentorum facultatibus* 2.38.4 (ed. Helmreich, 305, lines 17–19).

53. "with a decoction of thinning roots": Cf. Galen, *De alimentorum facultatibus* 2.67.2 (ed. Helmreich, 328, lines 18–19): καθ' ἑαυτό τε καὶ μεθ' ὑσσώπου καὶ ὀριγάνου μετρίως ἑψηθέντων ἐν αὐτῷ (on its own or with hyssop and oregano gently boiled in it).

54. Galen, *De alimentorum facultatibus* 2.67.2 (ed. Helmreich, 328, lines 13–19).

55. Galen, *De alimentorum facultatibus* 3.14.10 (ed. Helmreich, 347, lines 24–29).

56. "to strengthen their expulsive faculty": Cf. Galen, *De usu partium* 4.17 (ed. Helmreich, 1:242, line 15): σφοδρότητός τε γὰρ ἕνεκα; English translation in May, 1:239: "to allow for the violence of the expulsive faculty."

57. Galen, *De usu partium* 4.17 (ed. Helmreich, 1:242, lines 13–17, 25–p. 243, line 5).

58. "with the end of a sharp iron instrument": Cf. Galen, *De symptomatum causis* 1.2 (ed. Kühn, 7:100): γραφείῳ (with a pencil).

59. Galen, *De symptomatum causis* 1.2 (ed. Kühn, 7:100). Chauliac refers to the Latin translation of this text in his *Chirurgia Magna* (ed. McVaugh and Ogden, 1:190, lines 24–26; 2:160–61).

60. Galen, *De locis affectis* 3.11 (ed. Kühn, 8:195–96).

61. Galen, *De locis affectis* 4.11 (ed. Kühn, 8:290–91).

62. "until his life span was completed": Cf. Galen, *De locis affectis* 4.11 (ed. Kühn, 8:293): ἄχρι τῆς τελευτῆς ("until the end [of his life]"). The Arabic text seems to imply the Islamic concept of *ajal* (i.e., an appointed term of man's life); see *Encyclopaedia of Islam*, new ed., 1:204; and Maimonides, *Epistle on the Length of Life*.

63. Galen, *De locis affectis* 4.11 (ed. Kühn, 8:291–93).

64. "pulse": Lit. "vein."

65. Galen, *De locis affectis* 4.11 (ed. Kühn, 8:294–95). Cf. aphorism 23.79 above.

66. Cf. Galen, *De locis affectis* 6.3 (ed. Kühn, 8:394); Maimonides, *Medical Aphorisms* 8.68 (ed. and trans. Bos, 2:56); and Narboni, *Sefer Oraḥ Ḥayyim*, fol. 56a.

67. "Says Moses: This illness has never passed by me in the Maghreb, nor did any one of my elders tell me about it. But here in the land of Egypt, in a period of twenty years I have seen about twenty men and three women suffering from this illness. This prompts me to say: This illness only rarely occurs in cold countries but often in hot ones": Cf. Narboni, *Sefer Oraḥ Ḥayyim*, fol. 56a: "Says Moses: Similarly, I have never seen this illness in the Maghreb, nor did any one of the elders with whom I studied tell me that he saw it. But here today in the land of Egypt, in a period of ten years I have seen about twenty men suffering from this illness. This indicates that this illness mostly originates in a hot country. Perhaps the waters of the Nile are influential in this respect [as well]."

68. "Maghreb": For *gharb* used by Maimonides in the sense of *maghrib*, see Friedländer, *Arabisch-deutsches Lexikon*, XVIII–XIX n. 1; Maimonides, "Medicinischer Schwanengesang" (ed. Kroner, 89–90); and also *On Asthma* 4.4 (ed. and trans. Bos, 1:21, 127 n. 7).

69. "twenty": Ten (Narboni, *Sefer Oraḥ Ḥayyim*, fol. 56a).

70. "and three women": Omitted by Narboni, *Sefer Oraḥ Ḥayyim*, fol. 56a.

71. Galen, *De locis affectis* 6.3 (ed. Kühn, 8:394); see aphorism 24.39 above.

72. Galen, *De praesagitione ex pulsibus* 2.4 (ed. Kühn, 9:282–83).

73. Galen, *De simplicium medicamentorum temperamentis ac facultatibus* 10.1 (ed. Kühn, 12:252–53).

74. "together with some pork": Cf. Galen, *De simplicium medicamentorum temperamentis ac facultatibus* 10.1 (ed. Kühn, 12:254): ὡς ὕεια (as pork; i.e., they sold it as if it were pork).

75. Galen, *De simplicium medicamentorum temperamentis ac facultatibus* 10.1 (ed. Kühn, 12:254); cf. Galen, *De alimentorum facultatibus* 3.1 (ed. Helmreich, 333, lines 23–27); English translation in Grant, 155: "The similarity between the flesh of man and pig in taste and smell has been observed when certain people have eaten unawares human meat instead of pork. Such incidents perpetrated by unscrupulous restaurateurs and other such people have been witnessed in the past." See also Lieber, "Maimonides, the Medical Humanist," 59; Maimonides, *Medical Aphorisms* 20.19 (ed. and trans. Bos, 4:67–68); and aphorism 25.9 below.

76. "A treatise by Galen on the prohibition of the burial [of the dead] within twenty-four hours, translated by al-Biṭrīq": For this treatise see Steinschneider, "Griechische Ärzte," 461, no. 101; Steinschneider, *Hebräische Übersetzungen des Mittelalters*, 656–57; Meyerhof, "Echte und unechte Schriften Galens," 543, no. 64; Ritter and Walzer, "Arabische Übersetzungen griechischer Ärzte," 819; Ullmann, *Medizin im Islam*, 59, no. 95; and Sezgin, *Geschichte des arabischen Schrifttums*, 3:126–27, no. 93. This psuedo-Galenic treatise is currently being edited by Oliver Kahl as it is found on its own in MSS Istanbul Ayasofia 3724 and Paris 6734, and as part of the commentary by Ibn Bukhtīshū[c] (cf. Ullmann, *Medizin im Islam*, 110). Kahl's publication will include a supplement consisting of an edition (by Gerrit Bos) of Judah Alharizi's Hebrew translation of the treatise.

77. On the translators al-Biṭrīq and his son Yaḥyā al-Biṭrīq, see Dunlop, "Translations of al-Biṭrīq," 140–50, esp. 143; and Endress, "Arabische Übersetzungen von Aristoteles' *De Caelo*," 89–96. See as well aphorism 24.59 below.

78. "in his capacity of a translator": Lit. "in what he translated."

79. Cf. Maimonides' statement about his translation technique in his Letter to Samuel ibn Tibbon (Maimonides, *Igrot ha-RaMBaM*, ed. Shailat, 2:432), where Maimonides states that since al-Biṭrīq tried to translate literally while keeping up the word order of the original, his translations of Aristotle's works are questionable and corrupt. Maimonides' critical evaluation of al-Biṭrīq's translations is confirmed in Arabic bio-bibliographical literature; see the sources mentioned in Endress, "Arabische Übersetzungen von Aristoteles' *De Caelo*," 94–95. For a revaluation, see Ullmann, *Wörterbuch zu griechisch-arabischen Übersetzungen*, 35–47.

80. "Teaching the followers of Moses and Christ is easier and faster than teaching these physicians and philosophers": Cf. Galen, *De differentia pulsuum* 3.3 (ed. Kühn, 9:657): θᾶττον γὰρ ἄν τις τοὺς ἀπὸ Μωϋσοῦ καὶ Χριστοῦ μεταδιδάξειεν ἢ τοὺς ταῖς αἱρέσεσι προστετηκότας ἰατρούς τε καὶ φιλοσόφους (one might more easily teach novelties to the followers of Moses and Christ than to the physicians and philosophers who cling fast to their schools).

81. Galen, *De differentia pulsuum* 3.3 (ed. Kühn, 9:657); cf. Walzer, *Galen on Jews and Christians*, 14, 39.

82. Galen, *In Hippocratis Aphorismos commentarius* 6.18 (ed. Kühn, 18A:27–29). Cf. Maimonides, *Commentary on Hippocrates' Aphorisms* 6.18 (ed. and trans. Bos, forthcoming): "Says Hippocrates: if a tear occurs in the bladder or the brain or the heart or the kidneys or one of the smaller intestines or the stomach or the liver, it is fatal. Says the commentator: Galen says: Hippocrates uses the term "fatal" for that which kills necessarily [always] or kills in most cases. I have seen myself a man who was afflicted by a large, deep wound in his brain and [yet] he recovered. However, this only happens rarely."

83. "moved": Cf. Galen, *Doctrines of Hippocrates and Plato* 1.6 (ed. and trans. De Lacy, 80, line 8 [Greek text], 81, lines 7–8 [English translation]): καὶ πάντα ἐκίνει σφοδρῶς τὰ κῶλα ("and kept all its limbs in violent motion").

84. "the broken [fragments of a] bone": Cf. Galen, *Doctrines of Hippocrates and Plato* 1.6 (ed. De Lacy, 78, lines 34–35): τὰ κατεαγότα τῶν ὀστῶν.

85. Cf. Galen, *Doctrines of Hippocrates and Plato* 1.6 (ed. De Lacy, 78, lines 34–35; 80, lines 1–3).

86. "Slavs" (*ṣaqāliba*): Cf. *Encyclopaedia of Islam*, new. ed., 8:872: "the designation in medieval Islamic sources for the Slavs and other fair-haired, ruddy-complexioned peoples of Northern-Europe"; cf. Galen, *Doctrines of Hippocrates and Plato* 3.3 (ed. De Lacy, 186, line 1): Σκύθαι (Scyths).

87. "non-Arabs": Cf. Galen, *Doctrines of Hippocrates and Plato* 3.3 (ed. De Lacy, 186, line 1): Γάλαται (Gauls).

88. Galen, *Doctrines of Hippocrates and Plato* 3.3 (ed. De Lacy, 186, lines 1–3).

89. "of prattlers": Galen, *Doctrines of Hippocrates and Plato* 6.8 (ed. De Lacy, 426, line 1): τῶν φλυαρούντων.

90. "So-and-so who had shown his passion to the wife of so-and-so and committed adultery with her": Cf. Galen, *Doctrines of Hippocrates and Plato* 6.8 (ed. and trans. De Lacy, 424, line 28 [Greeek text], 425 [English translation]): Λητὼ γὰρ εἵλκυσε Διὸς κυδρὴν παράκοιτιν ("For he [i.e., Tityos] had assaulted Leto, glorious wife of Zeus").

91. "two kites": Cf. Galen, *Doctrines of Hippocrates and Plato* 6.8 (ed. De Lacy, 424, line 26: γῦπε (two vultures).

92. Cf. Galen, *Doctrines of Hippocrates and Plato* 6.8 (ed. De Lacy, 424, lines 21–35; 426, lines 1–2).

93. "he was so fond of conversation and talking that his body wasted away entirely": Following Rosner (Maimonides, *Medical Aphorisms* [ed. and trans. Rosner and Muntner, 2:169]). Larrain, ed., Galen, *Kommentar zu Platons Timaios*, 215, has the following corrupt translation: "And this occurred to him for the reason that he passed his time in the mountains listening to his own voice."

94. Cf. Galen, *In Platonis Timaeum* (ed. Schröder, 33; ed. and trans. Larrain, 214–15 ).

95. This aphorism and the next one are valuable quotations from the ancient translation by al-Biṭrīq that was lost, except for his translation of book six that survives in MS Istanbul, Ahmet III 2083, and in the quotations by Maimonides and Abū al-Rayḥān al-Bīrūnī. The translation that survived completely and was consulted by most Arab physicians is the one prepared by Ḥunayn (see Ullmann, *Wörterbuch griechisch-arabischen Übersetzungen*, 15–41; Ullmann has refuted the current theory that this translation was prepared by Ḥubaysh). The Arabic text of aphorisms 24.59–60 also appears in a synoptic table in Ullmann, *Wörterbuch griechisch-arabischen Übersetzungen*, 36–38, in which Ullmann compares the original Greek text with the translation prepared by Ḥunayn, and with that prepared by al-Biṭrīq as quoted by Maimonides. The MS consulted by Ullmann is **L**. On al-Biṭrīq see as well aphorism 24.44 above.

96. "spurge [*Euphorbia resinifera*]" (*farabiyūn*): Cf. Galen, *De simplicium medicamentorum temperamentis ac facultatibus* 3.18 (ed. Kühn, 11:601): κώνειον (hemlock [*Conium maculatum*]). The Arabic *farabiyūn* here originates from a misreading of the Arabic transcription *qūniyūn* for Greek κώνειον as *farabiyūn*. Ullmann, *Wörterbuch zu griechisch-arabischen Übersetzungen*, 37, mistakenly reads the version of **L** as *qūniyūn*.

97. "an old woman who lived in the land of Italy": Cf. Galen, *De simplicium medicamentorum temperamentis ac facultatibus* 3.18 (ed. Kühn, 11:601): ἡ Ἀττικὴ γραῦς (an old woman from Attica).

98. "spurge": Cf. Galen, *De simplicium medicamentorum temperamentis ac facultatibus* 3.18 (ed. Kühn, 11:601): hemlock.

99. Cf. Galen, *De simplicium medicamentorum temperamentis ac facultatibus* 5.6 (ed. Kühn, 11:724).

## The Twenty-Fifth Treatise

1. ʿAlī ibn Riḍwān (d. 1068), Abū al-ʿAlāʾ ibn Zuhr (d. 1130–31), and other physicians came to the defense of Galen against the attack of al-Rāzī and tried to solve the doubts raised by him (*ḥall al-shukūk*); see Averroës, "Contra Galenum," ed. and trans. Bürgel, 285; and Bos, "Medical Aphorisms: Towards a Critical Edition," 43.

2. For Maimonides' defense of Galen against al-Rāzī's criticism, see Averroës, "Contra Galenum," 289–90; Temkin, *Galenism: Rise and Decline*, 77–78; Stroumsa, "Al-Fārābī and Maimonides," 235–49, esp. 247; and Bos, "Medical Aphorisms: Towards a Critical Edition," 43–44.

3. "it may come either from a mistake that befell the ones who translated [Galen's] works into Arabic, or it may come from unmindfulness that happened to Galen, as nobody is free from these things except for exalted human beings, or the cause may be my bad understanding": Speaking about the possible causes of a corrupt textual tradition of Flavius Josephus' *Antiquities*, the Italian Jewish scholar Azariah de Rossi (sixteenth century) quotes these errors in a summarized form in his *Sefer Meʾor Enayim*, pt. 3 (*Imrei Binah*), sec. 4, ch. 53 (ed. Cassel, p. 442). See the English translation in Weinberg, ed., *Light of the Eyes*, 654: "Perhaps it was not Galen who was in error, but rather the translator, or I the reader," and adds two other possible errors of his own, namely, "of the scribes or the printers."

4. "exalted human beings": I.e., those human beings who are perfect in their rational and moral qualities and thus fit for receiving prophecy (cf. Maimonides, *Guide of the Perplexed* 2.32 [ed. and trans. Pines, 2:360–63]).

5. My translation of this aphorism is basically derived from Schacht and Meyerhof, "Maimonides against Galen," 64–65, with some corrections and adaptations.

6. "Only one extremely weak nerve is distributed through the whole liver because it does not need much sensation": Cf. Galen, *De usu partium* 5.10 (ed. Helmreich, 1:279, line 25–p. 280, line 1; English translation in May, 1:265): εἰς μέντοι τὸ ἧπαρ, οὕτω μέγα τε καὶ κύριον σπλάγχνον, ἐλάχιστον ἐνέφυ νεῦρον, ὡς ἂν μήτε κινούμενον, ὥσπερ οἱ μύες, μήτ' αἰσθήσεως περιττοτέρας δεόμενον, ὥσπερ τὰ ἔντερα (Yet a very small nerve is inserted into the liver, that large and important viscus, because it does not move like the muscles or need extra sensation like the intestines).

7. "Similarly, he explained in this treatise that the spleen, gallbladder, and kidneys have little sensation": Cf. Galen, *De usu partium* 5.10 (ed. Helmreich, 1:280, lines 3–10; English translation in May, 1:265): "And these four parts [i.e., two kidneys, spleen, and bladder] that purify the liver do not need a larger share of sensation because they would not be harmed by residues proper to them."

8. "As for nerves, we do not find any distributed and spread through the heart substance, just as we do not find this in the liver, kidneys, and spleen. But a small nerve reaches the membrane that surrounds the heart (i.e., pericardium). But in those animals that have large bodies, something of a nerve that is perceptible sometimes attaches to the heart": Galen, *De usu partium* 6.18 (ed. Helmreich, 1:364, lines 6–12).

9. Galen, *On the Natural Faculties* 2.9 (trans. Brock, 216–17).

10. Galen, *De locis affectis* 5.7 (ed. Kühn, 8:358–59).

11. Galen, *De causis pulsuum* 1.12 (ed. Kühn, 9:52–53).

12. "the quantitative dissolution of the psychical pneuma": Cf. Galen, *De sanitate tuenda* 2.11 (ed. Koch, 66, line 12): ἡ κατὰ τὴν ποσότητα τοῦ ψυχικοῦ πνεύματος ἀλλοίωσις (a quantitative alteration of the psychical pneuma).

13. Galen, *De sanitate tuenda* 2.11 (ed. Koch, 66, line 12).

14. Cf. the discussion in *De febribus differentiis* 1.7 (ed. Kühn, 7:294–300); cf. Anastassiou and Irmer, eds., *Hippokrateszitate in übrigen Werken Galens*, 92 (cf. Hippocrates, *Aphorismes* 4.55 [ed. and trans. Littré, 4:522, lines 8–9 (Greek text), 523, lines 9–10 (French translation)], and 165–66 (cf. Hippocrates, *Des Épidémies* 2.3.5 [ed. and trans. Littré, 5:108, line 7 (Greek text), 109, lines 9–10 (French translation)]).

15. Cf. Galen, *De causis morborum liber* 2 (ed. Kühn, 7:4–5).

16. Cf. Langermann, "Maimonides on the Synochous Fever," 186.

17. Galen, *De temperamentis* 2.2 (ed. Kühn, 1:594).

18. Galen, *De sanitate tuenda* 1.2 (ed. Kühn, 6:5).

19. Cf. Bos and Fontaine, "Medico-philosophical Controversies," 37–38.

20. Galen, *De methodo medendi* 7.5 (ed. Kühn, 10:470; ed. and trans. Johnston and Horsley, 2:256–57); cf. Maimonides, *Medical Aphorisms* 8.61 (ed. and trans. Bos, 2:54).

21. Galen, *De methodo medendi* 7.10 (ed. Kühn, 10:508–9; ed. and trans. Johnston and Horsley, 2:312–15).

22. Galen, *De compositione medicamentorum secundum locos* 4.1 (ed. Kühn, 12:700).

23. Galen, *De compositione medicamentorum secundum locos* 4.1 (ed. Kühn, 12:708); Galen does not speak about egg white in particular, but about eggs in general.

24. Galen, *De alimentorum facultatibus* 3.14 (ed. Helmreich, 345, lines 12–13): Camel's milk is most watery and least fatty; then comes horse's milk, and then ass's milk.

25. Galen, *De sanitate tuenda* 5.7 (ed. Koch, 149, 31): Donkey's milk is on the whole safer.

26. Galen, *De bonis malisque sucis* 4.25 and 6.8–9 (ed. Helmreich, 404, lines 4–7; 412, lines 27–29). See also Lieber, "Maimonides, the Medical Humanist," 58; Levinger, "Maimonides' Guide of the Perplexed on Forbidden Food," 201; and Maimonides, *Medical Aphorisms* 20.19 (ed. and trans. Bos, 4:67–68) and aphorism 24.43 above. For the contradictory element that is missing in our text, see the Hebrew translation by Zeraḥyah ben Yitsḥak ben She'altiel Ḥen, MS Florence, Biblioteca Mediceo-Laurenziana, MS Plut. 88.29, fol. 120b: "And in *De alimentorum* [*facultatibus*], book 1, he places pork among the other things that are thick and sticky and hard to dissolve"); see Galen, *De alimentorum facultatibus* 1.2.11 (ed. Helmreich, 220, line 29–221, line 4), which was quoted by Maimonides in his

*Medical Aphorisms* 20.62 (ed. and trans. Bos, 4:85–86): "Food that is hard to dissolve is that consisting of thick, sticky things such as pork and pure bread. If someone who does not exercise were to constantly eat this food, he would soon suffer from the illness of overfilling, just as if someone who practices bodily exercise were to constantly feed himself with vegetables and barley juice, his body would be destroyed and quickly waste away."

27. For the topic of revulsive bleeding, see Brain, *Galen on Bloodletting*, 135–44.

28. "repeatedly mentioned in the writings of Galen and Hippocrates": Cf. Galen, *De curandi ratione per venae sectione* 19 (ed. Kühn, 11:305); *De methodo medendi* 12.8 (ed. Kühn, 10:861; see Maimonides, *Medical Aphorisms* 8.42 [ed. and trans. Bos, 2:51]); *Ad Glauconem de methodo medendi* 1.4 (ed. Kühn, 11:91–93); *In Hippocratis Epidemiarum librum 2 commentarius* 6 (ed. Wenkebach and trans. Pfaff, 389, lines 9–21); and aphorism 25.15 below. Cf. Hippocrates, *Humours* 1 (ed. and trans. Jones, 4:65–66).

29. "severe illnesses of the eye": Cf. Galen, *De curandi ratione per venae sectionem* 16 (ed. Kühn, 11:297); and Maimonides, *Medical Aphorisms* 12.36 (ed. and trans. Bos, 3:36).

30. "angina": Cf. Galen, *De methodo medendi* 13.11 (ed. Kühn, 10:904).

31. Galen, *De curandi ratione per venae sectionem* 19 (ed. Kühn, 11:305–6).

32. Galen, *De curandi ratione per venae sectionem* 19 (ed. Kühn, 11:305–6); cf. Galen, *De methodo medendi* 13.11 (ed. Kühn, 10:904).

33. This quotation does not appear in the seventh book of *In Hippocratis Aphorismos commentarius*, but in book six (cf. ed. Kühn, 18A:57–58).

34. "vertigo or dizziness": Cf. Galen, *De curandi ratione per venae sectionem* 16 (ed. Kühn, 11:307): σκοτωματικούς; cf. Brain, *Galen on Bloodletting*, 82 n. 45: "Scomatic disease was characterised by giddiness and falling; as we say, 'blackouts.'"

35. Cf. marginal glosses in **L**: I say that the meaning of Galen's words, 'if someone suffers from epilepsy or vertigo or obstruction, he should especially be bled from the leg,' is that if the cause of the epilepsy or vertigo or obstruction is a retention of what usually is evacuated by the expulsive [force] of nature, as when a hemorrhoid is retained, and when one is afraid that [one of] these illnesses has occurred, then bleeding from the leg is one of the most appropriate treatments for these illnesses because it attracts [the matter] to the side that is far away and because it propels the blood that ascends to the brain towards the place from which it is usually evacuated by nature. This is as far as one can understand his words [when the illness] is caused by a retention and its explanation [...].

36. Galen, *In Hippocratis Epidemiarum librum 1 commentarius* 1 (ed. Wenkebach and trans. Pfaff, 29, lines 26–28); Latin translation in Deller, "Epidemienkommentare," 521, no. 1.

37. Galen, *In Hippocratis Epidemiarum librum 1 commentarius* 2 (ed. Wenkebach and trans. Pfaff, 88, line 27–89, line 1); not in Deller, "Epidemienkommentare."

38. "putrefies": Cf. Galen, *In Hippocratis Epidemiarum librum 1 commentarius* 2 (ed. trans. and Pfaff, 88, line 29): ἐκπυρωθῇ (becomes burning hot).

39. This pseudo-Galenic treatise is perhaps identical with *Maqāla fī l-ḥuqan wa-al-qūlanj* (*De clysteribus et colica*), cited by Ibn Abī Uṣaybiʿah, *ʿUyūn al-anbāʾ* (ed. Riḍā, 149); cf. Meyerhof, "Echte und unechte Schriften Galens," 543, no. 62;

Sezgin, *Geschichte des arabischen Schrifttums*, 3:128, no. 100; and Maimonides, *Medical Aphorisms* 7.65 (ed. and trans. Bos, 2:39, 115 n. 129).

40. Galen, *De simplicium medicamentorum [temperamentis ac facultatibus]* 7.48 (ed. Kühn, 12:42).

41. In his *Kitāb al-adwiya al-mufrada* (ed. and trans. Aguirre de Cárcer, 1:86), Ibn Wāfid actually remarks that it is drying to the first degree; on Ibn Wāfid (999–1067 CE), who served as a vizier in Toledo, see also Bos, introduction to Maimonides, *Medical Aphorisms* (ed. and trans. Bos); and Maimonides, *Medical Aphorisms* 21.67 (ed. and trans. Bos, 4:121–22).

42. Galen, *De bonis malisque sucis* 11.23 (ed. Helmreich, 425, lines 16–17); Galen adds: but only that they heat more or less.

43. Cf. Galen, *De febrium differentiis* 1.4 (ed. Kühn, 7:283); here, however, Galen describes these foods as bad (μοχθηρά) by their very nature and causing putrid and pestilential fevers.

44. The question is about the propriety of emesis over bleeding. Bleeding from a vein in the head would be nearer than emesis.

45. "by which they (i.e., the senses) [are well supplied] when [the nerves] are healthy": Cf. Galen, *De symptomatum causis* 1.5 (ed. Kühn, 7:112): ὡς ὑφ' ὧν ἕκαστα χορηγεῖται νεύρων ἐρρωμένων.

46. Galen, *De symptomatum causis* 1.5 (ed. Kühn, 7:112).

47. Galen, *De symptomatum causis* 1.1 (ed. Kühn, 7:86).

48. Galen's statement here, as paraphrased by Maimonides, can be schematized: If a sense becomes impaired, then (1) the principal organ through which it functions is impaired; (2) the faculty that impels this principal organ is impaired; or (3) [one of] the parts that was created for the use of this principal organ (such as a nerve) is impaired; or, If A, then B or C or D. Galen is reasoning from effect to causes. To reverse this (If B or C or D, then A) is normally invalid (fallacy of affirming the consequent) since we don't know enough about these causes to say whether any one of them acting alone can produce the impairment. We would have to verify this empirically, which is all Maimonides is saying in the last part. He is making a claim that damage to the nerve alone might be sufficient to impair the sense, which is a clear reversal of Galen's original argument. (I thank Dr. Glen Cooper for this explanatory note.)

49. Cf. Maimonides, *Medical Aphorisms* 15.3 (ed. and trans. Bos, 3:57): "One should not cauterize a part of the body that has depth or hollowness—all bodily parts have depth or hollowness except the hands, feet, and loins"; and **C**: One should also refrain from cauterization in the case of bodily parts that have depth, especially when the part has a deep hollowness, for all the parts have hollowness except the hands, feet, and thighs. (This quotation does not appear in Solomon ha-Meʾati's Hebrew translation of Galen, *Commentary on Airs, Waters, Places* [ed. and trans. Wasserstein]).

50. Galen, *In Hippocratis Epidemiarum librum 6 commentarius* 7 (ed. Wenkebach and trans. Pfaff, 421, lines 37–42); Latin translation in Deller, "Epidemienkommentare," 542, no. 109.

51. "an [inflammation in all parts of the body]": Cf. Galen, *De locis affectis* 2.8 (ed. Kühn, 8:96): τοῖς φλεγμαίνουσι μέρεσι.

52. "'phlegmone'": Cf. Galen, *De locis affectis* 2.8 (ed. Kühn, 8:97): φλεγμονή.

53. "a dissolution of continuity": Cf. Galen, *De methodo medendi* 12.6 (ed. Kühn, 10:852): συνεχείας λυσίς; cf. De Lacy, "Galen's concept of continuity."

54. Cf. Galen, *De inequali intemperie liber* 6 (ed. Kühn, 7:745); and *In Hippocratis librum de fracturis commentarius* 3 (ed. Kühn, 18B:586).

55. Cf. Galen, *De symptomatum causis* 1.2 (ed. Kühn, 7:87).

56. Galen, *De inequali intemperie liber* 6 (ed. Kühn, 7:745).

57. "first opinion": Namely, that there is only one cause of pain, i.e., a dissolution of continuity.

58. Cf. *De locis affectis* 2.5 (ed. Kühn, 7:80); English translation in Siegel, 46–47: "I know that I often spoke in other [lectures] about two principal types of pain, one [provoked] by an overwhelming change of the [humoral] mixture, and the other by the loss of continuity [of the tissues]. This does not contradict my previous statements."

59. Galen, "De puero epileptico consilium" 4 (ed. Keil, 16; ed. Kühn, 11:371).

60. Namely, from beets and cabbage; cf. Galen, "De puero epileptico consilium" 4 (ed. Keil, 10, line 17).

61. "mountain celery [*Peucedanum oreoselinum*]": Cf. Galen, "De puero epileptico consilium" 4 (ed. Keil, 10, line 19): σμυρμίον (*Smyrnium perfoliatum*).

62. "celery": Cf. Galen, "De puero epileptico consilium" 4 (ed. Keil, 13, line 16): σμυρμίον (*Smyrnium perfoliatum*).

63. "garlic": Cf. Galen, "De puero epileptico consilium" 4 (ed. Keil, 13, line 16): πετροσέλινον καὶ δαῦκος (parsley, parsnip).

64. Cf. Galen, "De puero epileptico consilium" 4 (ed. Keil, 13, lines 13–20).

65. Following the Greek text, Maimonides' doubt applies only to σμυρμίον (*Smyrnium perfoliatum*), i.e., mountain celery in the Arabic translation.

66. "garlic": Read: parsley or parsnip.

67. Galen, *De alimentorum facultatibus* 2.69 (ed. Helmreich, 329–30).

68. My translation of aphorisms 25.23–24 closely follows that of Langermann in his "Maimonides on the Synochous Fever," 184–88.

69. "abating [and attacking]": I.e., intermittent.

70. "For . . . beyond the cycle of quartan [fever]": This section appears only in **GS** and is thus missing in Langermann's translation, since he consulted **B**.

71. "and result in [a putrefying heat that affects] one thing after another over a longer period": Cf. Galen, *De febrium differentiis* 1.7 (ed. Kühn, 7:297): χρόνῳ πλείονι τὸ σηπεδονῶδες ἀνάπτειν θερμόν (so that they inflame the putrefying heat over a longer period).

72. Emendation based on Wernhard, "Galen: Über die Arten der Fieber in der arabischen Version des Ḥunain ibn Isḥāq," p. 60,13.

73. Galen, *De febrium differentiis* 1.7 (ed. Kühn, 7:297–99).

74. Galen, *De febrium differentiis* 2.2 (ed. Kühn, 7:336); and Maimonides, *Medical Aphorisms* 10.19–20 (ed. and trans. Bos, 3:5–6).

75. "For . . . continuous fevers": This section appears only in **GS** and is thus missing in Langermann's translation.

76. Galen, *De febrium differentiis* 2.13 (ed. Kühn, 7:379).

77. "[The putrefying humor] flows and moves through the entire body": Cf. this aphorism with an earlier statement in 25.23: "Intermittent fevers, that is, those that have a sensible abatement, occur only when the humor that produces the fever moves and flows throughout the entire body"; cf. also with aphorism 25.24 below: "But the gist of his second statement is that there is no sensible abatement unless the putrefying humor is outside the vessels and moves and flows throughout the entire body." This passage does not occur in Galen, *De febrium differentiis* 2.17 (ed. Kühn, 7:396).

78. Galen, *De febrium differentiis* 2.17 (ed. Kühn, 7:396–97).

79. "And this is most astonishing, how it can be outside the vessels in one place, without any doubt, but [also] streaming and moving throughout the entire body": Missing in Langermann's translation.

80. "those engaged in speculation" (*ahl al-naẓar*): Cf. Maimonides, *Guide of the Perplexed* 1.51 (ed. and trans. Pines, 1:113): "some people engaged in speculation"; and *Regimen of Health* 2.1 (ed. and trans. Bos, forthcoming).

81. A similar statement about the role of passion, and equally in the context of a critical attitude towards Galen, was made by Abū Bakr Muḥammad ibn Zakariyyā᾽ al-Rāzī (c. 860–923) in his *Kitāb al-shukūk* (ed. and trans. Mohaghegh, p. 2, line 23–p. 3, line 3 [Arabic text], 112–13 [English translation]): "Asked why modern scholars should attach [such critiques] to [the works of] the ancients, I cite several reasons. Among these is that error is inherent in human beings; and that passion overwhelms reason. For passion may perhaps affect the steady gaze of reason in the case of a certain man concerning some matter or other, to the extent that he may pronounce an error in regard to it, whether he be aware of that error or not." Al-Rāzī's monograph is also an important tool for reconstructing parts of Galen's lost *De demonstratione*, mentioned by Maimonides in this aphorism.

82. "*De demonstratione*": For this lost work by Galen, see Ullmann, *Medizin im Islam*, 62–63; see also aphorism 25.59 below.

83. "until he made them more eminent than the heart with his analogical reasoning": Cf. *On Semen* 1.15 (ed. and trans. De Lacy, 125, 127): "Thus the testicles surpass even the heart itself in this, that besides providing heat and strength to animals they also lead the way to the perpetuation of the race"; "By as much as living well is better than plain and simple living, by so much, among animals, are the testicles to be preferred to the heart"; cf. aphorism 25.26 below.

84. For Galen's lengthy discussion on the usefulness of the testicles and Aristotle's ignorance in this matter, see Galen, *On Semen* 1.12–17 (ed. and trans. De Lacy, 106-43).

85. Galen, *On Semen* 1.15 (ed. and trans. De Lacy, 126–27).

86. For the controversy concerning the function of the testicles, see Bos and Fontaine, "Medico-philosophical Controversies," 52–53.

87. "cold": Cf. Galen, *De symptomatum causis* 2.7 (ed. Kühn, 7:201): δυσκρασία (dyscrasia).

88. Galen, *De symptomatum causis* 2.7 (ed. Kühn, 7:201).

89. Galen, *De locis affectis* 3.11 (ed. Kühn, 8:193); English translation in Siegel, 94: "Almost all physicians have neglected to differentiate the three types of epilepsy. [. . .] All types [of epilepsy] have in common an affection of the brain,

[regardless of] whether this disease originates in the brain as is the case in most epileptics, or from the opening of the stomach. [. . .] Rarely another type of epilepsy [. . .] develops when the affection happens to start in some part [of the body] and then ascends to the head in a manner perceptible to the patient."

90. "and is guided from organ to organ": Cf. Galen, *De locis affectis* 3.11 (ed. Kühn, 8:194–95): ἀναδίδοσθαι ἀλλοιουμένων τῶν μορίων κατὰ τὸ συνεχές; English translation in Siegel, 95: "is transmitted through adjoining organs which had suffered a metabolic change." For the Arabic term بذرقة, see Ibn Janāh, *Kitāb al-Talkhīṣ* (forthcoming), no. 179: البَذْرَقة هو الدفع والإنفاذ، يقال بذرق الغذاء إذا دفعه وأنفذه وأوصله، قال أبو الفتوح: إنّما يقال للفرسان الذين يوصلون الرفقة من بلد إلى بلد ويَحْمُونَها من اللصوص والسلّابين بذرقة، ثمّ استُعِيرَ هذا الاسم للشيء الذي يوصل الغذاء إلى الأعضاء. *Badhraqa* (the escort) is the handing over and the delivery. One says "it escorts" (*badhraqa*) the nourishment, if it hands it over, delivers it, or conveys it. Abū al-Futūḥ: The knights, who convey a group of people from one place to another and protect them from robbers and raiders, are called *badhraqa*. This name was later used metaphorically for the things that convey the nourishment to the organs.

91. "or some vaporous substance that comes with this quality": Cf. Galen, *De locis affectis* 3.11 (ed. Kühn, 8:195): ἢ πνευματική τις οὐσία ("or that it is a vaporous substance").

92. Maimonides' account is not a fair reflection of the Galenic statement in this matter. In fact, Galen does not consider the third type of epilepsy to be merely a quality without any substance whatsoever. He raises the question whether types two or three are the result of an insubstantial quality or of some actual substance. Like Pelops, he believes in at least some substantial change, even if the result is achieved by a sort of sympathy. The cold breeze is thus something physical, a symptom of ongoing changes.

93. For this aphorism, see Ullmann, "Zwei spätantike Kommentare," 254–56.

94. Cf. Galen, *On Semen* 2.4 (ed. and trans. De Lacy, 176, lines 24–25 [Greek text], 177 [English translation]: "Indeed the female is wetter and colder, the male hotter and dryer." For other references in Galen, see De Lacy, ed. and trans., *On Semen*, 176.

95. Galen, *On Semen* 2.4 (ed. and trans. De Lacy, 176–79).

96. "growth": Ullmann, "Zwei spätantike Kommentare," 254, deriving **L** نشو from نشو, and not from نشأ, translates: "das Trunken werden" (intoxication).

97. For this lost commentary, see aphorism 24.1 above.

98. Galen's commentary is indeed based on Hippocrates, *Des maladies des femmes* 1.1 (ed. and trans. Littré, 8:12 [Greek text], 13, lines 24–25 [French translation]): "La femme a le sang plus chaud, et c'est pourquoi elle est plus chaude que l'homme" (A woman has hotter blood and is therefore hotter than a man).

99. "*De animalibus*": It is under this name that Aristotle's *Historia animalium* (10 bks.), *De partibus animalium* (4 bks.), and *De generatione animalium* (5 bks.) were known among the Arabs as one book. Thus the eighteenth book of *De animalibus* corresponds to *De generatione animalium* 4. The Arabic text of the relevant passage from Aristotle (765b16ff.), as quoted by Maimonides, differs considerably from the Arabic translation ascribed to Yaḥyā ibn al-Biṭrīq (Aristotle, *Generation of*

*Animals* [ed. Brugman and Drossaart Lulofs, 139, line 2ff.]); cf. Ullmann, "Zwei spätantike Kommentare," 255 n. 43.

100. Galen, *De bonis malisque sucis* 4.4.8 (ed. Helmreich, 398, lines 21–26); cf. Maimonides, *Medical Aphorisms* 20.41 (ed. and trans. Bos, 4:75–76); and Levinger, "Maimonides' Guide of the Perplexed on Forbidden Food," 207.

101. Galen, *De alimentorum facultatibus* 3.14.6 (ed. Helmreich, 346, lines 14–16).

102. Galen, *De victu attenuante* 12 (ed. Kalbfleisch, 451, lines 5–6).

103. Galen, *De simplicium medicamentorum temperamentis ac facultatibus* 10.8 (ed. Kühn, 12:266); cf. Maimonides, *Medical Aphorisms* 21.14 (ed. and trans. Bos, 4:101–2).

104. "again": Cf. Galen, *De alimentorum facultatibus* 3.14.5 (ed. Helmreich, 346, line 11): αὖθις.

105. Galen, *De alimentorum facultatibus* 3.14.5 (ed. Helmreich, 346, lines 9–13).

106. "All the partly alterative faculties": Cf. Galen, *On the Natural Faculties* 1.6 (ed. Brock, 24): Αἱ δὲ κατὰ μέρος ἅπασαι δυνάμεις [...] αἱ ἀλλοιωτικαί (Every single one of all the alterative faculties); the Arabic translator has clearly misunderstood the meaning of the Greek κατὰ μέρος.

107. Galen, *On the Natural Faculties* 1.6 (ed. and trans. Brock, 24 [Greek text], 25 [English translation]).

108. Galen, *On the Natural Faculties* 1.13 (ed. and trans. Brock, 50–53).

109. Galen, *On the Natural Faculties* 3.11 (ed. and trans. Brock, 280–81).

110. Galen, *De usu partium* 14.14 (ed. Helmreich, 332; trans. May, 2:652). In fact, Galen says the opposite, namely, that both the uteri and the urinary bladder have only one coat.

111. "copyists": Lit. "copying." Maimonides' conclusion that the inconsistency can possibly be explained as an error by the translator or copyist(s) does not hold true for **H**, fol. 257b, which provides a correct translation of the relevant Galenic text in *De usu partium* 14.14.

112. Galen, *De morborum differentiis* 5 (ed. Kühn, 6:851).

113. Galen, *Ad Glauconem de medendi methodo* 1.4 (ed. Kühn, 11:17).

114. Galen, *De alimentorum facultatibus* 2.37.2 (ed. Helmreich, p. 303, line 20–p. 304, line 1).

115. Galen, *De simplicium medicamentorum temperamentis ac facultatibus* 7.18 (ed. Kühn, 12:77).

116. Galen, *De alimentorum facultatibus* 3.38.7 (ed. Helmreich, p. 381, line 28–p. 382, line 6).

117. Galen, *De usu partium* 16.2 (ed. Helmreich, 2:382, lines 3–7; trans. May, 685); Arabic translation in Savage-Smith, 61 [Arabic text], and 115 [English translation]. This text also appears in aphorism 25.52.

118. Galen, *De locis affectis* 3.14 (ed. Kühn, 8:214).

119. Galen, *De morborum differentiis* 2 (ed. Kühn, 6:839); cf. Maimonides, *Medical Aphorisms* 2.12 (ed. and trans. Bos, 1:29–30).

120. Galen, *De causis morborum liber* 6 (ed. Kühn, 7:22); cf. Maimonides, *Medical Aphorisms* 2.12 (ed. and trans. Bos, 1:29–30).

121. Galen, *De atra bile* 3 (ed. Kühn, 5:112; ed. de Boer, 75); cf. Maimonides, *Medical Aphorisms* 6.25 (ed. and trans. Bos, 2:6).

122. Maimonides' quotation is not exact; Galen, *De atra bile* 3 (ed. Kühn, 5:112; ed. de Boer, 75), remarks: τὸν μὲν τῆς ἀκριβοῦς μελαίνης χολῆς χυμὸν ὀλεθρίως ἐκκρινόμενον ἐθεασάμην ἀεί, τὴν δὲ τῶν μελάνων κένωσιν οὐκ ὀλιγάκις ἐπ' ἀγαθῷ γινομένην (I have always seen that the excretion of juice consisting of pure black bile had a ruinous effect, but that the evacuation of [other] black [juices] was wholesome in not a few cases).

123. "ignorant": Galen, *De atra bile* 3 (ed. Kühn, 5:112; ed. de Boer, 75), speaks of inexperienced physicians; cf. Maimonides, *Medical Aphorisms* 6.26 (ed. and trans. Bos, 2:6).

124. Galen, *De atra bile* 3 (ed. Kühn, 5:112; ed. de Boer, 75); cf. Maimonides, *Medical Aphorisms* 6.26 (ed. and trans. Bos, 2:6).

125. Galen, *In Hippocratis Aphorismos commentarius* 4.22 (ed. Kühn, 17B:686).

126. "The instrument to measure this" (*sibār)*: Lit. "probe."

127. Galen, *De temperamentis* 2.3 (ed. Kühn, 1:603).

128. "That which pours must inevitably and unavoidably be moist and fluid in its appearance": Cf. Galen, *De causis morborum liber* 6 (ed. Kühn, 7:21): ἐνίοτε δὲ ἐμπίπλαται ῥεύματος ὑγροῦ μὲν πάντως τὴν ἰδέαν, οὐχ ὑγροῦ δὲ τὴν δύναμιν (but sometimes [the body] is full with liquids that are entirely moist in their appearance but not moist in their power).

129. "books": Cf. Galen, *De simplicium medicamentorum temperamentis ac facultatibus* 1–11 (ed. Kühn, 11:379–12:377).

130. Galen, *De causis morborum liber* 6 (ed. Kühn, 7:21–22).

131. "as it is measured with the sense [of touch]": Lit. "with the probe of the sense [of touch]."

132. "Hippocrates says over here": Cf. Hippocrates, *De la nature de l'homme* 7 (ed. and trans. Littré, 6:48 [Greek text], 49 [French translation]).

133. Galen, *In Hippocratis De natura hominis commentaria tria* 1.34 (ed. Mewaldt, 44, lines 3ff.).

134. "The matter is according to Hippocrates' statement": This is Maimonides' conclusion.

135. The Arabic translation of this text has a different version; cf. **C**: [Now I want to explain how Hippocrates, Aristotle, Athenaeus, and other eminent physicians agree that] spring is hot and moist. But this is not the case if one looks into the matter in a way that is sufficiently exact. [I have explained this matter and clarified it in the book *De temperamentis* where I said that there is no season, nature, or age that has a temperament that should be called hot and moist or cold and dry, since these things deviate from moderateness]. For an extensive discussion of this controversy, see Bos and Fontaine, "Medico-philosophical Controversies," 35–37.

136. "sumac [*Rhus coriaria*] juice": Cf. Galen, *De methodo medendi* 7.4 (ed. Kühn, 10:469; ed. and trans. Johnston and Horsley, 2:254 [Greek text], 255 [English translation]): ῥου χυλόν (the juice of pomegranate [*sic*]).

137. "all those medications": I.e., bitter asparagus, bulbs, quinces, apples, and pomegranate; cf. Galen, *De methodo medendi* 7.4 (ed. Kühn, 10:469; ed. and trans. Johnston and Horsley, 2:254–55).

138. "they made him like someone": Lit. "they put him into the category of someone." "They made him like someone whose body was wasted away and depleted of moisture until he was as if he were dead": Cf. Galen, *De methodo medendi* 7.4 (ed. Kühn, 10:469; ed. and trans. Johnston and Horsley, 2:254 [Greek text], 255 [English translation]): ὀλίγου δεῖν ἀπεφήναντο ἀλίβαντα (they pronounced him almost dead).

139. Galen, *De methodo medendi* 7.4 (ed. Kühn, 10:468–69; ed. and trans. Johnston and Horsley, 2:254–55).

140. Galen, *De methodo medendi* 7.6 (ed. Kühn, 10:472; ed. and trans. Johnston and Horsley, 2:260–61).

141. Cf. Galen, *De methodo medendi* 7.7 (ed. Kühn, 10:496; ed. and trans. Johnston and Horsley, 2:296 [Greek text], 297 [English translation]): διαμένειν γὰρ αὔτη καθ' ἑαυτὴν ἡ ξηρότης, ἀμέμπτου τῆς κατὰ τὸ θερμὸν καὶ ψυχρὸν ἀντιθέσεως ὑπαρχούσης, οὐ δύναται (It is impossible for dryness to remain pure in itself and to be uncontaminated by the opposition between hot and cold); i.e., the continual dryness is not just a result of an imbalance between wet and dry, but also requires some imbalance between hot and cold.

142. Galen, *De methodo medendi* 7.7 (ed. Kühn, 10:496; ed. and trans. Johnston and Horsley, 2:296–97); cf. Maimonides, *Medical Aphorisms* 3.15 (ed. and trans. Bos, 1:37).

143. Galen, *De methodo medendi* 7.7 (ed. Kühn, 10:496; ed. and trans. Johnston and Horsley, 2:296 [Greek text], 297 [English translation]): ἀλλ' ὅπερ ἐν ἀρχῇ λέλεκται, ξηρότητος ἴασιν ἐποιησάμεθα νῦν ἐξ ἀρχῆς τε συστάσης μόνης ἄχρι πλείστου τε μηδεμίαν ἀξιόλογον ἀκολουθοῦσαν ἐχούσης ψύξιν (But what I said at the start is that we effect a cure of dryness from the beginning when it exists alone to a great extent; there is no significant cooling that follows). What Galen wants to say is that he is only talking about curing dryness and is theorizing about it as if it were there from the very beginning (i.e., not caused by any other qualitative changes) and continued to be there in isolation. (I thank Vivian Nutton for this explanatory note.)

144. Galen, *De pulsibus libellus ad tirones* 12 (ed. Kühn, 8:483); cf. Maimonides, *Medical Aphorisms* 4.16 (ed. and trans. Bos, 1:64).

145. Galen, *De praesagitione ex pulsibus* 2.13 (ed. Kühn, 9:328); cf. Maimonides, *Medical Aphorisms* 4.7 (ed. and trans. Bos, 1:62).

146. Galen, *De totius morbi temporibus* 4 (ed. Kühn, 7:451); cf. Maimonides, *Medical Aphorisms* 11.2 (ed. and trans. Bos, 3:20).

147. Galen, *De crisibus* 1.4 (ed. Kühn, 9:561); cf. Maimonides, *Medical Aphorisms* 11.25 (ed. and trans. Bos, 3:25–26).

148. Maimonides' solution is incorrect because Galen definitely mentions epilepsy (ἐπιληψίαι) in *De crisibus* 1.4 (ed. Kühn, 9:561).

149. "yellow vitriol" (*qalqaṭār*): A kind of iron sulphate; cf. Maimonides, *Glossary of Drug Names* 140 (trans. Rosner, 107); and Galen, *De simplicium medicamentorum temperamentis ac facultatibus* 4.19 (ed. Kühn, 11:688): χαλκῖτις.

150. "green vitriol" (*zāj aḫḍar*): Green vitriol, imported from Cyprus, was considered to be the best kind of vitriol; cf. Maimonides, *Glossary of Drug Names*

140 (trans. Rosner, 107–8), no. 140; and Galen, *De simplicium medicamentorum temperamentis ac facultatibus* 4.19 (ed. Kühn, 11:688): μίσυ.

151. "red vitriol": Cf. Galen, *De simplicium medicamentorum temperamentis ac facultatibus* 4.19 (ed. Kühn, 11:688): σώρυ.

152. Galen, *De simplicium medicamentorum temperamentis ac facultatibus* 4.19 (ed. Kühn, 11:688).

153. Galen, *De methodo medendi* 11.15 (ed. Kühn, 10:785; ed. and trans. Johnston and Horsley, 3:186–87); Maimonides omits two conditions the patient should fulfill, namely, a certain age and sufficient bodily strength.

154. Cf. Galen, *De curandi ratione per venae sectionem* 10 (ed. Kühn, 11:282); Galen does not speak about pure phlegmatic fever, but simply about fever.

155. I could not retrieve this statement in Galen's works. Maimonides' text may be an adaptation of Galen, *De curandi ratione per venae sectionem* 12 (ed. Kühn, 11:287), where Galen remarks that when there is a *plethos* of seething blood, enkindling a very acute fever, there is need for copious evacuation.

156. Galen, *De simplicium medicamentorum temperamentis ac facultatibus* 6.13 (ed. Kühn, 11:817).

157. Galen, *De simplicium medicamentorum temperamentis ac facultatibus* 6.13 (ed. Kühn, 11:818).

158. Galen, *In Platonis Timaeum* 2 (ed. Schröder, 26; ed. and trans. Larrain, 216).

159. The text is incomplete since we do not have a second quotation from Galen's works whose conclusion—according to Maimonides—is opposite to that of the first one.

160. Galen, *De locis affectis* 3.13 (ed. Kühn, 8:206); cf. Maimonides, *Medical Aphorisms* 6.35 (ed. and trans. Bos, 2:8).

161. Galen, *De curandi ratione per venae sectionem* 7 (ed. Kühn, 11:268); cf. the English translation in Brain, *Galen on Bloodletting*, 75: "The quantity of any plethos is estimated from the magnitude of its characteristic signs. To whatever extent the patient has a sensation of heaviness, it is clear that dynamic plethos has increased to that degree; similarly, to whatever extent the sensation of tension has increased, to that extent also the other kind of plethos has increased, which, as I said, is called by some plethos by filling." See also Brain's explanation: "The essence of dynamic plethos is that the faculties are weak, so that the peccant humor oppresses them; hence the sensation of weight. The other variety, plethos by filling, physically distends the vessels, so that the patient feels swollen" (Brain, *Galen on Bloodletting*, 75 n. 24); and Maimonides, *Medical Aphorisms* 6.5 (ed. and trans. Bos, 2:2).

162. Galen, *De compositione medicamentorum secundum locos* 4.1 (ed. Kühn, 12:700).

163. "the vein at the inner side [of the arm]": I.e., the cubital vein; cf. Galen, *De methodo medendi* 5.8 (ed. Kühn, 10:341; ed. and trans. Johnston and Horsley, 2:54 [Greek text], 55 [English translation]): φλέβα κατ' ἀγκῶνα τὴν ἔνδον (a vein in the antecubital fossa).

164. Galen, *De methodo medendi* 5.8 (ed. Kühn, 10:341; ed. and trans. Johnston and Horsley, 2:54–55).

165. Galen, *In Hippocratis de humoribus commentarius* 1.18 (ed. Kühn, 16:175–76).

166. Galen, *De simplicium medicamentorum temperamentis ac facultatibus* 8.23 (ed. Kühn, 12:158).

167. Galen, *Ad Glauconem de medendi methodo* 2.3 (ed. Kühn, 11:86); cf. Maimonides, *Medical Aphorisms* 9.105–6 (ed. and trans. Bos, 2:82).

168. Galen, *De methodo medendi* 13.17 (ed. Kühn, 10:920–21; ed. and trans. Johnston and Horsley, 3:388 [Greek text], 389 [English translation]: ὁμοίων μὲν γὰρ δεῖται φαρμάκων κατὰ τὸ γένος ἀμφότερα τὰ σπλάγχνα· τοσούτῳ δ' ἰσχυροτέρων ὁ σπλήν, ὅσῳ παχυτέρᾳ χρῆται τροφῇ (Both viscera require similar medications in terms of class although, to the extent that the spleen is stronger, it uses thicker nutriment).

169. Galen, *De usu partium* 4.15 (ed. Helmreich, 1:235, lines 12–17; trans. May, 1:234).

170. "The language of the Greek is the most pleasant of all languages and the most universal for all people [endowed] with logic, the most eloquent and most human": Cf. Galen, *De differentia pulsuum* 2.5 (ed. Kühn, 8:586): τὴν ἡδίστην τε καὶ ἀνθρωπικωτάτην διάλεκτον (the most pleasant and most human language).

171. "green woodpecker" (*shaqirrāq*): See Freytag, Lexicon arabico-latinum, 2:415: "*Picus*, spec. *viridis*"; Lane, *Arabic-English Lexicon*, 1581: "green wood-pecker (*Picus viridis*); common roller (*Coracias garrula*)"; but cf. Dozy, *Supplément aux dictionnaires arabes*, 1:751: "mérops" (bee-eater). Galen, *De differentia pulsuum* 2.5 (ed. Kühn, 8:586), speaks about the sound of κολοιῶν (jackdaw, *Corvus monedula*) or κοράκων (raven, *Corvus corax*).

172. "whistle": Alternative reading: hiss; cf. Galen, *De differentia pulsuum* 2.5 (ed. Kühn, 8:586): συρίττουσιν.

173. Galen's theory of the superiority of the Greek language is contested by al-Rāzī, *Kitāb al-shukūk* (ed. Mohaghegh, 87); by the fifteenth-century mystical philosopher Johanan Alemanno (following Idel, *Language, Torah, and Hermeneutics*, 137–38); and by De Rossi, *Sefer Me'or Enayim* 3.4 (ed. Cassel, 464; trans. Weinberg, 689). The Spanish Hebrew poet and philosopher Moses Ibn Ezra (ca. 1055–after 1135) defends Galen against al-Rāzī's critique in his *Kitab al-muḥāḍara*, 40–41. For a general discussion, see Zwiep, *Mother of Reason and Revelation*, 193–96; and Eco, *Search for the Perfect Language*, 32.

174. See al-Rāzī, *Kitāb al-shukūk* (ed. and trans. Mohaghegh, 87); Pines, "Rāzī critique de Galien," 256; and Zwiep, *Mother of Reason and Revelation*, 195.

175. "conventional": But not natural, as Galen thought; cf. Maimonides, *Guide of the Perplexed* 2.30 (ed. and trans. Pines, 357–58): "Among the things you ought to know and have your attention aroused to is the dictum: And the man gave names, and so on (Gen. 2:20). It informs us that languages are conventional and not natural, as has sometimes been thought." On the medieval controversy of language being natural or conventional, see Zwiep, *Mother of Reason and Revelation*, 107–61; and Idel, *Language, Torah, and Hermeneutics*, 16–27.

176. See Zwiep, *Mother of Reason and Revelation*, 195–96.

177. Cf. al-Fārābī, *Kitāb al-ḥurūf* 118 (ed. Mahdi, 136–37). See Freudenthal, "Maimonides' Stance on Astrology," 83–84; and Zwiep, *Mother of Reason and Revelation*, 196. On al-Fārābī (870?–950), one of the foremost Islamic philosophers, see *Encyclopaedia of Islam*, new ed., 1:778–81.

178. "the climatic zone that is in the middle [of the earth]": I.e., the equatorial zone. One might think that, since they live in the middle of the earth, that is, the most moderate zone, they should speak perfectly.

179. For aphorisms 25.59–68, I have consulted and sometimes quoted from the translation by Schacht and Meyerhof, "Maimonides against Galen," which is based on **G**.

180. "It is a well-known saying of the philosophers that the soul can be healthy or ill just as the body can be healthy or ill": Cf. Maimonides, *Eight Chapters* (ed. and trans. Gorfinkle, 51): "The ancients maintained that the soul, like the body, is subject to good health and illness"; Maimonides, *On Asthma* 8.2–4 (ed. and trans. Bos, 1:37–39); Kranzler, "Maimonides' Concept of Mental Illness," 53–54; and Bos, "Maimonides on the Preservation of Health," 222–25.

181. "'human'": mental **EL**.

182. "human": mental **EL**.

183. "the philosophical, theoretical, or speculative sciences": Cf. Maimonides, *Treatise on Logic* 14 (trans. Efros, 61–64 [1938]; Judeo-Arabic text, ed. Efros, 38–42 [1966]); and Kraemer, "Maimonides on Philosophic Sciences," 85.

184. "conventional": Cf. Maimonides, *On Asthma* 13.13 (ed. and trans. Bos, 1:87, 136 n. 17); Schacht and Meyerhoff, "Maimonides against Galen," 65: "traditional."

185. The next section until the end of aphorism 25.59 has been translated and commented on by Steinschneider on the basis of the Hebrew translation prepared by Zeraḥyah ben Isaac ben She'altiel Ḥen, in *Al-Farabi*, 31–43.

186. "and to others in his time as well": Cf. **BKa**: but not to others in his time.

187. "and his discoveries of some of the conditions of the pulse, anatomy, and the usefulness and functions [of organs]—which are undoubtedly more correct than what Aristotle mentions in his books, if one looks at them impartially": This text is quoted by Ibn Falaquera in his *Moreh ha-moreh* (ed. Shiffman, 275, lines 100-102), a commentary on Maimonides' *Dalālat al-ḥā'irīn* (*Moreh ha-nevukim*; *Guide of the Perplexed*), which he completed around the year 1280.

188. "*On My Own Opinions*": Galen, *On My Own Opinions*, ed. and trans. Nutton.

189. "*On the Doctrines of Hippocrates and Plato*": Galen, *On the Doctrines of Hippocrates and Plato* (ed. and trans. De Lacy).

190. "*On Sperm*": Galen, *On Semen* (ed. and trans. De Lacy).

191. "a book on motion, time, the possible, and the first mover": Cf. Alexander of Aphrodisias, *Refutation of Galen's "Treatise on the Theory of Motion"* (ed. Rescher and Marmura, 3–4). The editors suggest that what we have here actually corresponds to the three treatises criticized by Alexander of Aphrodisias, namely, "On Place and Time" (not: "On Motion and Time"), "On the Possible," and "On the First Mover."

192. Maimonides recommended al-Fārābī's works to Samuel ibn Tibbon in his famous letter to the translator of the *Guide of the Perplexed* and stated that as far as books on logic are concerned, one should only study al-Fārābī's writings (Kraemer, "Maimonides on Philosophic Sciences," 81–82 n. 12). Kraemer remarks that "it would not be inaccurate to view the greater part of Maimonides' *Treatise on the Art of Logic* as an elementary textbook derived in the main from Alfarabi's introductions to logic."

193. "hyparctic": I.e., the 'assertoric' syllogism.

194. Cf. Aristotle, *Analytica priora* 1.1. Al-Fārābī's commentary on this section has been lost; see Lameer, *Al-Farabī and Aristotelian Syllogistics*, 7–9, 59–61.

195. "kinds": Lit. "shapes, forms"; cf. Steinschneider, *Al-Farabi (Alpharabius)* 34: "Beschaffenheit" (nature).

196. For an evaluation of Galen's competence in logic by other Islamic scholars, see Zimmermann, introduction to Al-Fārābi, *Commentary and Short Treatise on Aristotle's "De Interpretatione"* (trans. Zimmermann), lxxxi n. 2. For al-Fārābī's critique of Galen, see Averroës, "Contra Galenum" (ed. and trans. Bürgel, 287–89); Zimmermann, "Al-Farabi und die philosophische Kritik an Galen," 401; and Bos and Fontaine, "Medico-philosophical Controversies," 32–33.

197. Cf. Aristotle, *Analytica priora* 1.11. Al-Fārābī's commentary on this section has been lost; see Lameer, *Al-Fārābī and Aristotelian Syllogistics*, 7–9, 59–61.

198. "general premises": Cf. Al-Farabi's *Commentary and Short Treatise on Aristotle's "De Interpretatione"* (trans. Zimmermann, 77, lines 19–21 and n. 4: "'Mashhūr' [commonly known] is the technical term corresponding to Aristotle's ἔνδοχος. A premiss which deserves this predicate is not unquestionably true, but is supported by a respectable body of opinion"; Lameer, *Al-Fārābī and Aristotelian Syllogistics*, 206, translates the term as "generally accepted or plausible propositions."

199. The text may refer to *De usu partium* 10.12–14, where during a dream Galen is ordered by a divinity to reveal the mechanism of vision. Gersonides (1288–1344) remarks in *Wars of the Lord* 2.4 (trans. Feldman, 44) that Maimonides rejected Galen's account of how he obtained much medical knowledge through dreams and that Maimonides argued that this knowledge was acquired while awake but appeared to Galen as if it had originated in sleep. For the Galenic text, see Kudlien, "Galen's Religious Belief," 120.

200. For Galen's attack on Moses and the belief in an omnipotent God, and Maimonides' defense, see Walzer, *Galen on Jews and Christians*, esp. 11–13 and 33ff.; see also French, *Ancient Natural History*, 192–95. See also the letter by Solomon ben Abraham Adret (*Iggerot ʿim Iggeret ha-Bedershi*, fol. 19b) in which he explicitly refers to Maimonides' defense and strongly condemns Galen, introducing him as גאלינוס הרופא ישחקו עצמותיו (Galen, the physician, may his bones be ground [to dust]). The sections 25.62–66 are quoted by the philosopher Nachman Krochmal (1785–1840) in his magnum opus *Moreh Nevukhei ha-Zeman* (ed. Rawidowicz, 24–27) on the basis of the corrupt Lemberg 1804 Hebrew edition of the translation by Nathan ha-Meʾati. I thank Dr. Jack Rutner, who is preparing an annotated English translation of Krochmal's work, for this reference.

201. By adopting this material principle, Galen—in fact—denies two fundamental doctrines of the Mosaic and Christian religion, namely, that of God's omnipotence and that of the *creatio ex nihilo*.

202. "a million times": Cf. Galen, *De usu partium* 11.14 (ed. Helmreich, 2:159, line 7): μυριάκις.

203. "while greatly changing from their [initial] condition": Cf. Galen, *De usu partium* 11.14 (ed. Helmreich, 2:159, lines 8–9): τά τε γὰρ ἄλλα; English translation in May, 2:534: "As for the other requirements." Schacht and Meyerhof,

"Maimonides against Galen," 79, translate this phrase as "in spite of all his preference."

204. "foolish": weak **G**; cf. Galen, *De usu partium* 11.14 (ed. Helmreich, 2:159, line 18): μοχθηρός (wretched).

205. Cf. Galen, *De usu partium* 11.14 (ed. Helmreich, 2:158, line 2–p. 159, line 21); English translation in May, 2:532–34.

206. "a necessary consequence of the principle and basic rule": Lit. "a branch" (*farᶜ*), which is consequential upon the root (*aṣl*) and basis; these terms are common in the science of the religious law in Islam; the roots (*uṣūl*) are sources of legal knowledge, and the branches (*furūᶜ*) are the body of positive rules derived from them; see *Encyclopaedia of Islam*, new ed., 2:886–89.

207. "a necessary consequence of the difference in the principles": Lit. "a branch intrinsically connected to the difference in roots"; cf. note 206 above.

208. See Maimonides, *Guide of the Perplexed* 3.25 (ed. and trans. Pines, 2:503): "After having explained this, I shall say: A man endowed with intellect is incapable of saying that any action of God is in vain, futile, or frivolous. According to our opinion—that is, that of all of us who follow the Law of Moses our Master—all His actions are good and excellent."

209. See Maimonides, *Guide of the Perplexed* 3.19 (ed. and trans. Pines, 2:479): "Do you hold that it could have happened by chance that a certain clear humor should be produced, and outside it another similar humor, and again outside it a certain membrane in which a hole happened to be bored, and in front of that hole a clear and hard membrane?"

210. See Proverbs 3:19.

211. See Exodus 4:2–3; 7:10.

212. See Exodus 8:13.

213. See Maimonides, *Guide of the Perplexed* 2.29 (ed. and trans. Pines, 2:346): "Namely, we agree with Aristotle to one half of his opinion and we believe that what exists is eternal a parte post and will last forever with that nature which He, may He be exalted, has willed; that nothing in it will be changed in any aspect unless it be in some particular of it miraculously—although He, may He be exalted, has the power to change the whole of it, or to annihilate it, or to annihilate any nature in it that He wills."

214. See Exodus 7:20.

215. See Exodus 9:23.

216. See Exodus 4:6; and Maimonides, *Guide of the Perplexed* 2.29 (ed. and trans. Pines, 2:345).

217. See Numbers 11:8.

218. Cf. Maimonides, *Guide of the Perplexed* 2.21 (ed. and trans. Pines, 2:314–15): "Know that among the latter-day philosophers who affirm the eternity of the world there are some who maintain that God, may He be exalted, is the Agent of the world.[…] For the meaning of the assertion, as maintained by Aristotle, that this being proceeds necessarily from its cause and is perpetual in virtue of the latter's perpetuity—that cause being the deity—is identical with the meaning of their assertion that the world derives from the act of the deity […], but that it has always been and will always be as it is—just as the sunrise is

indubitably the agent of the day, though neither of them precedes the other in point of time."

219. Cf. Maimonides, *Guide of the Perplexed* 2.13 (ed. and trans. Pines, 2:284–85).

220. "skeptical about the principle but passes judgment in favor of [the possibility] of a necessary consequence": Lit. "Skeptical about the root but passes judgment in favor of a branch"; see aphorism 25.63, n. 206 above.

221. "the principles and their necessary consequences": Lit. "the roots and their branches"; see previous note.

222. See aphorism 25.59 above.

223. "My aim . . . that the only major organ is the heart" (aphorism 25.70): This section is quoted by Ibn Falaquera in his *Moreh ha-moreh* 2.22 (ed. Shiffman, p. 275, line 113–p. 276, line 122). This quotation continues with a citation from aphorisms 25.71–72, starting with "You know his constant argumentation . . ."

224. "eyes": Lit. "senses."

225. This positive evaluation by Maimonides is missing in Ibn Falaquera's quotation (*Moreh ha-moreh* 2.22 [ed. Shiffman, 276, line 120]).

226. For the controversy between Aristotle and Galen concerning the primacy of the heart alone or heart, brain, and liver together, see Kaufmann, *Sinne*, 64–65; Gätje, "'Innere Sinne' bei Averroes," 290–91; Temkin, *Galenism: Rise and Decline*, 120–21; Zimmermann, "Al-Farabi und die philosophische Kritik an Galen," 412; and Bos and Fontaine, "Medico-philosophical Controversies," 33, 46–52.

227. "You know . . . both statements at the same time" (aphorism 25.72): This section is quoted by Ibn Falaquera in his *Moreh ha-moreh* 2.22 (ed. Shiffman, 276, lines 122–32). It is followed by quoting the text starting with "if what he says is correct . . ."; see 25.72 at note 232 below.

228. "crush it": Cf. Galen, *Doctrines of Hippocrates and Platon* 2.4 (ed. and trans. De Lacy, 126, line 20): θλᾶν.

229. "altar": Lit. "the place of the sacrifices."

230. Galen, *Doctrines of Hippocrates and Platon* 2.4 (ed. and trans. De Lacy, 126, lines 18–25).

231. Galen, *De locis affectis* 5.2 (ed. Kühn, 8:303; trans. Siegel, 138); cf. Maimonides, *Medical Aphorisms* 3.97 (ed. and trans. Bos, 1:56).

232. "if what he says is correct . . . though their heart has stopped [beating]": This section is quoted by Ibn Falaquera in his *Moreh ha-moreh* 2.22 (ed. Shiffman, 276, lines 132–37); it continues with "Likewise, some animals . . ."; see following note.

233. "Likewise, some animals . . . nothing else": This text is quoted by Ibn Falaquera in his *Moreh ha-moreh* 2.22 (ed. Shiffman, 276, lines 136–38).

# Supplement

*Critical comparison of the Arabic text with the Hebrew translations and the translation into English*

**22.9**: حبّ القرع (tapeworms): This term is found twice in this sentence. The first time **N** translates: הדלועיים התולעים (worms in gourds), and the second time: גרגרי הדלעת (seeds of gourds). This last term is translated by **r** as: "gourd eggs." **Z** translates: התולעים הקטנים הדומים לזרע הדלעת (small worms resembling gourd seeds).

**22.23**: الركبة (the knee): Reading this term as: الرقبة **N** translates: הצואר and **r** translates: "the neck." **Z** translates correctly: הארכובה.

**22.36**: إسهال (diarrhea): **N** following the reading in **L**: آفة, translates this term as: פגע and **r** as: "damage." **Z** translates correctly: שלשול.

**22.40**: فصول (seasons): Reading this term as: فضول **N** translates: מותרים (superfluities). **Z** translates correctly: זמנים.

**22.49**: البزاة والصقور (hawks and falcons): **N** translates these terms as: הנץ והעוף הנקרא אלצאקור. **Z** does not give a translation but merely gives a general description of the kind of birds: אפרוחי העופות אשר יצודו בהם (young birds which are used for hunting).

**22.49**: طعم (taste): **N**'s correct version טעם is corrupted in **p** as: נגעים and translated by **r** as: "afflictions." **Z** has טעם just like **N**.

**22.54**: قمل (lice): **N**'s correct version כנים is corrupted in **p** as: עוות הפנים and translated by **r** as: "facial paresis." **Z** has כנים just like **N**.

**22.54**: غبيراء (sorb): **N** translates this term wrongly as: אגרינס, and **r** as: "larch fungus." **Z** has a correct version: העשב הנקרא גבירא.

**23.33**: كيس and أكياس (bag, bags): **N** wrongly translates these terms as: מחבת and **r** as: "frying pan." **Z** has a correct translation: כיס.

**23.34**: غرب (western side): **N** wrongly translates this term as: מזרח, and **r** as: "eastern side." **Z** has a correct translation: מערב.

**23.39a**: يحويها (surrounds them): **N**'s correct version יקיפם is corrupted in **p** as יקפיאם. **r** translates it as: "congeals them." **Z** has: מקיף.

**23.57**: أسماء مخترعة (invented terms): **N** wrongly translates this as: שמות נרדפים, and **r** as: synonyms. **Z** correctly translates: שמות בדויים.

**23.67**: تلك العلل (those diseases): **N**'s correct version אותה העלה is corrupted in **p** as: אותה הפעלה and translated by **r** as: "the maintenance." **Z** has a correct version: אותם החליים.

**23.68**: ضروبا (kinds): **N** corrupts this term as: כאב ראש, and **r** translates it as: "headache." **Z** translates the term as: מין (kind), following **L**: ضرب.

**23.70**: حدقة (pupil): N has שרפה (= حرقة), which is translated by **r** as: "burning." **Z** translates: (בבת העין =) בת העין.

**23.74**: لحم زائد (fleshy excrescence): Reading the term زائد as زيت, **N** translates: כזית בשר, and **r**: "an olive's size of flesh." **Z** correctly translates: בשר נוסף.

**23.75**: حرارة نارية (fiery heat): Corrupted by **N** as: חום עובר, **r** translates: "transient fever." **Z** correctly translates: חמימות אשי.

**23.91**: قيام (to relieve oneself): **N** understanding this term literally translates it as: לקום, and **r** as: "to stand erect." **Z** translates it correctly as: לקום לנקביו.

**24.5**: قصّ (breastbone): **N** translates this term incorrectly as: גרון, and **r** as: "throat." **Z** correctly translates: עצם החזה.

**24.33**: البقول الدنيئة (vegetables of poor quality): **N** translates this term incorrectly as: ירקות מדבריות, and **r** as: "wild vegetables." **Z** correctly translates: עשבים רעים.

**24.42**: طبيبان (two physicians): **N** reading this term as: طبيخان (two dishes), translates it as: שני תבשילים, and **r** as: "who were preparing a decoctum." **Z** correctly translates: שני אנשים רופאים.

**24.47**: ملتويا (tortuous): **N** translates this term correctly as: מקופל. However, **Z** reading it as: ممتلئا, translates: מלא (full).

**24.52**: المغترّين بالأهواء (who are deluded by heretic tendencies): **N** translates these terms incorrectly as: המשתדלים בלמודים, and **r** as: "who strive in their own school." **Z** translates the first term incorrectly but the second correctly as: המשנים בתאותם.

**24.57**: آبق (runaway): **N** transcribes the term as: מתאבק, and **r** reading it as a Hebrew term translates it as: "a chimney sweep" (Rosner, ed., *Medical Aphorisms,* 400n102). **Z** translates this term as: גנב (thief).

**24.58**: نَفْس (soul): Reading this term as نَفَس, **Z** translates it as: ניפוש (respiration). **N** translates it correctly as: נפש.

**24.60**: كماد (a hot compress): **N** translates this term incorrectly as: יין, and **r** as: "wine." **Z** translates it as: שאר הדברים (other things).

**25.1**: حلّ (to resolve): **N** reads this term as: حال, and consequently translates it as: ענין (matter). **Z** translates it correctly as: להתיר.

**25.1**: إمام (master): **N** reads this term as: أمام, and consequently translates it as: נכח (opposite). **Z** translates it correctly as: אדון.

**25.2**: انبثّ (to spread): Reading this term as: نبت, **N** translates it as: צמח, and **r** as: "growing." **Z** translates it correctly as: התפשט.

**25.6**: متناقص (diminishing): **N** translates this term correctly as: מתחסר. **Z** reading the term as: متناقض, translates it as: היה זה נגד זה (to be contradictory).

**25.11**: صَرْع (epilepsy): Probably reading this term as: صداع, **N** translates it as: כאב ראש, and **r** as: "headache." **Z** transcribes it as: צרע.

**25.17**: انضرّ (to be impaired): Reading this term as: نظر, **N** translates it as: ראה (to see). **Z** translates it correctly as: היה ניזק.

**25.20**: حذف (to cancel): Reading this term as: خفض, **N** translates it as: חיסר. **Z** translates it correctly as: עזב.

**25.23**: جار (flowing): Probably reading this term as: غار, **N** translates it as: שוקע̃, and **r** as: "settles." **Z** translates it correctly as: רץ.

**25.26**: جودة الحياة (living well): Reading جودة as: وجودة, **Z** translates this expression as: מציאות החיים. **N** translates it correctly as: החיים הטובים.

**25.26**: نقض (to refute): Reading this term as: نقص, **Z** translates it as: היה גרוע (to be deficient). **N** translates it correctly as: סתר.

**25.40**: أجفّ (drier): Reading this term as: أخفّ, **Z** translates it as: יותר קל (lighter). **N** translates it correctly as: יותר נגוב.

**25.40**: جار (flowing): Reading this term as: حارّ, **Z** translates it as: חם (hot). **N** translates it correctly as: נוזל.

**25.43**: على حدته (on its own): Reading this term as: على آخرته, **N** translates it as: באחריתו. **Z** translates it as: כמו שהוא.

**25.45**: برأ (to be cured): Reading this term as: بدأ, **N** translates it as: התחיל. **Z** translates it correctly as: התרפא.

**25.52**: استثقل (to feel heaviness): Reading this term as: استنقل **Z** translates it as: נעתק. **N** translates it as: כבד כובד.

**25.59**: هذى (to talk nonsense): **N** possibly reading the term as: هدى, translates it as: הלך, and **Z** reading it as: هدأ, translates it as: נח.

**25.59**: مهرة (experts): **N** translates this term incorrectly as: טעות; and **r** as: "err." **Z** translates it as: זריזות.

**25.63**: شرائع (divine laws): Possibly reading this term as: شرائط , **N** translates it as: תנאים. **Z** translates it correctly as: דתות.

**25.64**: كوّن (to form): Reading this term as: كون, **Z** translates it as: היות, while **N** translates it correctly as: הוה.

**25.67**: علم (knowledge): **Z** reads this term as: عالم, and consequently translates it as: עולם. **N** translates it correctly as: חכמה.

# Bibliographies

## Translations and Editions of Works by or Attributed to Moses Maimonides

*(arranged alphabetically by translator or editor)*

Bos, Gerrit, ed. and trans. *Commentary on Hippocrates' Aphorisms.* Provo, UT: Brigham Young University Press, forthcoming.

———. *On the Elucidation of Some Symptoms and the Response to Them.* Provo, UT: Brigham Young University Press, forthcoming.

———. *Medical Aphorisms.* 7 vols. Provo, UT: Brigham Young University Press, 2004–.

Bos, Gerrit, ed. and trans., and Michael R. McVaugh, ed. *On Asthma.* 2 vols. Provo, UT: Brigham Young University Press, 2002–8.

———. *On Hemorrhoids.* Provo, UT: Brigham Young University Press, 2012.

———. *On Poisons and the Protection against Lethal Drugs.* Provo, UT: Brigham Young University Press, 2009.

———. *The Regimen of Health.* Provo, UT: Brigham Young University Press, forthcoming.

Bos, Gerrit, et al., ed. and trans. *On Coitus.* Provo, UT: Brigham Young University Press, forthcoming.

Deller, K. H., ed. and trans., and K. Deichgräber, ed. "Die Exzerpte des Moses Maimonides aus den Epidemienkommentare des Galen." Supplement to Galen, *In Hippocratis Epidemiarum librum* 6 *commentaria* 1–8, edited by Ernst Wenkebach and Franz Pfaff. Corpus Medicorum Graecorum 5.10.2.2. Berlin: Akademie Verlag, 1956.

Efros, Israel, ed. and trans. *Maimonides' Treatise on Logic (Maḳālah fi-ṣinā'at al-manṭiḳ). The Original Arabic and Three Hebrew Translations.* New York: American Academy for Jewish Research, 1938.

Gorfinkle, Joseph I., ed. and trans. *The Eight Chapters of Maimonides on Ethics (Shemonah Peraḳim). A psychological and ethical treatise.* 1912. Reprint, New York: AMS Press, 1966.

Kroner, Hermann, ed. "Der medizinische Schwanengesang des Maimonides: *Fī bajān al-aʿrāḍ* (Über die Erklärung der Zufälle)." *Janus* 32 (1928): 12–116.

Meyerhof, Max, ed. and trans. *Sharḥ asmāʾ al-ʿuqqār (L'explication des noms des drogues). Un glossaire de matière médicale composé par Maïmonide.* Cairo: Imprimerie de l'Institut français d'archéologie orientale, 1940. (See also Rosner's translation below.)

Munk, Salomon, ed. *Dalālat al-ḥāʾirīn: Moreh ha-nevukim.* Judeo-Arabic text with variant readings by Issachar Joel. Jerusalem: J. Junovitch, 1930–31 (See also Pines' edition and translation below).

Muntner, Süssman, ed. *Pirḳe Mosheh bi-refuʾah.* Jerusalem: Mosad ha-Rav Ḳuḳ, 1959.

Pines, Shlomo, ed. and trans. *The Guide of the Perplexed.* 2 vols. Chicago: The University of Chicago Press, 1963. (See also Munk's edition above.)

Rosner, Fred, trans. *The Medical Aphorisms of Moses Maimonides.* Haifa: Maimonides Research Institute, 1989.

———. *Moses Maimonides' Glossary of Drug Names.* Haifa: Maimonides Research Institute, 1995. (See also Meyerhof's edition and translation above.)

Rosner, Fred, and Süssman Muntner, eds. and trans. *The Medical Aphorisms of Moses Maimonides.* 2 pts. in 1 vol. New York: Yeshiva University Press, Department of Special Publications, 1970–71.

Schliwski, Carsten, ed. and trans. "Sharḥ fusūl Abūqrāṭ. Kommentar zu den Aphorismen des Hippokrates." PhD diss., University of Cologne, 2002.

Shailat, Isaac, ed. *Igrot ha-RaMBaM.* 2 vols. Jerusalem: Hotsaʾat Maʿaliyot le-yad Yeshivat "Birkat Moshe" Maʿaleh Adumim, 1987–88.

Stern, Samuel Miklos, ed. and trans. "Maimonides' *Treatise to a Prince, Containing Advice on Sexual Matters.*" In *Maimonidis Commentarius in Mischnam e codibus Hunt, 117 et Pococke 295 in Bibliotheca Bodleiana Oxoniensi servatis et 72–73 Bibliothecae Sassooniensis Letchworth*, edited by Samuel Miklos Stern, 17–21. Copenhagen: Ejnar Munksgaard, 1956–66.

Weil, Gotthold, ed. and trans. *Über die Lebensdauer.* Basel: Karger, 1953. Reedited by M. Schwartz as *Teshuvat ha-Rambam bi Sheʾelat ha-Qets ha-qatsuv la-Ḥayyim.* Tel Aviv: Papyrus, 1979.

## Editions of Galenic Works

*(arranged alphabetically by translator or editor)*

Alexanderson, Bengt, ed. and trans. *Peri Kriseōn Galenos (De crisibus).* Göteborg: Almquist & Wiksell, 1967.

Baumgarten, Hans, ed. "Galen über die Stimme. Testimonien der verlorenen Schrift Περὶ φωνῆς. Pseudo-Galen, *De voce et hanelitu.*" PhD diss., University of Göttingen, 1962.

Boer, Wilko de, ed. *Galeni de propriorum animi cuiuslibet affectuum dignotione et curatione, de animi cuiuslibet peccatorum dignotione et curatione, de atra bile.* Corpus Medicorum Graecorum 5.4.1.1. Leipzig: Teubner, 1937.

Bos, Gerrit, Michael McVaugh, and Joseph Shatzmiller. *Transmitting a Text through Three Languages: The Future History of Galen's "Peri Anomalou Dyskrasias."* Philadephia: The American Philosophical Society, 2014.

Brock, Arthur John, ed. and trans. *On the Natural Faculties.* London: Heinemann, 1916. Reprint, Cambridge, MA: Harvard University Press, 1979.

De Lacy, Phillip, ed. and trans. *On the Doctrines of Hippocrates and Plato.* Vol. 1, bks. 1–5. Corpus Medicorum Graecorum 5.4.1.2. Berlin: Akademie-Verlag, 1978.

———. *On Semen.* Corpus Medicorum Graecorum 5.3.1. Berlin: Akademie Verlag, 1992.

Grant, Mark, trans. *Galen on Food and Diet.* London: Routledge, 2000. (See also Helmreich's edition below.)

Green, Robert Montraville, trans. *A Translation of Galen's "Hygiene" (De sanitate tuenda).* Introduction by Henry E. Sigerist. Springfield, IL: Thomas 1951. (See also Koch's edition below.)

Helmreich, Georg, ed. *De alimentorum facultatibus.* Corpus Medicorum Graecorum 5.4.2. Leipzig: Teubner, 1923. (See also Grant's translation above.)

———. *De bonis malisque sucis.* Corpus Medicorum Graecorum 5.4.2. Leipzig: Teubner, 1923.

———. *In Hippocratis de victu acutorum commentaria quattuor.* Corpus Medicorum Graecorum 5.9.1. Leipzig: Teubner, 1914.

———. *De usu partium corporis humani.* 2 vols. Bibliotheca Scriptorum Graecorum et Romanorum Teubneriana. Leipzig: Teubner, 1907–9. Reprint, Amsterdam: Adolf M. Hakkert, 1968. (See also May's translation below.)

Iskandar, Albert Z., ed. and trans. *On Examinations by Which the Best Physicians Are Recognized* [*De optimo medico cognoscendo*]. Corpus Medicorum Graecorum, Supplementum Orientale 4. Berlin: Akademie-Verlag, 1988.

Johnston, Ian, and G. H. R. Horsley, eds. and trans. *Method of Medicine.* 3 vols., 14 bks. Harvard: Loeb Classical Library, 2011.

Kalbfleisch, Karl, ed. *De victu attenuante.* Corpus Medicorum Graecorum 5.4.2. Leipzig: Teubner, 1923.

Keil, Winfried, ed. and trans. "De puero epileptico consilium: Galeni Puero epileptico consilium." PhD diss., University of Göttingen, 1959.

Klein-Franke, Felix, ed. and trans. "The Arabic Version of Galen's Περὶ ἐθῶν." *Jerusalem Studies in Arabic and Islam* 1 (1979): 125–50. (See also Schmutte's edition with Pfaff's translation below.)

Koch, Konrad, ed. *De sanitate tuenda.* Corpus Medicorum Graecorum 5.4.2. Leipzig: Teubner, 1923. (See also Green's translation above.)

Kühn, Karl Gottlob, ed. *Claudii Galeni opera omnia.* 20 vols. 1821–33. Reprint, Hildesheim, Germany: Georg Olms, 1964–65.

Larrain, Carlos J., ed. and trans. *Galens Kommentar zu Platons Timaios.* Stuttgart: Teubner, 1992.

May, Margaret Tallmadge, trans. *Galen on the Usefulness of the Parts of the Body.* 2 vols. Ithaca, NY: Cornell University Press, 1968. (See also Helmreich's edition above.)

Mewaldt, Johannes, ed. *In Hippocratis De natura hominis commentaria tria.* Corpus Medicorum Graecorum 5.9.1. Leipzig: Teubner, 1914.

Meyerhof, Max, and Joseph Schacht, eds. and trans. *Galen über die medizinischen Namen.* Arabisch und deutsch herausgegeben. Berlin: Akademie der Wissenschaften, 1931.

Nutton, Vivian, ed. and trans. *On My Own Opinions.* CMG 5.3.2. Berlin: Akademie Verlag, 1999.

Nutton, Vivian, and Gerrit Bos, eds. *On Problematic Movements.* Cambridge: Cambridge University Press, 2011.

Richter-Bernburg, Lutz, trans. "Eine arabische Version der pseudogalenischen Schrift *De Theriaca ad Pisonem.*" PhD diss., University of Göttingen, 1969.

Savage-Smith, Emilie, ed. and trans. "Galen on Nerves, Veins and Arteries." PhD diss., University of Wisconson, 1969.

Schmutte, Joseph M., ed. *Galeni de consuetudinibus.* With a German translation of Ḥunayn's Arabic version by Franz Pfaff. Corpus Medicorum Graecorum, Supplement 3. Leipzig: Teubner, 1941. (See also Klein-Franke's edition and translation above.)

Schröder, Heinrich Otto, ed. *In Platonis Timaeum commentarii fragmenta.* Corpus Medicorum Graecorum, Supplement 1, Leipzig: Teubner, 1934.

Siegel, Rudolph E., trans. *Galen on the Affected Parts: Translation from the Greek Text with Explanatory Notes.* New York: Karger, 1976.

Singer, Peter N., trans. *Galen: Selected Works.* New York: Oxford University Press, 1997.

Wasserstein, Abraham, ed. and trans. *Galen's Commentary on the Hippocratic Treatise "Airs, Waters, Places": In the Hebrew Translation of Solomon ha-Meʾati.* Jerusalem: Israel Academy of Sciences and Humanities, 1983.

Wenkebach, Ernst, and Franz Pfaff, eds. *Galeni in Hippocratis Epidemiarum librum 1–3 commentaria* 5. *In Hippocratis Epidemiarum commentaria* 1–8, *Indices.* Corpus Medicorum Graecorum 5.10.1, 5.10.2.1; 5.10.2.2, 5.10.2.4. Leipzig and Berlin: Teubner-Akademie Verlag, 1934–56.

Wernhard, Matthias, ed. and trans. "Galen. Über die Arten der Fieber in der arabischen Version des Ḥunain ibn Isḥāq." PhD diss., Munich, 2004.

## General Bibliography

Adret, Solomon ben Abraham. *Iggerot ʿim Iggeret ha-Bedershi.* Edited by Samson Bloch ha-Levi. Lemberg: Uri Zevi Rubinstein, 1809.

Alexander of Aphrodisias. *The Refutation by Alexander of Aphrodisias of Galen's "Treatise on the Theory of Motion."* Edited by Nicholas Rescher and Michael E. Marmura. Islamabad: Islamic Research Institute, 1965.

Álvarez Millán, Cristina. "Actualización del corpus médico-literario de los Banū Zuhr: Nota bibliográfica." *Al-Qanṭara: Revista de estudios árabes* 16, no.1 (1995): 173–80.

Anastassiou, Anargyros, and Dieter Irmer, eds. *Hippokrateszitate in den übrigen Werken Galens einschließlich der alten Pseudo-Galenica*. Pt. 2, vol. 2 of *Testimonien zum Corpus Hippocraticum*. Göttingen: Vandenhoeck & Ruprecht, 2001.

Aristotle. *Aristotle's "De anima." Translated into Hebrew by Zeraḥyah ben Isaac ben She'altiel Ḥen*. Edited with an introduction and index by Gerrit Bos. Leiden: Brill, 1994.

———. *Generation of Animals. The Arabic Translation commonly ascribed to Yaḥyā ibn al-Biṭrīq*. Edited with an introduction and glossary by Jan Brugman and Hendrik J. Drossaart Lulofs. Leiden: Brill, 1971.

Aubaile-Sallenave, Françoise. "*Al-Kishk*: The Past and Present of a Complex Culinary Practice." In *Culinary Cultures of the Middle East*, edited by Sami Zubaida and Richard Tapper, 105–39. London: Tauris, 1994.

Averroës. "Averroes 'contra Galenum': Das Kapitel von der Atmung im Colliget des Averroes als ein Zeugnis mittelalterlich-islamischer Kritik an Galen." Edited and translated by J. Christoph Bürgel. *Nachrichten der Akademie der Wissenschaften in Göttingen: Philologisch-Historische Klasse* 9 (1967): 263–340.

Baron, Salo Wittmayer. *A Social and Religious History of the Jews*. 18 vols. 2nd ed. New York: Columbia University Press, 1952–83.

Beit-Arié, Malachi, comp., and R. A. May, ed. *Catalogue of the Hebrew Manuscripts in the Bodleian Library: Supplement of Addenda and Corrigenda to Vol. 1 (A. Neubauer's Catalogue)*. Oxford: Clarendon, 1994. (See also Neubauer's catalogue below.)

Blau, Joshua. *The Emergence and Linguistic Background of Judaeo-Arabic: A Study of the Origins of Middle Arabic*. London: Oxford University Press, 1965. Reprint, Jerusalem: Ben Zvi Institute for the Study of Jewish Communities in the East, 1981.

Bos, Gerrit. "Maimonides' Medical Aphorisms: Towards a Critical Edition and Revised English Translation." *Ḳorot* 12 (1996–97): 35–79.

———. "Maimonides' Medical Works and Their Contributions to His Medical Biography." *Maimonidean Studies* 5 (2008): 243–66.

———. "Maimonides on the Preservation of Health," *Journal of the Royal Asiatic Society. Third Series* 4, no. 2 (1994): 213–35.

———. *Novel Medical and General Hebrew Terminology*. 3 vols. *Journal of Semitic Studies*, Suppl. 27, 30, 37. Oxford: Oxford University Press, 2011–2016.

———. "R. Moshe Narboni, Philosopher and Physician: A Critical Analysis of Sefer Oraḥ Ḥayyim." *Medieval Encounters* 1 (1995): 219–51.

Bos, Gerrit, Martina Hussein, Guido Mensching, and Frank Savelsberg. *Medical Synonym Lists from Medieval Provence: Shem Tov ben Isaac of Tortosa: Sefer ha-Shimmush, Book 28. Part 1: Edition and Commentary of List 1 (Hebrew-Arabic-Romance/Latin)*. Leiden: Brill, 2011.

Bos, Gerrit, and Resianne Fontaine. "Medico-philosophical Controversies in Nathan b. Yo'el Falaquera's *Sefer Ṣori ha-Guf*," *Jewish Quarterly Review* 90, no. 1–2 (1999): 27–60.

Bouros-Vallianatos, Petros. "Galen's Reception in Byzantium: Symeon Seth and his Refutation of Galenic Theories on Human Physiology," *Greek, Roman, and Byzantium Studies* 55 (2015): 431–69.

Brain, Peter. *Galen on Bloodletting: A Study of the Origins, Development and Validity of His Opinions, with a Translation of the Three Works*. Cambridge: Cambridge University Press, 1986.

Brockelman, Carl. *Lexicon Syriacum*. Hildesheim, Germany: Olms, 1966.

Cano Ledesma, Aurora. *Indización de los manuscritos árabes de El Escorial*. Madrid: Ediciones Escurialenses, Real Monasterio de El Escorial, 1996.

Chauliac, Guy de. *Inventarium sive Chirurgia Magna*. 2 vols. Vol 1: *Text*. Edited by Michael R. McVaugh. Vol.2: *Commentary*. Prepared by Michael R. McVaugh and Margaret S. Ogden. Leiden: Brill, 1997.

Colin, Gabriel. *Avenzoar: Sa vie et ses oeuvres*. Paris: Leroux, 1911.

De Lacy, Phillip. "Galen's Concept of Continuity." *Greek, Roman and Byzantine Studies* 20, no. 1 (1979): 355–69.

De Rossi, Azariah. *The Light of the Eyes by Azariah de' Rossi*. Translated with an introduction by Joanna Weinberg. New Haven, CT: Yale University Press, 2001.

———. *Sefer Meʾor Enayim*. Edited by David Cassel. Vilna: Romm, 1866.

Dols, Michael W. *Majnūn: The Madman in Medieval Islamic Society*. Edited by Diana E. Immisch. Oxford: Clarendon, 1992.

Deichgräber, Karl. *Hippokrates' De humoribus in der Geschichte der griechischen Medizin*. Mainz: Verlag der Akademie der Wissenschaften und der Literatur, 1972.

Derenbourg, Hartwig, comp., and Henri Paul Joseph Renaud, ed. *Médecine et histoire naturelle*. Vol. 2, fasc. 2 of *Les manuscrits arabes de l'Escurial*. Paris: LeRoux, 1939.

Dietrich, Albert. *Medicinalia Arabica. Studien über arabische medizinische Handschriften in türkischen und syrischen Bibliotheken*. Göttingen: Vandenhoeck & Ruprecht, 1966.

Dioscurides. *Dioscurides triumphans: Ein anonymer arabischer Kommentar (Ende 12. Jahrh. n. Chr.) zur Materia medica*. Edited and translated by Albert Dietrich. 2 vols. Göttingen: Vandenhoeck & Ruprecht, 1988.

———. *Pedanii Dioscuridis Anazarbei De materia medica, libri quinque*. Edited by Max Wellmann. 3 vols, 5 bks. 1906–14. Reprint, 1 vol., Berlin: Weidmann, 1958.

Dols, Michael W. *Majnūn: The Madman in Medieval Islamic Society*. Edited by Diana E. Immisch. Oxford: Clarendon, 1992.

Dozy, Reinhart Pieter Anne. *Supplément aux dictionnaires arabes*. 2nd ed. 2 vols. Leiden: Brill, 1927.

Dunlop, D. M. "The Translations of al-Biṭrīq and Yaḥyā (Yuḥannā) b. al-Biṭrīq." *The Journal of the Royal Asiatic Society of Great Britain and Ireland* 3–4 (1959): 140–50.

Durling, Richard J. "Excreta as a Remedy in Galen, his Predecessors and his Successors." In *Tradition et traduction. Les textes philosophiques et scientifiques grecs au Moyen Âge latin. Hommage à Fernand Bossier*, edited by Rita Beyers, Jozef Brams, Dirk Sacré, and Koenraad Verrycken, 25–35. Leuven: Leuven University Press, 1999.

Eco, Umberto. *The Search for the Perfect Language*. Translated by James Fentress. London: Fontana Press, 1997.

*Encyclopaedia of Islam*, new edition. 12 vols. Leiden: Brill, 1960–94.

Endress, Gerhard. "Die arabischen Übersetzungen von Aristoteles' Schrift *De Caelo*." PhD diss., Johann Wolfgang Goethe-Universität, Frankfurt am Main, 1966.

Fārābī, Abū Naṣr al-. *Al-Farabi's Commentary and Short Treatise on Aristotle's "De Interpretatione."* Translated with an introduction and notes by Friedrich W. Zimmermann. Oxford: Oxford University Press, 1981.

———. *Alfarabi's Book of Letters (Kitāb al-ḥurūf). Commentary on Aristotle's Metaphysics.* Edited with an introduction and notes by Muhsin Mahdi. Beirut: Dar El-Mashreq, 1969.

French, Roger. *Ancient Natural History: Histories of Nature.* London: Routledge, 1994.

Freudenthal, Gad. "Maimonides' Philosophy of Science." In *The Cambridge Companion to Maimonides*, edited by Kenneth Seeskin, 134–66. New York: Cambridge University Press, 2005.

———. "Maimonides' Stance on Astrology in Context." In *Moses Maimonides. Physician, Scientist, and Philosopher,* edited by Fred Rosner and Samuel S. Kottek, 77–90. Northvale, NJ: Jason Aronson, 1993.

———. "Les sciences dans les communautés juives médiévales de Provence: Leur appropriation, leur rôle." *Revue des études juives* 152, no. 1–2 (1993): 29–136.

Freytag, Georg Wilhelm. *Lexicon Arabico-Latinum. Praesertim ex Djeuharii Firuzabadique et Aliorum Arabum Operibus Adhibitis Golii Quoque et Aliorum Libris Confectum. Accedit Index Vocum Latinarum Locupletissimus.* 4 vols. Halle, Germany: C. A. Schwetschke and Son, 1830–37.

Friedenwald, Harry. *The Jews and Medicine: Essays.* 2 vols. 1944. Reprint, New York: Ktav, 1967.

Friedländer, Israel. *Arabisch-deutsches Lexikon zum Sprachgebrauch des Maimonides: Ein Nachtrag zu den arabischen Lexicis.* Frankfurt am Main: J. Kauffmann, 1902.

Gätje, Helmut. "Die 'inneren Sinne' bei Averroes," *Zeitschrift der Deutschen Morgenländischen Gesellschaft* 115 (1965): 255–93.

Gersonides. *The Wars of the Lord* [Sefer Milḥamot ha-Shem]. Translated by Seymour Feldman. 3 vols. Philadelphia: The Jewish Publication Society, 1987.

Ghāfiqī, Aḥmad ibn Muḥammad al-. *The Abridged Version of "The Book of Simple Drugs" of Aḥmad ibn Muḥammad al-Ghāfiqī by Gregorius Abuʾl-Farag (Barhebraeus).* Edited and translated by Max Meyerhof and G. P. Sobhy. Cairo: The Egyptian University, 1932.

Grmek, Mirko D. *Diseases in the Ancient Greek World.* Translated by Mireille and Leonard Muellner. Baltimore: Johns Hopkins University Press, 1989.

Hinz, Walther. *Islamische Maße und Gewichte: Umgerechnet ins metrische System.* 1955. Photomechanical reprint, Leiden: Brill, 1970.

Hippocrates. *Humours.* In *Hippocrates.* Vol. 4: *Heracleitus on the Universe.* Edited and translated by W. H. S. Jones, 61–95. Loeb Classical Library. Cambridge, MA: Harvard University Press 1931.

———. *Œuvres complètes d'Hippocrate.* Edited and translated by É. Littré. 10 vols. 1839–61. Reprint, Amsterdam: Hakkert, 1973–82.

Hopkins, Simon. *The Languages of Maimonides.* In *The Trias of Maimonides/Die Trias des Maimonides*, edited by Georges Tamer, 85–106. Berlin: de Gruyter, 2005.

Ibn Abī Uṣaybiᶜah. *ᶜUyūn al-anbāʾ fī ṭabaqāt al-aṭibbāʾ*. Edited by Nizār Riḍā. Beirut: Dār Maktabat al-Ḥayah, 1965.

Ibn al-ᶜAbbās al-Mājūsī, ᶜAlī. "Livre royal (*al-malaki*) par ᶜAlī ibn al-ᶜAbbās. Texte et traduction. Deuxième section de la première partie." Edited and translated by Pieter de Koning. In *Trois traités d'anatomie d'arabes par Muḥammed ibn Zakkariyyā al-Rāzī, ᶜAlī ibn al-ᶜAbbās et ᶜAlī ibn Sīnā*, edited by Pieter de Koning, 90–431. Leiden: Brill, 1903.

Ibn al-Bayṭār, ᶜAbd Allāh ibn Aḥmad. *Al-Jāmiᶜ li-mufradāt al-adwiya wa-l-aghdhiya*. 4 pts. in 2 vols. Beirut: Dār al-Kutub al-ᶜIlmīyah, 1992.

———. *Traité des simples par Ibn el-Beïthâr*. Translated by Lucien Leclerc. 3 vols. 1877–83. Reprint, Paris: Institut du monde arabe, 1987.

Ibn al-Jazzār. *Ibn al-Jazzār on Sexual Diseases and Their Treatment: A Critical Edition of "Zād al-musāfir wa-qūt al-ḥāḍir" (Provision for the Traveller and the Nourishment of the Sedentary), Book 6*. Edited and translated by Gerrit Bos. New York: Kegan Paul International, 1997.

Ibn al-Tilmīḏ. *The Dispensatory of Ibn at-Tilmīdh*. Edited and translated by Oliver Kahl. Leiden: Brill, 2007.

Ibn Ezra, Abraham. *Sefer Hanisyonot: The Book of Medical Experiences attributed to Abraham ibn Ezra*. Edited, translated, and commented on by Joshua O. Leibowitz and Shlomo Marcus. Jerusalem: Magnes Press, 1984.

Ibn Ezra, Moses. *Kitāb al-muḥāḍara wa-al-mudhākara. Liber Discussionis et Commemorationis* (Poetica Hebraica). Edited with Hebrew translation by Abraham S. Halkin. Jerusalem: Mekize Nirdamim, 1975.

Ibn Falaquera, Shem Tov ben Joseph. *Moreh ha-moreh*. Edited by Yair Shiffman. Jerusalem: World Union of Jewish Studies, 2001.

Ibn Janāḥ, Abū al-Walīd Marwān. *Kitāb al-Talkhīṣ*. Edited by Gerrit Bos, Fabian Käs, Guido Mensching, and Maylin Lübke. Forthcoming.

Ibn Isḥāq, Ḥunayn. *Ḥunain ibn Isḥāq über die syrischen und arabischen Galen-Übersetzungen: Zum ersten Mal herausgegeben und übersetzt*. Edited by Gotthelf Bergsträsser. Leipzig: Brockhaus, 1925.

Ibn Lūqā, Qusṭā. *Qusṭā ibn Lūqā's Medical Regime for the Pilgrims to Mecca: The Risāla fī tadbīr safar al-ḥajj*. Edited and translated by Gerrit Bos. Leiden: Brill, 1992.

Ibn Sahl, Sābūr. *Dispensatorium parvum (al-Aqrābādhīn al-ṣaghīr)*. Edited by Oliver Kahl. Leiden: Brill, 1994.

Ibn Sayyār al-Warrāq. *Annals of the Caliphs' Kitchens. Ibn Sayyār al-Warrāq's Tenth-Century Baghdadi Cookbook*. Translated with an introduction and glossary by Nawal Nasrallah. Leiden: Brill, 2007.

Ibn Wāfid. *Kitāb al-adwiya al-mufrada (Libro de los Medicamentos Simples)*. Edited and translated by Luisa Fernanda Aguirre de Cárcer. 2 vols. Madrid: Consejo Superior de Investigaciones Científicas, Agencia Española de Cooperación Internacional, 1995.

Ibn Zuhr, Abū l-ᶜAlāʾ. *La Teḏkira d'Abū al-ᶜAlāʾ*. Edited and translated by Gabriel Colin. Paris: Ernest Leroux, 1911.

Ibn Zuhr, Abū Marwān ᶜAbd al-Malik. *Kitāb al-aghdhiya (Tratado de los Alimentos)*. Edited and translated by Expiración García Sánchez. Fuentes Arábico-

Hispanas 4. Madrid: Consejo Superior de Investigaciones Científicas, Instituto de Cooperación con el Mundo Árabe, 1992.

———. *Kitāb al-taysīr fī al-mudawāt wa-al-tadbīr.* Edited by Muḥammad al-Khouri. Damascus: Dār al-Fikr, 1983.

Idel, Moshe. *Language, Torah, and Hermeneutics in Abraham Abulafia.* Translated from the Hebrew by Menahem Kallus. Albany, NY: State University of New York Press, 1989.

Isrā'īlī, Isḥāq Ibn Sulaymān al-. *Kitāb al-aghdhiya wa-al-adwiya.* Edited by Muḥammad al-Ṣabbāḥ. Beirut: Mu'assasat ʿIzz-al-Dīn, 1992.

Kahle, Paul. "Mosis Maimonidis Aphorismorum praefatio et excerpta." In *Galeni in Platonis Timaeum commentarii fragmenta*, edited by Heinrich Otto Schröder, Appendix 2. Corpus Medicorum Graecorum, Supplement 1, 89–99. Leipzig: Teubner, 1934.

Kaufmann, David. "Le neveu de Maïmonide." *Revue des études juives* 7 (1883): 152–53.

———. *Die Sinne. Beiträge zur Geschichte der Physiologie und Psychologie im Mittelalter aus hebräischen und arabischen Quellen.* Leipzig: Brockhaus, 1884.

Keyser, Paul T. "Science and Magic in Galen's Recipes (Sympathy and Efficacy)." In *Galen on Pharmacology, Philosophy, History, and Medicine. Proceedings of the Vth International Galen Colloquium, Lille, 16–18 March 1995,* edited by Armelle Debru, 175–98. Leiden: Brill, 1997.

Kraemer, Joel L. "Maimonides on the Philosophic Sciences in his Treatise on the Art of Logic." In *Perspectives on Maimonides: Philosophical and Historical Studies,* edited by Joel L. Kraemer, 77–104. Littman Library. Oxford: Oxford University Press, 1991.

———. "Six Unpublished Maimonides Letters from the Cairo Genizah." *Maimonidean Studies* 2, no. 1 (1991): 61–94.

Kranzler, Harvey N. "Maimonides' Concept of Mental Illness and Mental Health." In *Moses Maimonides. Physician, Scientist, and Philosopher,* edited by Fred Rosner and Samuel S. Kottek, 49–57. Northvale, NJ: Jason Aronson, 1993.

Krochmal, Nachman. *Moreh Nevukhei ha-Zeman.* Kitvei RaNaQ. Nachman Krochmals Werke. Edited by Simon Rawidowicz, based on Leopold Zunz's edition, Lemberg 1852. Berlin: Ajanoth, 1924.

Kudlien, Fridolf. "Galen's Religious Belief." In *Galen: Problems and Prospects. A Collection of Papers submitted at the 1979 Cambridge Conference,* edited by Vivian Nutton, 117–30. London: The Wellcome Institute for the History of Medicine, 1981.

Kuhne Brabant, Rosa. "Abū Marwān b. Zuhr: Un professionel de la médecine en plein XIIème siècle." In *Actes du VII Colloque universitaire tuniso-espagnol sur le patrimoine andalous dans la culture arabe et espagnole, Tunis, 3–10 février 1989*, 129–41. Tunis: Université de Tunis, CERES, 1991.

Lameer, Joep. *Al-Farabi and Aristotelian Syllogistics: Greek Theory and Islamic Practice.* Leiden: Brill, 1994.

Lane, Edward William. *Arabic-English Lexicon.* 8 vols. London: Williams and Norgate, 1863–93.

Langermann, Y. Tzvi. "Arabic Writings in Hebrew Manuscripts: A Preliminary Listing." *Arabic Sciences and Philosophy* 6, no. 1 (1996): 137–60.

———. "Gersonides on the Magnet and the Heat of the Sun." In *Studies on Gersonides: A Fourteenth-Century Jewish Philosopher-Scientist,* edited by Gad Freudenthal, 267–84. Leiden: Brill, 1992.

———. "Maimonides on the Synochous Fever." *Israel Oriental Studies* 13 (1993): 175–98.

———. "Perusho shel Shelomo ibn Yaᶜish le-Qanun shel Ibn Sina." *Kiryat Sefer* 63 (1990–91):1331–33.

Levinger, Jacob. "Maimonides' Guide of the Perplexed on Forbidden Food in the Light of His Own Medical Opinion." In *Perspectives on Maimonides: Philosophical and Historical Studies,* edited by Joel L. Kraemer, 195–208. Littman Library. Oxford: Oxford University Press, 1991.

Liddell, H. G., and R. Scott. *A Greek-English Lexicon.* Revised by H. S. Jones, with a Supplement, 1968. Reprint, Oxford: Clarendon Press, 1989.

Lieber, Elinor. "Maimonides, the Medical Humanist." *Maimonidean Studies* 4 (2000): 39–60.

Marx, Alexander, ed. "Texts by and about Maimonides." *Jewish Quarterly Review* 25 (1934): 321–428.

Meyerhof, Max. "The Medical Work of Maimonides." In *Essays on Maimonides: An Octocentennial Volume,* edited by Salo Wittmayer Baron, 265–99. New York: Columbia University Press, 1941.

Meyerhof, Max. "Über echte und unechte Schriften Galens, nach arabischen Quellen." *Sitzungsberichte der Preußischen Akademie der Wissenschaften zu Berlin: Philosophisch-historischen Classe* 28 (1928): 533–48.

Narboni, Moses. *Sefer Oraḥ Ḥayyim.* MS Munich 276, fols. 1–141.

Neubauer, Adolf. *Catalogue of the Hebrew Manuscripts in the Bodleian Library and in the College Libraries of Oxford.* 2 vols. 1886–1906. Reprint, Oxford: Clarendon, 1994. (See also Beit-Arié's supplement above.)

Nutton, Vivian. "Galen on Theriac: Problems of Authenticity." In *Galen on Pharmacology: Philosophy, History and Medicine. Proceedings of the Vth International Galen Colloquium, Lille, 16–18 March 1995* , edited by Armelle Debru, 133–51. Leiden: Brill, 1997.

Oberhelman, Steven M. "Dreams in Graeco-Roman Medicine." In *Aufstieg und Niedergang der römischen Welt.* Part 2, 37.1. Edited by Hildegard Temporini and Wolfgang Haase, 121–56. Berlin: De Gruyter, 1993.

Perry, Charles, trans. *Kitāb al-Ṭibākha: A Fifteenth-Century Cookbook.* In *Medieval Arab Cookery: Essays and Translations,* by Maxime Rodinson, A. J. Arberry, and Charles Perry, 467–75. Blackawton, Totnes, Devon, England: Prospect, 2001.

Pertsch, Wilhelm. *Die arabischen Handschriften der herzoglichen Bibliothek zu Gotha.* 5 vols. Gotha, Germany: Perthes, 1877–92.

Pines, Shlomo. "Rāzī critique de Galien." In *The Collected Works of Shlomo Pines.* Vol. 2: *Studies in Arabic Versions of Greek Texts and in Mediaeval Science,* 256–63. Jerusalem: Magnes Press, 1986.

Ravitzky, Aviezer. "Mishnato shel Rabi Zeraḥyah ben Yitshak ben Sheᶜaltiᵓel Ḥen veha-hagut ha-maimonit-tibonit ba-meᵓah ha-13." PhD diss., Hebrew University, 1977.

Rāzī, Abū Bakr Muḥammad ibn Zakarīyā' al-. *Kitāb al-Ḥāwī fī al-ṭibb*. Vols. 1–23. Hyderabad, India: Da'iratu al-Ma'arifī al-Osmania (Osmania Oriental Publications Bureau), Osmania University, 1952–74.

———. *Kitāb al-shukūk ʿalā Jālīnūs*. Edited by Mehdi Mohaghegh. Tehran: Institute of Islamic Studies, Tehran University, 1993.

Richter, Paul. "Über die allgemeine Dermatologie des ʿAlī ibn al-ʿAbbās (Haly Abbas) aus dem 10. Jahrhundert unserer Zeitrechnung." *Archiv für Dermatologie und Syphilis* 118, no. 1 (1913): 199–208. Reprinted in *Beiträge zur Geschichte der arabisch-Islamischen Medizin. Aufsätze*. Vol. 3: *Aus den Jahren 1909–1913*. Edited by Fuat Sezgin. Frankfurt am Main: Institut für Geschichte der Arabisch-Islamischen Wissenschaften an der Johann Wolfgang Goethe-Universität, 1987.

Ritter, Hellmut, and Richard Walzer, "Arabische Übersetzungen griechischer Ärzte in Stambuler Bibliotheken." *Sitzungsberichte der preussischen Akademie der Wissenschaften. Philosophisch-historische Klasse, Berlin* (1934): 801–18.

Schacht, Joseph, and Max Meyerhof. "Maimonides against Galen, on Philosophy and Cosmogony." *Bulletin of the Faculty of Arts of the University of Egypt* 5, no. 1 (1937): 53–88 (Arabic Section).

Schmucker, Werner. *Die pflanzliche und mineralische Materia medica im "Firdaus al-Ḥikma" des ʿAlī ibn Sahl Rabban aṭ-Ṭabarī*. Bonn: Selbstverlag des Orientalischen Seminars der Universität Bonn, 1969.

Schönfeld, Jutta. *"Über die Steine": Das 14. Kapitel aus dem "Kitāb al-Muršid" des Muḥammad ibn Aḥmad al-Tamīmī, nach dem Pariser Manuskript*. Freiburg: Klaus Schwarz Verlag, 1976.

Schwartz, Dov. "Magiyah, madda' nisyoni u-metodah madda'it be-mishnat ha-RaMBaM: Gishah u-parshanutah bime ha-benaim" ["Magic, experimental science and scientific method in Maimonides' teachings). In *Me-Romi l-Yirushalaim: Sefer Zikkaron le-Yoseph-Barukh Sermoneta (Joseph Baruch Sermoneta Memorial Volume)*, edited by Aviezer Ravitzky, 25–45. Jerusalem: The Hebrew University, 1998.

Sezgin, Fuat. *Geschichte des arabischen Schrifttums*. Vol. 3: *Medizin-Pharmazie-Zoologie-Tierheilkunde bis ca. 430 H.* Leiden: Brill, 1970.

Sirat, Colette. "Une liste de manuscrits: Préliminaire à une nouvelle édition du *Dalālat al-Hāyryn*." *Maimonidean Studies* 4 (2000): 109–33.

Steingass, F. *A Comprehensive Persian-English Dictionary*. 1963. Reprint, London: Routledge and Kegan Paul, 1984.

Steinschneider, Moritz. *Al-Farabi (Alpharabius), des arabischen Philosophen Leben und Schriften, mit besonderer Rücksicht auf die Geschichte der griechischen Wissenschaft unter den Arabern*. St. Petersburg: Kaiserliche Akademie der Wissenschaften, 1869.

———. *Die arabischen Übersetzungen aus dem Griechischen*. 1889–96. Reprint, Graz, Austria: Akademische Druck- und Verlagsanstalt, 1960.

———. "Die griechischen Ärzte in arabischen Übersetzungen." *Virchows Archiv* 124 (1891): 115–36, 268–96, 455–87.

———. *Die hebräischen Handschriften der K. Hof- und Staatsbibliothek in München*. 2nd ed. Munich: Commission der Palm'schen Hofbuchhandlung, 1895.

———. *Die hebräischen Übersetzungen des Mittelalters und die Juden als Dolmetscher*. 1893. Reprint, Graz, Austria: Akademische Druck- und Verlagsanstalt, 1956.

Strohmaier, G. "Der syrische und der arabische Galen." In *Aufstieg und Niedergang der römischen Welt*. Part 2, 37.2. Edited by Hildegard Temporini and Wolfgang Haase, 1987–2017. Berlin: de Gruyter, 1994.

Stroumsa, Sarah. "Al-Fārābī and Maimonides on Medicine as a Science." *Arabic Sciences and Philosophy* 3, no. 2 (1993): 235–49.

Temkin, Owsei. *The Falling Sickness. A History of Epilepsy from the Greeks to the Beginnings of Modern Neurology*. Baltimore: Johns Hopkins University Press, 1945.

———. *Galenism: Rise and Decline of a Medical Philosophy*. Ithaca, NY: Cornell University Press, 1973.

Thies, Hans-Jürgen. *Erkrankungen des Gehirns insbesondere Kopfschmerzen in der arabischen Medizin*. Beiträge zur Sprach- und Kulturgeschichte des Orients 19. Walldorf, Hessen, Germany: Verlag für Orientkunde, 1968.

Ullman, Manfred. *Islamic Medicine*. Translated by Jean Watt. Edinburgh: Edinburgh University Press, 1978.

———. *Die Medizin im Islam*. Leiden: Brill, 1970.

———. *Wörterbuch zu den griechisch-arabischen Übersetzungen des 9. Jahrhunderts*. Wiesbaden: Harrassowitz, 2002.

———. "Zwei spätantike Kommentare zu der hippokratischen Schrift 'De morbis muliebribus.'" *Medizinhistorisches Journal* 12 (1977): 245–62.

Vajda, Georges. *Index général des manuscrits arabes musulmans de la Bibliothèque nationale de Paris*. Paris: Éditions du Centre national de la recherche scientifique, 1953.

Vogelstein, Hermann, and Paul Rieger. *Geschichte der Juden in Rom*. 2 vols. Berlin: Mayer und Müller, 1895–96.

von Krzowitz, Wenzel Trnka. *Historia ophtalmiae omnis aevi observata medica continens*. Vienna: Graeffer, 1783.

Voorhoeve, Petrus, comp. *Handlist of Arabic Manuscripts in the Library of the University of Leiden and Other Collections in the Netherlands*. 2nd ed. The Hague: Leiden University Press, 1980.

Vullers, Johann August. *Lexicon persico-latinum etymologicum*. 2 vols. 1855–64. Reprint, Graz, Austria: Akademische Druck-und Verlagsanstalt, 1962.

Waines, David. "*Murrī*: The Tale of a Condiment." *Al-Qanṭara* 12, no. 2 (1991): 371–88.

Walzer, Richard. *Galen on Jews and Christians*. Oxford: Oxford University Press, 1949.

*Wörterbuch der klassischen arabischen Sprache*. Edited by Deutsche Morgenländische Gesellschaft et al. Wiesbaden: Harrassowitz, 1957–.

Zimmermann, Friedrich W. "Al-Farabi und die philosophische Kritik an Galen von Alexander zu Averroes." In *Akten des VII. Kongresses für Arabistik und Islamwissenschaft, Göttingen, 15. bis 22. August 1974* , edited by Albert Dietrich, 401-414. Göttingen: Vandenhoeck & Ruprecht, 1976.

Zonta, Mauro. "A Hebrew Translation of Hippocrates' *De superfoetatione:* Historical Introduction and Critical Introduction." *Aleph: Historical Studies in Science and Judaism* 3 (2003): 97–143.

Zotenberg, Hermann, ed. *Manuscrits orientaux: Catalogues des manuscrits hébreux et samaritains de la Bibliothèque impériale*. Paris: Imprimerie impériale, 1866.

Zwiep, Irene E. *Mother of Reason and Revelation: A Short History of Medieval Jewish Linguistic Thought*. Amsterdam Studies in Jewish Thought 5. Amsterdam: Gieben, 1997.

# Subject Index to the English Translation

on heart as only major organ, 25.70
syllogisms of, 25.60
armpits, 23.56
arms, 25.11, 25.53, 232n40
arsenic, 23.101
arthritis, 23.14, 25.45
artichoke, 22.56
arum, root of, 22.62
asafetida, 22.19
ascites, 23.50
ashes, 22.29, 23.109, 25.24, 25.62, 25.64
ass, wild, 22.37, 238n24
asthma, 22.30, 23.78, 23.79, 24.38
Athens, 24.22, 24.29
Avenzoar. *See* Abū Marwān ibn Zuhr

back, 22.26, 22.41, 25.72
balsam of Mecca, 22.52
barbarians, 24.56
barley, 23.33, 23.100, 228n238, 238n26
basil, sweet, 25.14
bat, brain of, 22.4
bean, broad, 22.54, 23.3, 23.100
bear, 24.28
bed-wetting, 22.59
beef, 22.58
belly, 22.9, 24.57
bile, 23.10, 221n120
black, 22.66, 23.46, 23.48, 23.63, 24.46, 25.39, 25.40, 25.48
green, 23.48, 25.35
of bull, 23.99
red, 23.10
thin, 24.37
yellow, 22.52, 22.58, 23.2, 23.10, 23.41, 25.12, 25.35, 25.40
Biṭrīq, al-, xxv, 24.44, 235n79, 236n95
bitter vetch, 23.33, 23.100
bladder, urinary
Galen's description of, 25.32, 244n110
illness of, 23.94
injury to, 235n82
neck of, 24.54
remedies for ailments of, 22.10, 22.51
stones, 22.10, 22.69
bleeding, 23.8, 24.22, 24.24, 24.37, 25.53, 25.72. *See also* bloodletting
blister, 23.38, 223n162
blood, 25.51, 25.53, 25.55, 25.64, 220n117, 239n35

# Addenda and Corrigenda to *Medical Aphorisms*, Volumes 1–4

## Medical Aphorisms: Treatises 1–5

***Arabic text:***

1.31 (p. 14, line 14): تعيا. Read: تعبا

1.66 (p. 23, line 11): مرئ. Read مريء

***English translation:***

3.15 (p. 37, line 11); 3.20 (p. 38, line 6); 3.30 (p. 40, lines 19–20): "main organs" (Ar. الأعضاء الأصلية). Read "elementary parts" (i.e., the homogeneous [homoeomerous] parts, such as arteries, veins, nerves, bones, cartilages, membranes, ligaments, and the various coats)

3.72 (p. 51, lines 25–26): "(namely, the other things which change its temperament)" Read: "(namely, the other things which change its temperament or dissolve its continuity)"

## Medical Aphorisms: Treatises 6–9

***Arabic text:***

6.10 (p. 3, line 11): يعتد به. Read: يعتدّ به

6.13 (p. 4, line 5): الرمص. Read: الرمض

7.63 (p. 39, line 10): أربغة. Read: أربعة

7.65 (p. 39, line 15): أذا. Read: إذا

7.73 (p. 41, line 16): تمثل. Read: تمثّل

8.17 (p. 46, line 2): تجذب الفضول نحو. Read: تجذب الفضول التي مالت نحو

9.11 (p. 61, line 14): على أصل. Read: على أصل اللسان

9.94 (p. 79, line 5): مائ. Read: مائي

9.113 (p. 83, line 13): يغتة. Read: بغتة

***English translation:***

6.10 (p. 3, lines 20–21): "and neither pain nor fever develops." Read: "and no considerable pain nor fever develops"

6.29 (p. 15, line 29); 7.11 (p. 26, line 15); 8.14 (p. 45, line 12); 8.58 (p. 54, line 12): "main organs" (Ar. الأعضاء الأصلية). Read "elementary parts" (i.e., the homogeneous [homoeomerous] parts, such as arteries, veins, nerves, bones, cartilages, membranes, ligaments, and the various coats)

8.17 (p. 46, lines 3–4): "attract the superfluities towards." Read: "attract the superfluities that tend towards"

9.11 (p. 61, line 25): "[of the tongue]." Read: "of the tongue"

9.53, 88 (p. 71, line 3; p. 78, line 1): "peppermint [*Mentha piperita* and var.]." Read "mint [*Mentha* spp.]"

9.79 (p. 76, line 13): "and the soul becomes upset." Add footnote to "the soul": I.e., the stomach; cf. aphorisms 9.51, 55.

9.108 (p. 82, line 23): "marshmallow." Read: "mallow"

## Medical Aphorisms: Treatises 10–15

***Arabic text:***

12.24 (p. 34, line 6): لألطف. Read: بألطف

13.5 (p. 41, line 4): مرئ. Read: مريء

13.36 (p. 47, line 16): يغري. Read: يغرّي

13.38 (p. 48, line 3): استفراغه أوّل. Read: استفراغ هؤلاء

13.43 (p. 48, line 16): ومغرية. Read: ومغرّية

13.52 (p. 51, line 5): يغري. Read: يغرّي

15.19 (p. 60, line 8): المحلوق. Read: المخلوق

15.22 (p. 61, line 1): مضرّة. Read: مضرّة من وجه آخر

15.70 (p. 71, line 3): ثلاثة أصابع. Read: ثلاثة أصابع أو أربع

***English translation:***

10.61 (p. 16, line 16): "main organs" (Ar. الأعضاء الأصلية). Read "elementary parts" (i.e., the homogeneous [homoeomerous] parts, such as arteries, veins, nerves, bones, cartilages, membranes, ligaments, and the various coats)

13.38 (p. 48, line 5): "Such a person should be, first of all, evacuated." Read: "Such a person should be evacuated"

15.15 (p. 59, line 13): "a site that has tendons and nerves." Read: "a site that has tendons and nerves or veins"

15.22 (p. 61, line 2): "will not come to any harm because of that." Read: "will not come to any harm in another aspect because of that"

15.41: (p. 64, lines 26–27): "We are forced to cauterize if the hemorrhage is caused by corrosion or putrefaction affecting it." Read: "We are forced to cauterize if the hemorrhage is caused by corrosion or putrefaction affecting the organ"

15.70 (p. 71, lines 4–5): "three thumbs." Read: "three or four thumbs"

## Medical Aphorisms: Treatises 16–21

***Arabic text:***

18.3 (p. 40, line 3): بالكَرّة. Read: بالكرة

***English translation:***

21.72 (p. 123, line 32): "*ṣeqāqul* [*Malabaila secacul*]." Read "sekakul parsnip [*Pastinaca sekakul DC.* (synonym: *Malabaila pumila Boiss*)]."

21.80 (p. 129, lines 24–25): "peppermint [*Mentha piperita* and var.]." Read "mint [*Mentha* spp.]"

## *About the Editor/Translator*

GERRIT BOS was born in the Netherlands and educated there and in Jerusalem and London. He is proficient in classical and Semitic languages, as well as in Jewish and Islamic studies. He has been a research assistant at the Free University in Amsterdam, a research fellow and lecturer at University College in London, a tutor in Jewish studies at Leo Baeck College in London, a Wellcome Institute research fellow, and chair of the Martin Buber Institute of Jewish Studies at the University of Cologne. He currently resides in the Netherlands with his wife and three children.

Professor Bos is widely published in the fields of Jewish studies, Islamic studies, Judeo-Arabic texts, and medieval Islamic science and medicine, having many books and articles to his credit. In addition to preparing the Medical Works of Moses Maimonides, Professor Bos is also involved with a series of medical-botanical Arabic-Hebrew-Romance synonym texts written in Hebrew characters, an edition of Ibn al-Jazzār's *Zād al-musāfir* (Viaticum), and an edition of Marwān Ibn Janāḥ, *Kitāb al-Talkhīṣ*. He is a Member of Honor of the Argentinean Society for the History of Medicine.